03 Comm

39^{50}
T

Secure Speech Communications

MICROELECTRONICS AND SIGNAL PROCESSING

Series editors: **P. G. Farrell,** University of Manchester, U.K.
J. R. Forrest, University College London, U.K.

About this series:
The topic of microelectronics can no longer be treated in isolation from its prime application in the processing of all types of information-bearing signals. The relative importance of various processing functions will determine the future course of developments in microelectronics. Many signal processing concepts, from data manipulation to more mathematical operations such as correlation, convolution and Fourier transformation, are now readily realizable in microelectronic form. This new series aims to satisfy a demand for comprehensive and immediately useful volumes linking microelectronic technology and its applications.

Key features of the series are:
• Coverage ranging from the basic semiconductor processing of microelectronic circuits to developments in microprocessor systems or VLSI architecture and the newest techniques in image and optical signal processing.
• Emphasis on technology, with a blend of theory and practice intended for a wide readership.
• Exposition of the fundamental theme of signal processing; namely, any aspect of what happens to an electronic (or acoustic or optical) signal between the basic sensor which gathers it and the final output interface to the user.

1. *Microprocessor Systems and Their Application to Signal Processing:* C. K. YUEN, K. G. BEAUCHAMP, G. P. S. ROBINSON
2. *Applications of Walsh and Related Functions: With an Introduction to Sequence Theory:* K. G. BEAUCHAMP
3. *Secure Speech Communications:* H. J. BEKER AND F. C. PIPER

In preparation

4. *Transform Coding of Images:* R. J. CLARKE

Secure Speech Communications

Henry J. Beker

Racal Research Ltd., Reading, and Royal Holloway College, University of London, Egham, United Kingdom

Fred C. Piper

Royal Holloway College, University of London, Egham, United Kingdom

1985

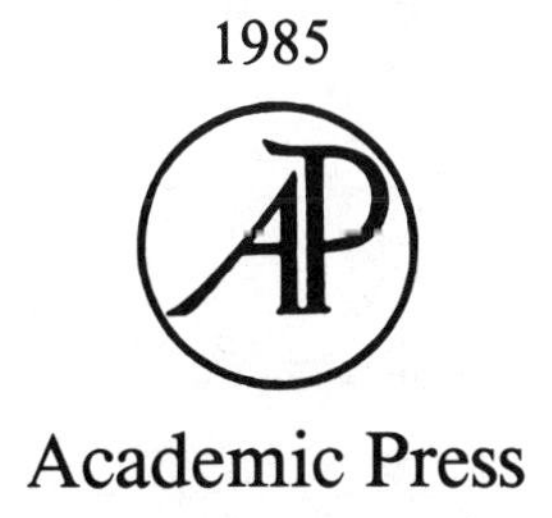

Academic Press

(Harcourt Brace Jovanovich, Publishers)

London Orlando San Diego New York
Toronto Montreal Sydney Tokyo

ACADEMIC PRESS INC. (LONDON) LTD.
24–28 Oval Road
LONDON NW1 7DX

United States Edition published by
ACADEMIC PRESS, INC.
Orlando, Florida 32887

British Library Cataloguing in Publication Data

Beker, H. J.
Secure speech communications.
1. Scrambling systems (Telecommunication)–
Design and construction
I. Title II. Piper, F. C.
658.4'7 TK6471

Library of Congress Cataloging in Publication Data

Beker, Henry.
Secure speech communications.

Bibliography: p.
Includes index.
1. Scrambling systems (Telecommunication)
I. Piper, F. C. (Frederick Charles), DATE .
II. Title.
TK5102.5.B354 1985 621.38 84-21528
ISBN 0–12–084780–9 (alk. paper)

PRINTED IN THE UNITED STATES OF AMERICA

85 86 87 88 9 8 7 6 5 4 3 2 1

Preface

Speech is a fundamental facet of our ability to communicate and the ability for speech communications to take place at a distance is more or less fundamental to our modern society. For instance, telephones, radios and televisions are all accepted and important parts of our everyday life. However, many means for communicating speech are susceptible to interception and/or intentional corruption, and this susceptibility has increased as modern technology has led to the introduction of new methods of speech transmission. One simple example of this phenomenon is provided by satellite communications. When a message is broadcast from a satellite it is usually receivable over a very large area called the 'footprint'. The footprint might typically be a large part of Western Europe. Thus, interception of a satellite transmission can take place 'from the comfort of your own armchair' and, unlike the situation with earlier methods of transmission, there is no need to dig up cables or even to move to a particular location to intercept a message. Nevertheless the latter is, of course, still possible and crimes depending on such techniques have certainly occurred. Many popular television crime stories are centred around the innocent bank manager or security man who checks a person's credentials by making telephone calls to various referees. Meanwhile, a collaborator of the person being refereed has already found the telephone cables from the building and is in position to intercept the calls and impersonate the referee. This is, unfortunately, a realistic situation. Furthermore, interception is likely to become easier since recent developments mean that it is no longer true that all telephone calls are transmitted over cables. For instance, in many countries an increasing number of mobile radio networks are being adopted. With these networks, calls are transmitted by radio and, hence, are relatively open to interception.

As speech communications become more widely used and even more vulnerable, the problems of providing some form of privacy or, in some cases, a high level of security are dramatically increasing in importance. The art of securing these communications has a number of names, the most common being cryptophony, encryption or scrambling. We will tend to use the last word since it is probably the most popular. So, for us, any device which attempts to secure speech communications against interception and/ or corruption is called a scrambler.

The aim of this book is to discuss both the techniques and principles underlying current scrambler design. Although we inevitably discuss many aspects of the more general problems of speech communications, we have not been able to cover this fascinating topic in as much detail as we would like. Our emphasis is definitely, as the title suggests, on security.

Chapter 1 considers the problems from the user's point of view. In particular, we discuss how he can identify his requirements, prepare a specification and then evaluate proposals. Chapters 2 and 3 contain the necessary background from speech communications and cryptography in order to understand the various scrambler designs. Chapters 4, 5 and 6 are devoted to analogue scramblers and consider, respectively, frequency based techniques, time based techniques and combinations of both. They also contain discussions of the general implementation problems, e.g., synchronization. In Chapter 7 we concentrate on the security of digital speech communications. In many ways this is not dissimilar to the handling of data. However, the user/designer should appreciate some of the aspects of this type of scrambler which are influenced by the fact that the data being encrypted was originally speech and that the people speaking expect their communications to be as for normal speech.

There has recently been a welcome increase in the number of female engineers. We very much hope they will not be put off by the fact that we refer to our readers and users as 'he' rather than 'he/she' or 'it'. Please regard this as a deficiency of the English language (or our use of it!) and not as male chauvinism on our part!

Acknowledgments

Many people have helped us during the preparation of this book. We are particularly indebted to Dave Alexander, Ted Beddoes, Tony Bromfield, Whitfield Diffie, Marion Kimberley, Chris Mitchell and Edward Stansfield for many useful discussions and their helpful criticisms of early versions of the manuscript. We must also thank Edward Stansfield for his advice and suggestions regarding sections on speech processing and analogue to digital conversion.

We would also like to thank both Racal Electronics Plc and Westfield College for their support and assistance.

Contents

1. The User's Perspective

I. Introduction

Speech provides a natural and simple method for individuals to exchange information and ideas. In fact speech is probably the most fundamental form of communication available to us. It is so important that our society has become highly dependent on our ability to transmit spoken messages quickly and accurately. The dependence is for both business and pleasure purposes, and there are many possible channels for the transmission of these messages. Obvious examples are the worldwide telephone network and the large number of private and military radio communications systems. The volume of traffic across these networks is enormous and is growing at an ever increasing rate.

When someone uses a communications system his main requirements are usually to send the message as quickly, accurately and cheaply as possible. He may, in certain instances, have to decide an order of priority for these three criteria. For instance he often has to choose between the speed of a telephone conversation and the economy of a letter. Even within the same network there may still be a choice. One illustration of this is the fact that a user of the British telephone system can chose between a number of charge rates with the knowledge that a choice of the lower rate will almost certainly restrict his usage to certain times during the day. As well as requiring speed, accuracy and low cost there are a number of situations where the information being transmitted is confidential and the communicators may not want any third party to understand their message. Their reasons for this may vary. They might, for instance, merely want some privacy and prefer no one else to know their business. They might, on the other hand, be transmitting very important, confidential information which, if discovered by a third party, could be used to their serious disadvantage. Whatever the reason, the communicators must, in this type of situation, take steps to conceal and protect the content of their message. Of course the amount of protection required will vary. If, as in our first example, a little privacy is all that is required, then it may be sufficient merely to prevent the casual eavesdropper from understanding the message. On the other hand, for important information it is crucial that even the most determined interceptor must not be able to deduce its content.

One of the many problems facing the designer of a speech scrambler arises from the fact that, as we have already mentioned, there exists a great variety of communications channels. A user might wish to use any one of them. However, each of these channels has its own characteristics and a scrambling technique which is ideal for one may not be suitable for another. Many of the ciphering techniques available to the designer of speech security equipment restrict the choice of communications channel. Furthermore, both the designer and user must never forget that almost all speech security systems reduce the audio quality of the voice transmission. In fact, cynical users often regard a speech scrambler as an expensive way of degrading the quality of the transmission! There is some truth in this. It is, of course, important that the designer ensures that the level of degradation is not too high. If the link is so bad that the listener has to ask for the message to be repeated, then any would-be eavesdropper is given another chance to determine the message. Clearly this cannot increase the security level. Thus it is necessary to seek some sort of compromise between the need for security and the desire to maintain good audio quality. It is also necessary, when deciding on this compromise, to consider the type of transmission link that might be used.

In practice a third, and usually equally important, consideration is the cost, where cost means both the financial cost and the complexity of the equipment. (Of course, these two aspects are not unrelated!) The restraints imposed by financial considerations are obvious and we need say no more about them. The effects of complexity may not be so obvious. However, if a piece of equipment is unduly complex then its maintenance is likely to be difficult and expensive. Furthermore, it is likely to be more prone to failure. An even more important consideration, at least in certain specific situations, is that increasing the complexity of a system is likely to result in a corresponding increase in the weight and size of the unit. There are many situations, for example if it has to be carried by a policeman on patrol or a soldier 'in the field', when this is unacceptable. Deciding on the right balance between audio quality, security and cost is one of the hardest problems facing both a designer and a potential user.

We will consider the problems facing a designer in later chapters, when we will also look at the techniques available to him. Meanwhile in this chapter we will try to look at the problems and decisions from the user's point of view. During the chapter we will occasionally use undefined technical terms.

The context should indicate their meaning and we will give rigorous definitions later on. Our aim in this chapter is to be as informal as possible. One obvious reason for this is that a user is likely to be a non-expert with some difficult decisions to make, He needs a clear, non-technical description of his options and does not want to be 'blinded by science'. The designer, on the other hand, has to be an 'expert', and he will need precise definitions.

A user may wish to add speech security to an existing communications system or to purchase a new system with speech security in it. In either case he will have a number of tasks to perform. We will consider them in an order which we think is logical. He should

(a) identify his requirements,
(b) determine the range of equipment available,
(c) evaluate the proposals from various manufacturers and designers,
(d) evaluate the installed equipment and rectify any faults.

II. Identifying the Requirements

As we have already hinted, there can be a considerable trade-off between the security level, the audio quality and the cost. Clearly the user will not want to pay for a higher security level than is required. Equally he will not want to accept anything but the minimum possible degradation of the audio quality. It is, therefore, absolutely crucial that a prospective user of speech security equipment determines his priorities and the degree to which he is prepared to be flexible. In practice he will probably need to rank his requirements and then, having made this ranking, must be prepared to make minor adjustments after determining what equipment is available. Unless he is prepared to design and manufacture his own equipment, a user will almost certainly fail to find a device satisfying his precise requirements in every detail. We will ignore the restriction of financial cost, which, although important, cannot possibly be quantified in a book of this type, and discuss four of the other areas which he will have to consider. They are

(a) the security level,
(b) performance and audio quality,
(c) intended use of the equipment and
(d) the assistance and support available.

A. The Security Level

The security level required is almost totally determined by the type of application which the user envisages. Users and their security needs vary considerably. Speech security equipments are used to secure the strategic contents of conversations between heads of nations. They are also used by diplomats at various levels, by the military, by various government and law enforcement agencies, by banks and by other commercial users. In fact, the list is almost endless. Clearly there is going to be considerable variation in the levels of security required. A secret conversation between two heads of nations may need to be protected 'forever'. In contrast, a specific instruction to a law officer to go to a certain destination and arrest an offender need only be secure until he actually gets there.

The level of security required by a user in a particular situation will depend not only on the user's needs but on the ability and determination of a would-be eavesdropper. This latter consideration probably depends, in turn, on the rewards available to the eavesdropper if he breaks the system. Thus the user needs not only to consider his personal needs but also to try to identify the 'enemy' and assess his capabilities. With this in mind he should ask himself a few questions.

1. *From whom do I need to protect my communications?*
The answer to this question is important. It might, for instance, be a foreign government or military adversary, a well-organised and wealthy crime syndicate, a business competitor, a casual eavesdropper or merely the general public. Once the potential interceptor has been identified this information can be used to determine the appropriate level of security. Within a military environment the identity of the enemy is usually clear and it is very likely that a high level of security is necessary. Within the police environment there are many potential uninvited listeners, and the threats presented by them vary. We will list two extreme examples.

(a) The criminals who listen in to monitor police activities so that they will know when they have been detected and can escape before the police arrive. Clearly the messages need protection from these people.
(b) Some of the general public who listen to the police broadcasts out of idle curiosity. It is probably safe to assume that a minimal amount of security will be sufficient to prevent most of them from understanding the messages.

Within the commercial world there are, as in the police environment, many different reasons for wishing to secure spoken communications. An obvious one may be that the managing director of a company wishes to protect his communications with his chairman and fellow directors from both his competitors and his own staff.

Once the potential eavesdropper has been identified the user must then assess whether or not this interceptor is likely to launch a serious attack on his system. (In the police environment, for instance, it is probably reasonable to assume that any member of the public who merely listens to the broadcasts out of idle curiosity will not be able, or even want, to break the system. However, the professional criminal will certainly want to break it and might be prepared to invest some money in having it broken).

2. *How capable is the interceptor of breaking the system and how determined is he likely to be?*
Clearly, if the user knows precisely, or even approximately, the cryptanalytic capability of his opponents he can assess his own requirements far more accurately than he could otherwise. In fact if the user has no idea of the interceptor's capabilities and determination he must assume the worst, i.e., he must assume that his foe is as able as the most competent cryptanalyst alive and that he has virtually limitless resources at his disposal. In this situation all users should always assume that the cryptanalyst is considerably more clever than they are.

When trying to assess the interceptor's capabilities the user will have to exercise his judgment; he will never know for sure. To answer with authority he needs to know if the interceptor has, or is likely to obtain, equipment similar to his own, and if he has recording devices, computers and spectrum analysing equipment. Even more important, does the potential interceptor have access to an experienced team of cryptanalysts? We stress that when in doubt the user should always assume the worst.

Let us now see how various answers to this type of question might influence the user's choice of system. Suppose, for instance, the user accepts that it is highly likely that the interceptor will be able to obtain some of his equipment. (This might be because it could be stolen or captured while in service. It might, on the other hand, be because it was commercially available). It is crucial that this must not increase, to an unacceptable level, the danger of the system being broken. We will have to wait until the later chapters before we can discuss the detailed practical implications of this, but it certainly means that the equipment must be reasonably complex. Now suppose, looking on the 'bright side' from the user's point of view, that he knows the interceptor does not have direct access to a computer and analysis equipment, but that the intercepted messages have to be delivered to a third party before they can be studied. (This may well be the situation in certain military environments where intercepts made in forward areas may have to be passed to rear areas for processing and analysis.) This would assure the user that it would be some time before his messages could be broken and so, if messages only had to be secure for short periods, he might be prepared to accept a comparatively low security level as a trade-off for some other consideration.

Although the material resources of the interceptor are important, we cannot over emphasize the importance of the personnel at his disposal. It must not be forgotten that, even if the interceptor has access to large powerful computers, computers cannot crack ciphers on their own. Any sophisticated cryptanalytic attack will require suitably qualified people. If the interceptor does not have immediate access to such a team it is likely to take him a considerable amount of time and money to train one.

It is, of course, impossible to judge precisely how much time and money an interceptor might be prepared to spend in order to break a given system. But it seems reasonable to assume that it will bear some relation to the rewards or advantages which he will gain if he is successful. The rewards from monitoring and breaking the user's traffic must justify the interceptor's efforts. (This justification may, of course, be measured in political or financial terms, depending on the situation.) Clearly there are occasions where it is worthwhile for the interceptor to spend 'endless' time and money to break a system. (However, we must hope that the users of such systems have no need to read a book like this!) On the other hand there are many situations where this is not the case, and in these the user must judge for himself the 'value' of his messages. We will now consider a situation which illustrates the user's dilemmas and how he might reach a decision. Suppose that a user has assigned a 'value' to his message and has estimated the capabilities of his opponent. He will then have some idea of whether, for instance, the interceptor is likely to be aware that certain ciphering techniques have the weakness that listeners can be trained to understand the scrambled messages. If he decides that the interceptor knows this, he must then decide if it is worth the interceptor's while to hire a trained person or to train himself. If the user feels confident that the interceptor does not know of these 'weak' systems, cannot learn these techniques or cannot afford to hire someone who can, he may feel that it is safe to use one of them.

We have just mentioned the possibility of agreeing to use 'weak systems'. This is not as bad as it may seem and the word 'weak' may be misleading. In our example the systems under consideration were only weak if the cryptanalyst had certain expertise. Most systems are theoretically breakable if the cryptanalyst is well trained and has unlimited resources and time. In most situations, once he has estimated the interceptor's probable resources and determination, the user needs some idea of the length of time it will take a cryptanalyst to break his system. (Again, we emphasize this time will depend on many factors including, for instance, the facilities available.)

The user must then determine the length of time for which he needs his messages to be secure. He will then decide if there is a sufficient safety margin (i.e. a sufficient difference in the two times) for him to use the system.

3. *How many of the messages is the opponent likely to intercept?*
We will consider this more fully when we consider the usage of equipment. However, it should be clear that the amount of intercepted traffic obtained

by the cryptanalyst affects the user's security level. Each extra intercepted message gives the interceptor further information and assists his attack on the system. If the user is unable to assess the likelihood of his messages being intercepted, then he must assume the worst and accept that the interceptor will obtain every scrambled message.

4. *What are the consequences should an interceptor break the system and read the traffic?*

Before we consider these consequences we make a very important observation. If an interceptor is able to break a system and to obtain useful information from traffic which the communicators believe to be secure, he will go to extraordinary lengths to keep it from them. It is clearly to the interceptor's advantage that the communicators believe their system to be secure and continue to transmit their messages. Having made this point, we can now look at the consequences of a system being broken. To do this we must distinguish between tactical and strategic communications because the security levels needed for the two environments are different. The French mathematician and cryptographer Anoine Rossignol reputedly said, 'A secret message must be safe enough for it to be too late to be of use to an enemy by the time he gets it solved'. Whether or not Rossignol actually said this, it is an extremely accurate assessment of the security needed in any given situation.

In a tactical environment the situation changes quickly. If the time taken for the message to be understood is long enough that the situation has changed, then the consequences are minimal. Thus in a tactical situation messages need only be secure for a short time. In strategic situations, however, the position is totally different. The consequences of a user's traffic being read may be extremely far reaching and disastrous for him. In these situations it is necessary that the user feels confident that his messages will be secure for a very long time. It is worth noting here that in practice high level strategic communications almost certainly use data links and not voice. It has been reported, for instance, that the hot line between Washington and Moscow is one such link. One reason for using data links is that, at the present time, data transmissions lend themselves more easily to high security than, for example, analogue speech systems.

Another important consideration when assessing the security level is that, to satisfy demands which conflict with security requirements, a lower grade security equipment than is ideal may be put into operation. This can be disastrous and can result in a system which is worse than having no security device at all. The reason for this is clear. If communicators know that they have no security equipment but feel that some aspects of their conversations are sensitive, they will often disguise the important terms by using codewords, insinuations, etc. However, if they believe their system to be secure, they will rely on it to provide all the secrecy. Thus, a sub-standard security system is worse than no security at all. It results in a false sense of security.

It might seem logical to deduce from our discussion so far that every user should simply assume the worst and opt for the highest security level available to him. Were it true that all systems offered the same performance and audio quality at the same cost, then this would clearly be the correct decision. However, this is not the case. The user has many other parameters to consider before making his choice. We will now discuss the second of these, the performance and audio quality.

B. Performance and Audio Quality

Unfortunately the majority of the current communications systems were not designed to support scramblers. As scramblers become cheaper and more commonly used this situation may change. However, at the present time most users will, in practice, want to retrofit scramblers to existing communications systems. When this is done one result is that the noise or distortion caused by any source in the communications system will become far more destructive. It simply must be accepted that there is a price to be paid for introducing security and that, in general, the addition of most scramblers will degrade the performance of the majority of the existing communications systems. A consequence of this is that if a scrambler is added to a communications system which offers only a marginally acceptable audio quality the resulting system may be totally unacceptable.

It is, in practice, difficult to specify and to judge the performance of a scrambler. (This is true both with respect to the level of security it offers and the audio quality. However, in this section we restrict our attention to the audio quality.) No matter what the designer thinks of it, most operators will be critical of a scrambler's performance. If the scrambling is some form of manual coding process which replaces certain important words by codewords, then the operators are likely to object to the time taken to 'translate' from the clear message to the coded version and back again. If, to take another possibility, the security is obtained by an automatic scrambling of the analogue signal, then the operator will probably be critical of the audio quality. It is almost certainly true that no matter what is done the operator will raise some objection. Furthermore, in each case he will probably have some justification. In practice the best attitude to adopt when assessing the performance of a scrambler is that one is trying to estimate the degradation caused by the scrambler and assessing whether or not it is acceptable.

There are very few well-accepted criteria for specifying the performance and audio quality of a system. In practice a user may simply demand that the system performs 'satisfactorily' or even 'not too badly'. Thus the user is really accepting the fact that scramblers degrade the system and is really saying he will accept the best performance and audio quality that he can find. It may well be that when he comes to evaluate various proposals he will realise just how diverse manufacturers' assessments of 'satisfactorily' can be. Once again we must mention the importance of the trade-off between security level and performance. There are, as we have already seen, many factors which affect this compromise, and the user's environment is obviously one of them. There is no doubt, for instance, that, in order to increase his security level, a military user in the field will accept a much poorer audio quality than the average telephone user.

Obviously it is to the user's advantage if he has some idea of how badly his communications are likely to be affected by the scrambler. We will look at this problem in some of the later chapters and will consider how the various scramblers under consideration are likely to affect different communications systems. For the moment, however, we will restrict ourselves to making general comments about the factors which influence a scrambler's performance.

Speech is highly redundant in the sense that it is certainly not necessary to hear every syllable of every word in order to understand a spoken communication. Anyone who has spoken on a crackling telephone line (and who has not?) will be aware that one can 'miss' an astonishingly large proportion of a conversation and yet still understand it. The redundancy of the language, plus the amazing decoding capabilities of the human brain and ear, allow speech communications to take place despite atrociously bad transmission conditions. Unfortunately scramblers, and in particular descramblers, tend to remove some of this capability. One way in which this might happen is that any ambient noise like, for instance, a moment's crackling on a telephone line, will be descrambled with the speech. This is quite likely to result in the descrambler producing, for a comparatively long period, a totally unintelligible signal at the receiver. The intelligibility of the descrambled signal is also dependent on the audio bandwidth of the system. We will discuss this type of problem in detail in the later chapters. For the moment we merely observe that most of the energy of a speech signal is contained within a bandwidth of about 3000 Hz. This suggests that it might not be unreasonable to use a bandwidth of roughly this size for the transmission of analogue speech signals. Indeed, this is precisely what happens in many networks including, for example, telephone systems. But, as we shall also see later, many scramblers perform by rearranging the voice frequencies. So if, for example, the scrambler moves many of the frequencies which contain the intelligence to the high end of the band and if high frequencies are lost because of the use of a limited bandwidth, then the descrambler may be unable to recover some of the intelligence contained in those higher frequencies. Consequently the signal may be partially, or even totally, lost.

A communications system may incorporate a variety of transmission media and components, for example, open wires, cables, radio relays, multiplexers, repeaters, satellites and echo suppressors, to mention but a few. These various elements may introduce delays and phase distortions, each of which may adversely affect the possibility of the descrambler reconstructing the signal successfully. Scrambling and descrambling are even likely to be hindered by some of the desirable characteristics of modern transceivers. Examples of such characteristics are pre-emphasis, de-emphasis and limiting, which all help to improve the quality, intelligibility and efficiency of normal voice transmissions but, nevertheless, may seriously degrade the scrambler/descrambler performance.

Another consideration for the user is synchronization. Many scramblers employ some form of synchronization but, if it is not particularly robust, this may be affected by various channel conditions. As well as those mentioned earlier, other conditions which may have a bad effect include a poor signal-to-noise ratio or multipath fading on a radio channel. For radio communications any scrambling system which is seriously degraded by a poor signal-to-noise ratio will result not only in low intelligibility but also in a decrease in the effective range of the radio accompanied by unreliable synchronization. Other sources of noise and distortion which may become more noticeable if scramblers are introduced include corroded switch and fuse contacts, poor ground contacts, power supply ripple, ignition noise and alternator whine.

If a prospective user, or reader, has not sufficient technical background to understand the meaning of each of the terms used, it does not really matter. The message should be clear. Any fault in a communications system is likely to cause a more serious degradation to the signal when scramblers are introduced.

One final and very important observation is that the introduction of scramblers/descramblers to a communications system is likely to cause a dramatic deterioration in the ability of the listener to recognise the speaker.

The conclusions of this section may be summarised as follows:

(1) The primary forms of degradation resulting from the incorporation of a scrambler are loss of (a) audio quality, (b) range for radio communications and (c) speaker recognition.

(2) Usually, but certainly not always, (a) increasing the complexity of the scrambling technique results in an increase in the degradation and (b) increasing the complexity of the communications systems also results in an increase in the degradation.

C. Intended Use of Equipment

Two more important factors for consideration while the user is deliberating about his choice of systems are the environment in which the equipment will be used and the way in which the scramblers will be deployed in this environment. In order to investigate these points we will adopt the same format as when assessing the security level, i.e., we will discuss some of the questions which the user needs to answer.

1. *Is the equipment to be used in a strategic or tactical environment?* The relevance of the question is likely to vary greatly with different types of user. For a commercial user there is probably no real purpose in even trying to distinguish between tactical and strategic situations. For a military user, on the other hand, the difference between the two environments is enormous. The requirements of most other users will fall somewhere between these two extremes.

In a military environment tactical devices are normally regarded as those which will be used in forward areas. Consequently they will need to be compact and light enough to be carried long distances, often by operators with limited technical skills. Furthermore it is likely to be extremely difficult to repair or physically maintain them in these forward areas. Other consequences of the environment are that they are likely to be captured by the enemy and that they will only be used to transmit information which needs to be secret for a comparatively short time. All these facts lead to more questions for a potential military user.

a. Will the security of the entire system be affected if a machine is tampered with or captured? Clearly it is desirable, in fact probably imperative, that the answer to this question is no. The user will probably, therefore, want some tamper-proofing (or in practice maybe tamper-resistance) capability built into the device. The efficiency of this tamper-resistance may be a principal factor in determining the final choice.

b. How bulky and heavy is the device? There is not much more to be said of this. Clearly as the distances which the device is likely to have to be carried increase so the relevance of the size and weight also increases.

c. How rugged is the device? This is important. If the operator is likely to have to move quickly while carrying the device than it is quite likely to get knocked, dropped etc. Consequently the user will probably require that it is built to the relevant military specifications including, for instance, waterproofing and the ability to withstand adequate levels of shock and vibration. If the device is battery operated, then the user should investigate how long the battery lasts.

d. How simple is it to operate the device? In almost all tactical environments simplicity of operation is a primary requirement. It is obviously pointless to choose equipment which offers a high level of security but which is too complex to be operated by non-technical operators. In most tactical situations the operator is unlikely to have had much training at operating complex equipment and this invariably results in lax operation of the devices. Furthermore there is always the possibility that the operator will become incapacitated and that a completely untrained operator will have to replace him. History has shown that, in practice, a system is more likely to be broken as a result of operator error than as a consequence of a cryptanalyst 'cracking' the cipher system.

e. How difficult is it to connect the scrambler to the transceiver? If this is too difficult then the operator may have to resort to transmitting unscrambled messages with potentially disastrous consequences.

f. How easily can the device be repaired or maintained? In the present context this probably means asking whether, if one of the transceiver or scrambler were to become defective, it could be replaced without needing to readjust the other.

g. How easily can the cryptographic keys be changed? A scrambler has to be able to scramble any given message in many different ways. The particular scrambling method to be used at any given time is determined by a cryptographic key. If any key is used for too long an interceptor may be able to deduce that particular scrambling pattern and will be able to understand all further messages for which the same key is used. Thus it is crucial that the key is changed frequently. Obviously if the key change has to be effected by an unskilled operator 'in the field', then key changing must be a straightforward task.

This list of questions is certainly not exhaustive. However, it is indicative of the kind of qualities which a military user will demand of any speech security equipment which is to be used in the field. Any other user who has to operate in a tactical environment will certainly need to consider some, if not all, of these points.

In a strategic system, however, the situation is almost certain to be totally different. Whereas a tactical device tends to be used in a hostile environment, the surroundings for a strategic device are normally friendly. It should no longer be necessary to pay so much attention to the possibilities of theft or tampering as the device is almost certainly housed and operated within a physically secure environment. Furthermore it is normally kept in a fixed location so that size and weight are less important. There is usually ample time for installing the equipment and the operators are likely to be well trained with sufficient time to perform tasks like changing the keys. In fact the entire physical conditions are so much better that the overriding factor will normally be the security level.

Of course, as we indicated earlier, these two environments are opposite extremes and most situations fall somewhere between them. For example, although a law enforcement agent may have to operate in a hostile environment, he will, usually, have more time for operating the device than his military counterpart. Furthermore his equipment will not be treated quite so roughly and, as a consequence, will not need to be so rugged. (It should be remembered, however, that for a non-waterproofed device a spilt cup of coffee may be as disastrous as any drenching in the field!) Another example of a requirement which we have not yet considered is that within a commercial environment, the user may want his system to be 'transparent' to the operator. (This merely means that the operator should not even be aware that a scrambler is being used.) This, of course, limits the tasks which the operator need be asked to perform.

2. *Is the device likely to be used in an environment where spoofing and/or jamming are likely to occur?*

First of all we must explain what we mean by 'spoofing' and 'jamming'. Both are terms given to specific methods of trying to disrupt communications. For *spoofing* the disruption is achieved either by inserting spurious messages which the receiver will accept as genuine or by replaying genuine messages which have already been transmitted. *Jamming*, on the other hand, is the name given to attempting to prevent the genuine messages from reaching their intended destination. This is, typically, achieved by using the same channel as the genuine transmitter but sending a signal which is considerably more powerful than his.

Obviously, if such attacks are likely, the user will want to take steps to protect his system against them. As we shall see, some systems are more prone to this type of attack than others.

3. *How are the scramblers to be deployed within the communications system?*

The type of question which might be asked in this context is: does the system need to have the same number of scramblers as transceivers? The user might, for example, have hopes of having a telephone system in which some, or all, of the telephones share the same scrambler. If this is to be considered, then the first priority is to decide upon a protocol which decides who has access to the scrambler at any given moment and to ensure that this protocol fits in with the expected overall operation of the system. Although such a scheme has the advantage that it may reduce the total cost of the system, it introduces a number of handicaps. For instance it necessitates that a number of users must share the same cryptographic keys which, of course, means it is not possible for the key used between each pair of communicators to be unique to them. Thus two communicators know that some of the other users will be able to understand their messages. This may not be acceptable. In addition users may have excessively long waiting times to make a secure call.

Another, equally important, question in this context is whether or not the entire communications system is to be secured. If the answer to this question is no then there are a number of consequences to consider. If, for instance, the scrambler is required to be able to transmit in clear (i.e., transmit unscrambled messages), then there is the potential danger that the operator might mistakenly send in clear an important message which should have been scrambled. So if the user wants the scrambler to be able to transmit in clear, then it should be so difficult for the operator to do so that he is unlikely to do it through forgetfulness or by mistake. Similarly if the user wants the scrambler to be able to receive clear communications, then the equipment should have the facility of *clear voice override*. (This means that the receiver can detect whether a communication is clear or scrambled and then decide whether or not it is necessary to switch on the descrambler). Similarly it is advantageous in this situation for the operator to have some means of distinguishing between clear and secure transmissions so that he can answer in the same mode.

If cost is an important consideration, then the user may wish to consider whether or not to reduce the number of scrambled messages in a network. Clearly, limiting the use of the scramblers means that the interceptor has fewer opportunities and less information with which to crack the security system. Further if the communications system is fairly complex, it may be very difficult to secure all the links. In this case it may be necessary to limit the scramblers to certain critical links which, of course, also decreases the cost of the system. Despite all these apparent advantages, limiting the use of scramblers may prove to be an unwise economy. There are also a number of important disadvantages. The first obvious one is that, if an operator is only scrambling the occasional message, he may forget how to use the scrambler or may use it incorrectly. Furthermore he may become lazy and be tempted to leave unscrambled one of the important messages which should be secured. A second, possibly more important, disadvantage is that if only a few of the links are secure, then the interceptor will quickly discover which are the important links. This may enable him to discover some of the more important locations. If he then notices that messages from some of these sources are changed from clear to scrambled, he will immediately be alerted that something unusual is happening, even if he does not know precisely what. There is a third disadvantage. If all messages, whether important or not, are scrambled then the interceptor will need to attack them all. If, on the other hand, only the important ones are scrambled then the interceptor's work will be considerably reduced. Suppose, for instance, that an interceptor can break a one-minute scrambled message in twenty-four hours. If only the important messages, say ten minutes' worth per day, are scrambled, then the interceptor can listen to one-tenth of the secure traffic per day. If, on the other hand, all the messages are scrambled, say four hours worth per day, then he can only listen to one-two hundred and fourtieth of the traffic. Furthermore, this small fraction will almost certainly be an unimportant message. This last point is so important that, in many situations, the communicators agree to transmit continuously and merely send bogus messages when they have nothing to say. This process is called *traffic flow security* and its presence inhibits the interceptor from performing any meaningful traffic analysis.

To summarise, it is usually advantageous, when possible, to secure all transmissions in a network, thereby limiting the important information which an interceptor will obtain.

4. *Is end-to-end encryption, link-by-link encryption or single-key encryption to be used in the network?*

We have already said a little about this but will give a brief explanation of each term and mention a few of the consequences of using them. *End-to-end encryption* occurs when the two parties concerned, the originator and recipient of the message, are the only two people with access to the cryptographic key (or keys) used to encipher or decipher the message. If the two parties concerned feel that they cannot trust any third party then they must insist on end-to-end encryption. With a *link-by-link* system intermediate parties will have access to the keys. In fact in this case the originator and receiver need not share the same key. Furthermore neither need know the key used by the other. The reason for this is simple. The originator of the message may send his encrypted message to a third party who can then decipher it and re-encipher with a different key before forwarding it. If this technique is used, then the number of third parties between originator and recipient can be as large as they choose. This type of communications may be useful if, for example, the sender and receiver either do not know or do not trust each other. The third parties might be solicitors, bankers or any other professional person in whom they both have confidence. A *single key network* is one in which all users share the same key or keys. Thus the users must all trust each other or need to share a large volume of common knowledge. Here one obvious example might be the board of directors of a company.

Clearly the mode of operation selected by the user will have important implications for his choice of equipment.

5. *How much traffic will the system support?*

As we have already seen, the success of an attack on a system is likely to depend on the amount of traffic which the interceptor obtains. Consequently it is important that the user has some idea of the volume of traffic which he expects to be scrambled within the network. He will then have an estimation of the maximum amount of scrambled speech which an interceptor might obtain. This knowledge is likely to affect many of his managerial decisions like, for instance, the frequency with which he will need to change his keys. The significance of these managerial decisions will be discussed in later chapters.

6. *What type of communications channel is to be employed?*
In our discussion of the user's requirements for performance and audio quality we gave a seemingly unending list of factors which affect the quality of a received descrambled message. To make matters even worse some of the scrambling techniques cannot even be employed over certain types of channel. We will explain why later. However, it is important that, even if he does not understand why, the user realises that the type of channel over which his scrambled speech is transmitted may restrict his choice of scrambler.

7. *Are communications to be simplex, half-duplex or duplex?*
We are all familiar with the fact that various communications systems operate in different ways. In a telephone network, for instance, the two communicators can usually talk to each other simultaneously. If, on the other hand, they are using hand-held 'walkie-talkies', then each communicator must press the appropriate button on his device in order to communicate, and then, when it is possible to communicate, messages can only be sent in one direction at a time. Examples of yet another type of system are provided by radio and television. No matter how loudly the infuriated listener shouts back, the commentator cannot hear him. In this system the messages can only travel one way. We shall assign to each of these types of system a technical name. However, we must point out that our terminology is not universally accepted. A *duplex*, or sometimes *full-duplex*, system is one in which messages may be transmitted both ways simultaneously. If messages can travel both ways, but not simultaneously, the system is called *half-duplex* and a *simplex* system is one in which all messages have to be sent in the same direction.

The choice between these three options is yet another important decision facing the user. As we shall see later, many scrambling schemes do not lend themselves to full-duplex operation. Half-duplex systems are far more popular and are normally much cheaper. One reason for the price difference is easy to understand. In order to decrease both the size and cost of the unit, many scramblers are designed so that the scrambler and descrambler employ the same basic hardware. But if the scrambler and descrambler occupy the same basic hardware, then, clearly, this may prevent the device from operating in transmit and receive modes simultaneously.

All that we have done in this section is list a few of the many choices and decisions which the user has to make. Our list is in no way complete but should be long enough to establish that the user may have a difficult time identifying his requirements and establishing his priorities.

D. Assistance and Support Available

In this context the user has a number of decisions to make. One of the first, and possibly the most important, is to what extent he will have to rely on the supplier of the equipment for his support and how much he is prepared to provide for himself. Although the user will, hopefully, feel that he needs a sufficient grasp of the fundamentals to make a sensible choice of equipment, it may still be true that neither he nor his staff has the mathematical/engineering capability to fully understand the cryptographic techniques involved. Of course one would expect military users to have the necessary expertise at their disposal. But within the commercial world this is unlikely to be the case. A book such as this will (we hope!) help the non-technical user to specify his needs and also enable the technical user to grasp the basis of the cryptography. This, in turn, will help him to make his own assessment of the security offered. But it will not make him an expert and he may still feel that he needs the extra assurance of specialised expert support.

To give some idea of the types of expert assistance which the user may need we will list six crucial topics for consideration. These may affect the choice of equipment since, if the supplier of the 'best' system cannot offer the right 'back-up' service, the user may feel he has to compromise and accept a slightly inferior system for which he is guaranteed suitable support. It is no use purchasing an excellent system if you cannot install it or operate it! The six points are

(1) mathematical and engineering assistance,
(2) installation of equipment,
(3) repair and maintenance of equipment,
(4) training of operators,
(5) documentation and
(6) key change.

We have already mentioned the need for mathematical and engineering assistance. If the user does not feel he has sufficient expertise at his disposal, then he must find out whether it can be supplied by either the equipment supplier or some third party. In fact if the user feels that he is unable to assess the security levels of the equipment being proposed, then he should consider consulting an independent expert to do it for him.

The installation of the equipment is obviously important. If the environment is strategic, then the user will probably want the equipment to be installed in a secure area. Is he prepared to allow someone from 'outside' into this area? If not, and if he is only prepared to allow certain approved staff into the installation area, then he must ensure that adequate training is provided for some of these selected personnel. The same type of problems may arise over the repair and maintenance of the equipment. If the equipment is in a secure area, then even more training may be necessary to enable the approved staff to carry out repairs and maintenance. If, on the other hand, the equipment is to be used in a tactical environment, then, as we have already seen, it may be necessary to ensure that faulty equipment can be replaced by an unskilled operator. If this is the case, then the simplicity of repairs and the time they take may become very important considerations. Other considerations in this context include deciding whether the user wants to be able to repair at module level and summon outside assistance for the component level faults or to repair to component level himself. If the user feels that his staff need operator and maintenance training, then he must determine precisely which facilities the equipment supplier is capable of supplying and the type of service which is available from independent sources. He must also inspect the documentation provided for the user and make sure it is sufficient for his requirements.

Apart from a few of the very simple privacy systems, most speech scramblers employ cryptographic keys. The keys are crucial to the overall security of the system, and the user must take extreme care to study all the problems involving keys. He must make sure that he knows the arrangements for the changing of keys. He must also look, in great detail, at the schemes for key generation, key distribution and key management. These are all absolutely vital considerations and his whole system will be at risk if any one of the three schemes is inefficient. It must never be forgotten that if an interceptor has a similar device (and we should always assume that he has!) and knows the keys being used, then he will be able to descramble the message. In most systems the entire security will probably depend on the interceptor not knowing, or being able to deduce, which keys are being used. Since the keys are so important, we will look at the problems relating to them in some detail.

A cryptographic key will normally consist of a number of characters which may be in various forms such as alphabetic, alphanumeric or numeric, including binary, octal, decimal and hexadecimal. The number of characters in a key can vary from one or two, which are likely to be sufficient in a privacy system, to perhaps as many as forty-plus for the more secure systems. To obtain a reasonable level of security, the number of possibilities for the complete set of keys must be sufficiently large that it will not be possible for an interceptor to determine the correct key simply by trying all possibilities. If each key consists of only a few characters, then, clearly, this limits the number of possible keys. Hence the desirability of having a large number of characters per key. Once the keys are chosen, there are many ways of entering the chosen set of characters into the equipment. They may, for instance, be entered via a key-pad or a set of dials, switches or hard-wired links.

We will now look at three of the major problems associated with keys.

a. Key generation. The first of these problems which confronts the user is how to generate his keys. If he decides to allow an operator to 'invent' the keys, then there is a danger that they will be predictable. People have a tendency to use words and numbers which have some special significance for them. For instance, they may use the telephone numbers and/or names of close friends and relatives. Thus, once the interceptor has discovered the identity of the appropriate operator, there is a distinct likelihood that, after a fairly small number of guesses, he will discover the correct key. This method of key generation is not recommended.

It is also undesirable to have a sequential method for generating keys. The reason for this is simple. If the interceptor knew the sequential method and then discovered just one key, he would know them all.

The most advantageous scheme for obtaining keys is to generate them randomly. However, the user may not have access to a random number generator. We will discuss some of the desirable properties of random number generators later. For the moment we merely stress that the user must pay serious attention to the method of generating the keys which he needs in order to secure his scramblers. His security depends on the interceptor not being able to determine the key being used at any given moment.

b. Key distribution. Once the keys have been generated they have to be distributed to the various receivers and transmitters throughout the system. If the system is large, or if the keys are to be changed frequently, then this is a non-trivial problem. In a secure communications network it is necessary to ensure that all communicators who share the same key actually have that key in their possession at the appropriate time. Furthermore no one else should have that key. This can be a sizeable logistics problem and if, for instance, it is performed manually, then it might involve the use of a considerable number of staff. It is, of course, not sufficient merely to ensure that each key is in the right place at the right time. It is also necessary to guarantee that it is entered correctly into the relevant devices. This may sound obvious, and indeed it is, but it is not always achieved. If the operator forgets the key as he is about to enter it or fails to enter it correctly for any other reason, then, to put it mildly, he has a problem. "Did you hear about the radio operator who failed to enter his key correctly? He resorted to clear communication and shouted down the hand set 'What was the key setting, Joe?' " Funny? Not really. Unfortunately there are occasions when it is too near to the truth!

It is possibly worthwhile, at this stage, to say a little in defence of operators. A well-trained qualified operator is highly skilled and unlikely to make elementary mistakes. But, as we have repeatedly mentioned, it is not always possible to ensure that all the equipment is manipulated by trained operators. Human error is still probably the most common contributory factor in the breaking of security systems. Thus, in an attempt to minimise this risk, it is usually best to assume that the operator is unskilled and to design the system such that it is very difficult for him to make any mistakes.

Key distribution can also be expensive. If, for instance, it involves a number of staff carrying keys from one location to another, then it is advisable to provide some means of ensuring that these staff are trustworthy. Furthermore, it may also be necessary to provide them with a certain amount of physical protection. Even if the protection required is minimal, the cost of 'checking' and protecting the couriers can be considerable.

There are, fortunately, alternatives to the manual distribution of keys. These include the automatic schemes which are becoming available as modern electronics increases the processing power available. If the user decides to adopt such a scheme, then he is entering a different process of identifying requirements, determining the range of equipment available, etc. We will postpone discussion of these problems.

c. Key management. By key management we mean the process of keeping accounts on all the keys used in the system. (The reader should be aware that some authors use the term "key management" to include what we have called generation and distribution as well as what we are calling management.) Key management is a complicated procedure which includes, for instance, ensuring that there is a record of precisely which keys are at each terminal at any given moment, that all lists of keys are accounted for (in the sense that none of them is lost, in which case, of course, one would have to assume that the enemy had it) and that all used keys are successfully destroyed. Clearly this is not a trivial task. The user must specify a key management procedure which is compatible with the security level he requires. There is no point whatsoever in deciding that you need a high level of security and then failing to control the key management.

Although our list is not complete, we have tried to give a reasonably comprehensive account of how a user might attempt to identify his requirements. Hopefully we have said enough to indicate that the user's task is never easy and that it will depend on various parameters such as the environment in which the system will operate. Once he has specified these requirements, but certainly not beforehand, the user can then begin investigating the various types of scramblers which are available.

III. Determining the Range of Equipment Available

Research into the design of speech scramblers is a very active area and, furthermore, is increasing rapidly. Thus there is no way in which we can possibly cover the complete range of equipment available. Indeed it is almost certain that by the time this book appears scrambling techniques will exist which, at the time of writing, have not yet been conceived. Our aim is to provide sufficient background information on the subject of scramblers that the reader will feel he knows how to begin his selection of a piece of equipment or even how to begin to actually design a system. It is not our intention to survey the scrambler market or to compare rival pieces of equipment. Instead we will try to evaluate and compare the various techniques which are currently in use.

If the introduction which we give in this chapter is too brief and/or too non-technical, then the reader need not despair. Each of the techniques discussed here will be explained in more detail in the subsequent chapters. Furthermore, each scheme will be analysed in detail. Its performance, both in terms of cryptographic security and audio quality, will be assessed and this evaluation will, of course, involve some discussion of the possible methods of implementing the scheme.

In general, people tend to refer to two basic scrambler modes: analogue and digital. It is often assumed, quite incorrectly, that these two terms refer to the way in which the signal is encrypted. In fact most, although not all, of today's more sophisticated scramblers utilize the advantages of digital signal processing. They convert the audio signal to a digital one before scrambling it. There are some totally analogue systems, i.e., systems which actually scramble the analogue signal, but they tend to be less secure.

The distinction between analogue and digital systems concerns the form in which the transmitter intends to send the scrambled signal. In an *analogue scrambler system* the aim is to transmit the message as a continuously varying, i.e., analogue, signal. In a *digital scrambler system*, on the other hand, the intention is to transmit the message as a signal which, at any given time, can take only one of a finite number of discrete values. Thus an analogue scrambler is one which *transmits* an analogue signal while a digital scrambler *transmits* a digital signal. The following three figures should help to clarify the situation.

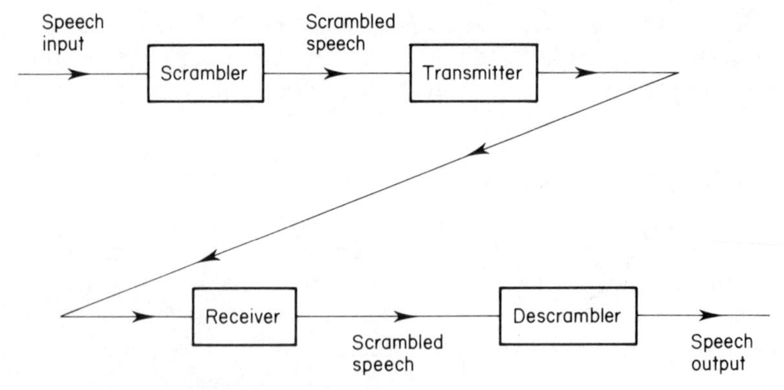

FIG. 1.1. Analogue speech scrambler with no digital signal processing.

Figures 1.1 and 1.2 both illustrate analogue scramblers. The difference between the two is the form of the signals when they are actually scrambled. In Fig. 1.1 the signal remains in analogue form throughout the entire process. In the system of Fig. 1.2, however, the signal is converted to digital form before it is scrambled. It is then reconverted to an analogue form before transmission. After transmission it is converted to digital again, descrambled and finally re-converted to an analogue signal. This is the type of scheme used in most of the current more sophisticated scramblers.

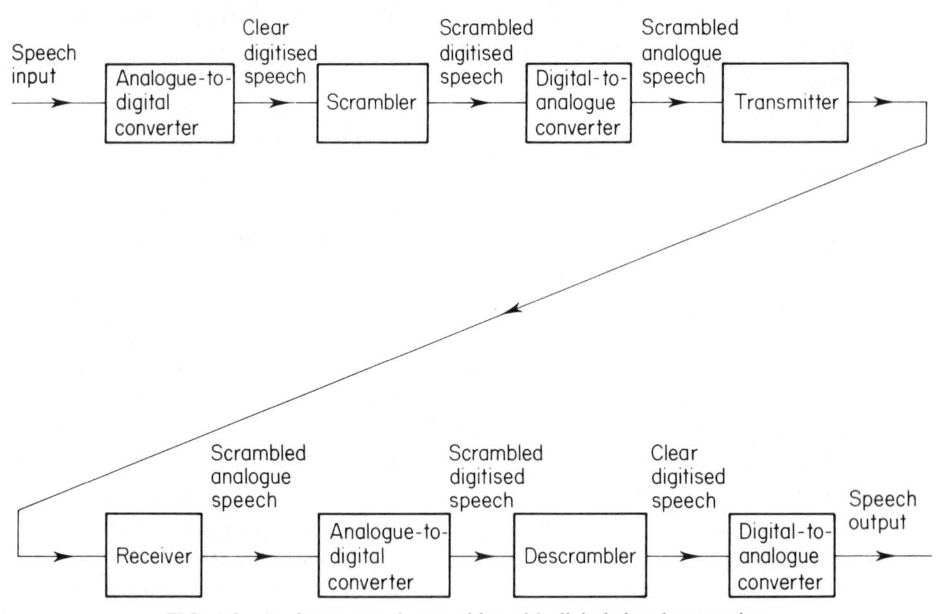

FIG. 1.2. Analogue speech scrambler with digital signal processing.

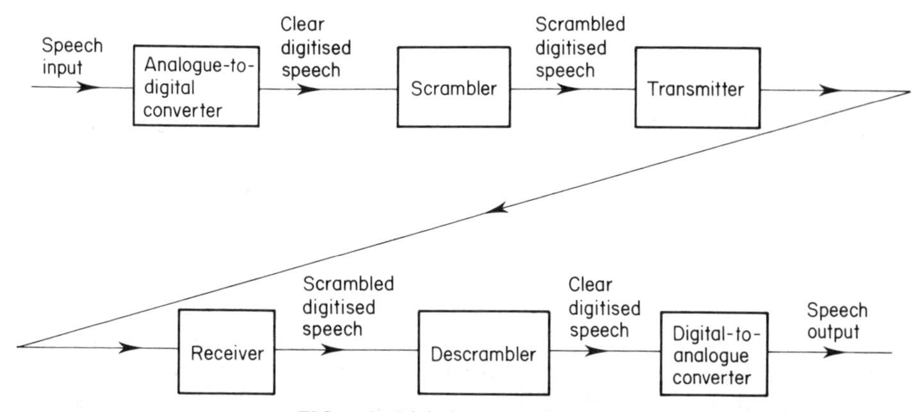

FIG. 1.3. Digital speech scrambler.

Figure 1.3 shows a typical digital system. The fundamental difference between this and the system of Fig. 1.2 is the lack of a digital to analogue (D/A) converter immediately prior to the transmitter and, similarly, the lack of an analogue to digital (A/D) converter immediately after the receiver.

From the diagrams and from our discussion so far, it should be apparent that the digital speech scrambler system of Fig. 1.3 is likely to be somewhat simpler than the analogue system of Fig. 1.2. In many circumstances it is also true that the digital system can be made considerably more secure than either of the analogue systems. Nevertheless there are many situations where it is highly desirable, possibly even necessary, to use an analogue scrambler. We will explain why in considerable detail when we discuss the effects of limited-channel bandwidth. However, in order to make this chapter 'self-sufficient', we include a brief discussion here.

We have already pointed out that our spoken signals are likely to be concentrated within a limited bandwidth. If, in a digital system, the A/D and D/A converters are not sophisticated enough to ensure that the numbers of bits per second which represent the analogue signal are sufficiently small, then the transmitted signal may occupy a larger bandwidth than that occupied by the original speech input. The same will be true if the transmitter and receiver are not sufficiently sophisticated. Furthermore, and probably more importantly, either of these 'faults' may result in the bandwidth required by the transmitted signal being too large for the chosen communications channel. Thus, as with so many other decisions, the final choice between using an analogue or digital system will depend on the individual requirements of the user. His answers to the questions of the earlier sections, like 'How important is audio quality?' and 'What type of channel is to be used?', will obviously affect this choice.

One obvious, straightforward technique for replacing one analogue signal by another is to use a codebook or some other similar means to replace certain selected sensitive words by suitably chosen codewords. Unfortunately, if a large part of the message is considered sensitive and has to be scrambled, the preparation involved can be time consuming. Furthermore the actual process of scrambling is likely to be laborious. One variation on this theme, which was almost certainly used by the United States of America in both world wars, was to employ communicators who translated the messages into obscure languages known by almost no one else in the world. (This of course avoided actually compiling a codebook and certainly avoided any delay in the actual scrambling process.) There are a number of possibilities for these languages and the Americans are reputed to have adopted some of those spoken by the American Indians. One example, quoted by David Kahn in his excellent book "The Codebreakers", involved the use of eight Choctaws of Company D, 141st Infantry, to transmit orders by field telephone in 1918. Clearly they were confident that the enemy forces did not include any Choctaws. Of course the security of such a system would have been jeopardized if one of these Indians had been captured. So, generally, the user is likely to require a rather more transportable and easily replaceable system. Indeed an analogue signal is normally thought of in terms of one or more of the following fundamental parameters: time, frequency or amplitude. Most scramblers then attempt to mask or scramble by operating on one or more of these parameters.

In one of the earlier types of scramblers, known as a *speech inverter*, the aim was simply to convert each frequency component of the speech signal to a new frequency. This new frequency was obtained by taking the difference between the original frequency and some chosen reference frequency. Thus, if the reference frequency was higher than the highest frequency of the speech signal, the result was an inverted frequency spectrum.

The principle behind a speech inverter is very simple. A more sophisticated idea, which still used the frequency domain, was to split the frequency domain of the speech signal into a number of sub-bands and then permute these sub-bands. This was improved still further by periodically changing the permutation.

There are a few techniques for trying to scramble the amplitude of the signal. In one of them, called *tone masking*, a tone or tones, sometimes even noise, is inserted into the signal in order to destroy the syllabic content of the speech.

One technique for scrambling in the time domain is to divide the speech into time frames, sub-divide each frame into a number of segments and then permute the segments within a frame. This technique is called *time element scrambling* and its security can be increased by applying different permutations to different frames.

In subsequent chapters, we will discuss each of these individual scrambling techniques in detail and also look at a number of possibilities for combining them in order to destroy the characteristics of speech in the transmitted signal. While doing this we will also have to remember the obvious, but crucial, fact that the original speech signal must be reconstructed at the receiver. As a general rule one must accept that the more the signal is distorted prior to transmission, the harder it will be to reconstruct it at the receiver. However, if the signal is not distorted enough, then, at least for analogue systems, the designer is faced with the problems of the redundancy of the language and the human brain's remarkable capacity to deduce the correct message from insufficiently scrambled signals. Clearly the designer of analogue scramblers has a difficult task.

For the designer of digital systems things are, in many ways, much easier. Here the aim is to encipher a number of digits, i.e., the intended values of the transmitted signal. To do this we can, as we shall see, use some of the algorithms and techniques that have been developed for data security. Most of these have been mathematically analysed and many of their properties are well understood. However, it can be imprudent to use even these sophisticated techniques without considering the effects they might have on the characteristics of a digital speech signal.

In this section we have given some idea of the type of equipment which might be available. Our discussion was brief but we will give more details in later chapters. This information will help the user to choose his equipment, but, unlike transmitters, receivers etc., there are very few generally accepted standards for scramblers. Thus it is usually the responsibility of the user to make the manufacturer as aware as he can of his particular requirements. He should send a general outline of his requirements to a number of prospective suppliers and invite them to submit proposals showing which of his requirements they can satisfy. The user should anticipate that no supplier will meet them all and he will have to evaluate the various proposals to see which is the most satisfactory.

IV. Evaluating Proposals from Various Manufacturers and Designers

In addition to any financial considerations, the evaluation procedure involves assessing three different aspects:

(a) the supplier,
(b) the performance and audio quality,
(c) the security level.

We will consider each of these in turn.

A. The Supplier

When the user is trying to assess the ability of a particular supplier to provide the equipment plus the level of support which he feels is necessary, he should be prepared to examine the company itself as closely as he scrutinizes their proposal. In this context he should investigate

(1) the company's reputation as a supplier of scramblers,
(2) the history and financial growth of the company,
(3) the technical ability and resources of the company,
(4) the willingness of the company's senior management and technical staff to cooperate with him and/or his own personnel.

The need to look at these four aspects of the company is more or less self-evident. Indeed the points raised would have to be considered in many other business transactions which are totally unrelated to speech scramblers. However, there is one special point which, although we have already mentioned it, we must stress yet again. In many communications environments it may be necessary to retrofit a scrambling network to an existing communications system. This may not be a simple matter and, consequently, the user must convince himself that he can rely on the support of the supplier.

B. Performance and Audio Quality

The user must convince himself that the equipment will come close to satisfying his requirements. However, he must be realistic and must not expect every one of his requirements to be completely satisfied. If, for instance, he has previously decided that no degradation is acceptable then he may find himself rejecting all proposals until he acknowledges the need to lower his sights a little. Deciding just how far one should be prepared to compromise is always difficult. The user obviously has to have some idea of the best levels of performance and audio quality which are obtainable. With this in mind it is essential that he obtains from all potential suppliers some of their units on which he can conduct some trials.

The user's first, and possibly easiest, task is to evaluate the ergonomics of the device. Are the size and weight appropriate? Is the power supply appropriate to the way in which he intends to use the device? In particular is there a battery back-up for the memory holding the cryptographic keys or, alternatively, some other method of ensuring key retention? If not this might mean that the key needs re-entering each time the unit is switched off. If there is such a back-up, for how long will it last? How appropriate is the man-machine interface? How long will it take to train an operator to use the device? All these questions should now be familiar. Essentially the user must

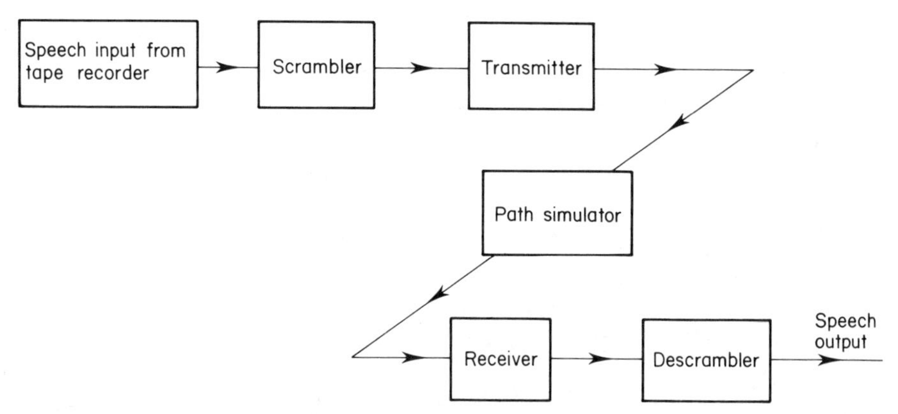

FIG. 1.4. Experimental set-up for evaluation.

work through his list of performance criteria and evaluate how closely each one is satisfied.

His next objective may be to evaluate the audio quality of the recovered message and, in particular, to perform user acceptability and/or intelligibility tests. To do this he will usually set up a laboratory experiment of the type illustrated in Fig. 1.4. By varying the characteristics of the path simulator he will be able to evaluate the quality of the recovered speech signal under various channel conditions.

The normal method of evaluating the intelligibility for this type of system is to have some standard words and phrases transmitted through the system and to measure the success rate of a number of selected listeners. These tests need to be performed carefully in order to ensure that the various scramblers are being compared fairly. Thus, for instance, a tape recorder is usually employed at the input since this ensures that all listeners will hear scrambled and recovered versions of exactly the same original message. Similarly, in order to eliminate individual differences between them, a large number of listeners should be used and all the listeners should test each scrambler. The idea behind this type of test is to obtain an average score giving the percentage of the message heard correctly by the listeners when there is no scrambler in the system and to compare it with their average score when the scramblers are operating. For a good communications channel the first score should, of course, be high and, conversely, for a good scrambler, the second should be low no matter which communications channel is used. Similar tests need to be performed on the recovered speech to evaluate the user acceptability of the system. By carrying out these tests over various simulated paths it should be possible to give a reasonably accurate indication of the limitations of the scramblers. For completeness we will list a typical set of path degradations which may be simulated in order to test a scrambler. (Any reader who is unfamiliar with some of the communications terminology should be prepared to 'skip' through the list and refer back to it after reading Chapter 2.)

(1) Introduce various signal-to-noise ratios into the communications path, i.e., by introducing increasing levels of broadband audio noise ('white' noise) increase the average noise power in relation to the average speech signal power.

(2) Alter the bandwidth of the path, i.e., insert filters in the path to decrease the bandwidth of the transmitted signal. (This tests the scrambler's susceptibility to poor audio frequency response between transmitter and receiver.)

(3) Introduce audio frequency tones and gradually increase their power levels to test the scrambler's susceptibility to interfering tones.

(4) Delay the signal in the path in order to test the effect of time delay. (This is particularly important for a full-duplex circuit.)

(5) Introduce phase delays and non-linear group delays to test their effects. This also tests the effect of a sudden change in the path length. (The latter might occur, for instance, in a voting system of receivers, if, during a continuous transmission, the signal is captured by a receiver other than the one which had originally captured it.)

(6) Systematically increase and decrease the attenuation between the transmitter and receiver, thereby reducing and increasing the signal level at the receiver, to test the effect of fading or signal loss.

(7) Introduce ignition noise into the path to simulate the effect of noise radiated from a vehicle and to test the scrambler's susceptibility to ignition noise.

In addition it may be advisable to test some other features which are not directly related to the path—for instance

(8) the effects of variations in the supply voltage,
(9) the effect of continuous transmission,
(10) the effect of variations in the temperature.

As well as performing these tests individually it may also be necessary to look at the combined effects of a number of the above degradations. Furthermore the user should be prepared to check for any of the standard problems associated with most scramblers. For a typical system using radio transmission, these include factors such as a reduction in the transmission range, the introduction of a time delay and a significant loss of speaker recognition.

We have listed a large number of tests and their implementation is likely to require a long time. Even so, the evaluation process is still not finished. No amount of laboratory testing can replace actual field trials in the environments where the scramblers will operate. In this context it is crucial to test the scramblers using the poorest transceivers with which they are likely to operate. Testing them with better equipment will obviously give misleading results. In these field tests all interfacing problems must be explored and, if the network is to use various types of communications equipment, the devices must be tested with each one. If there are likely to be any problems at all then obviously it is better to discover them before purchasing the equipment.

C. The Security Level

Although we have listed testing the security level as the third stage, we must stress that we are not proposing any particular priority or order for the evaluation process. Indeed in practice the three evaluation processes may take place simultaneously since the personnel performing each of the three stages will normally be different. Furthermore if an equipment is obviously unsatisfactory in any one aspect, than it will be unacceptable and the entire evaluation can be stopped. There are, for example, many equipments which can be dismissed on the security level offered and there is then no need to waste time evaluating their performance.

One of the main problems in evaluating the security level used to be the unwillingness of manufacturers to divulge the relevant information. However, this problem is gradually being eased and most manufacturers now appear willing to supply sufficient information for an assessment to be made. Before we list some of the ways of assessing security we must point out that, of course, the security level is not independent of either the level of performance or, in fact, the evaluation of the company. Thus assessing the security is bound to overlap with certain parts of the other evaluations.

There are various levels at which the security can be evaluated. The first is simply to listen to the scrambled speech and assess its intelligibility. Anyone who listens to a scrambled message for the first time will probably understand nothing. He should not draw any conclusions from this! If he listens a few more times, he will probably begin to recognise odd syllables and may even begin to understand small parts of the message. The human brain tends to adjust and learn very quickly and eventually, by a combination of careful listening and intelligent guessing, the listener may well understand the entire message. In fact, after a while, he may even actually 'hear' the correct message. It must not be forgotten that, just as parents can understand their child's 'speech' long before anyone else can, there are experts at understanding scrambled messages. Apparently some of these experts can even 'understand' messages that have been scrambled using a speech inverter. As in all other spheres, the ability of the experts will vary but the cryptographer should never underestimate the ability of the human brain to unscramble messages and must, therefore, be wary of the listener's descrambling capabilities, even if he does not have access to any sophisticated electronic equipment. To emphasize this we will, when we analyse scramblers, discuss their susceptibility to being broken by the human listener as well as discussing their security from a mathematical point of view. In this context it is perhaps worth noting that in assessing the intelligibility of a scrambled speech signal it is not normally necessary to try for a precise 'information theoretic' qualification. It is normally sufficient simply to decide whether or not an interceptor is likely to be able to understand more of a scrambled message that one would expect him to obtain by intelligent guesswork.

A speech signal contains two distinct types of information. As well as the verbal content of the actual message it also reflects the personality of the speaker, i.e., the intonations, speech rhythms and general characteristics which identify him. Thus, for the interceptor of a scrambled message, there is a considerable amount of intelligence information that has nothing to do with the actual words being spoken. Clearly one would like a scrambler to conceal both types of information. Many modern scramblers do not satisfy this requirement. However that does not necessarily completely rule them out of consideration for use. Their suitability will again depend on the user's precise requirements.

Thus to summarise, the first test of security level is to collect together a number of people to listen, probably many times, to a large number of scrambled messages and to decide whether or not they are understanding an unacceptable proportion of them. The second level of evaluation is much more analytical. It is to assess the security and sophistication of the algorithms used within the scrambler. We must postpone a discussion of this until we have discussed the types of algorithms which exist.

A possible third level of evaluation may be to assess the physical security of the device. A great deal of time, effort and money has been spent on trying to create a tamper-proof box, and such a device would be very important to many areas of security, not just to scramblers. Almost any form of tamper-proofing is likely to be costly and, unless it is considered absolutely necessary, may be best ignored. The lack of success in this area is reflected by the fact that manufacturers tend to avoid the term tamper-proof and talk about the tamper-resistance of their modules. The majority of the scramblers on today's market offer little or no form of tamper-resistance.

As should be apparent from our discussion, the overall evaluation procedure is a time consuming and complicated study. It is not unusual for it to take many months or even years. During this time new, improved products are likely to appear and there is a danger that the user may spend his whole time evaluating equipment and never actually buy anything!

V. Evaluating the Installed Equipment and Rectifying Any Faults

If the first three phases have been performed successfully then there should be virtually nothing to do. Unfortunately unforseen snags are always likely to arise. As an obvious example one should always expect some installation problems. Having gone through so much detailed evaluation of security, etc., the user must now resist all temptation to 'bodge-in' a 'patch' to the system in order to make it functional. He must not compromise his security by slackness at this late stage. It must not be forgotten that the *only* reason for installing a scrambler system is to obtain security. As we said at the beginning of the chapter it can be an expensive way of degrading communications. To degrade the communications and still not be secure would be disastrous!

2. Speech Communications

I. Introduction

One of our main aims is to make this book comprehensible to electronics engineers and to mathematicians. Consequently, in this chapter and the next we concentrate on providing the telecommunications and electronics which the mathematician will need together with the mathematics required by the engineer. Thus, all readers will probably find many sections of material which are familiar to them. Although, naturally, they will be able to read these sections more quickly than the others we nevertheless recommend that no one completely avoids any section. No matter how familiar the actual material, it is possible that the particular applications will be new. For instance, although all the mathematical results needed for our discussion of sequence generators may be familiar, most mathematicians will not have used them in this particular way. Similarly, our discussion on the properties of speech will almost certainly not be familiar to the majority of engineers. We are compelled to include these next two 'background chapters' because the study of speech scramblers involves both engineering and mathematical expertise. The former is needed to understand the practical constraints imposed on the scrambler's designer and to facilitate the avoidance of many design pitfalls. The mathematics is needed for the analysis of the security level, especially for the more sophisticated scramblers.

We begin with a general discussion of the various transmission media for voice signals.

II. The Transmission of Spoken Messages

The word *telecommunications* is used to describe communications at a distance which involve some form of equipment. Thus, a conversation over a telephone system is certainly a telecommunication whereas two people shouting at each other is not. For a telephone conversation the telecommunication equipment is both mechanical and electrical. Although this is true of most of the systems which we will consider, it is certainly not a prerequisite for a telecommunications system. For instance a conversation using a voice tube, i.e., an acoustic system, would also be classed as a telecommunication. For most of the book we will concentrate on electrical systems.

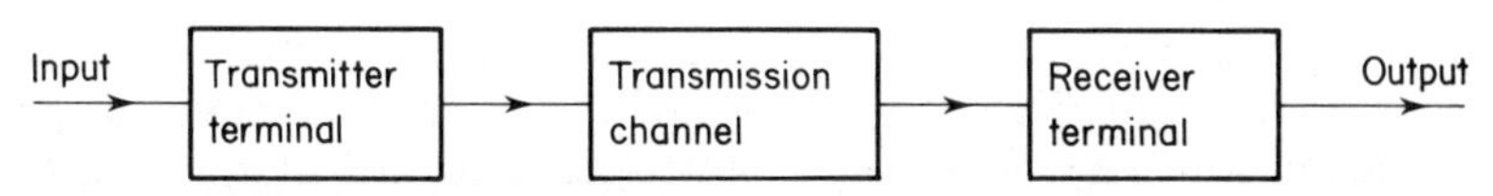

FIG. 2.1. Simple telecommunications system.

Figure 2.1 shows a simple telecommunications system. Note that this particular system only permits simplex communications, i.e., messages can only be sent in one direction. Furthermore, the input source and output destination are not shown. In general we will not include either the input source or output destination in our diagrams. We shall always assume that the input source is a human voice and that the input is speech. Similarly we shall assume that the output is always speech and its destination is another human. (The reader should be aware that considerable research is being done into systems for which, instead of speech, the output is a printed version of the message. This topic, called *speech recognition*, is extremely interesting but we will not discuss it here.)

In a typical system the transmitter terminal will contain an input transducer which converts the speech pressure waves in the air into an electrical signal. This input transducer is commonly called a *microphone*. Similarly, within the receiver terminal is a *loudspeaker*, i.e., an output transducer which converts the received electrical signal back into sound. The *transmission channel* is the medium by which the electrical signal is conveyed from the transmitter terminal to the receiver terminal. The people who provide the input sound by speaking into the microphone and receive the sound after transmission by listening to the loudspeaker are called the *communicators*. In practice the transmitter or receiver terminal will probably contain an *amplifier*. This then guarantees that even a small sound at the input to the transmitter microphone will produce a sound at the output of the receiver loudspeaker. In order to discuss examples and illustrate their properties we must introduce some extra terminology and make some definitions. We begin by looking at the electrical signals which will be conveyed through our telecommunications system.

A. Electrical Signals and Power

An electrical signal consists of varying voltages and currents. However it is convenient to consider the power of the signal rather than its voltage or current. *Power* is defined as the rate of doing work or, equivalently, as the rate of change of energy. The unit of electrical power is the watt and, if the voltage across a resistive network is v volts and the current is i amps, the power p in watts is given by $p = vi$. (Thus 1 *watt* (W) is the work done in 1 sec when a current of 1 A passes through a resistive network with a voltage of 1 V across it.) If the power is varying then the power at any particular moment is called the *instantaneous power*. Thus, the instantaneous power is the rate at which energy is being transferred at a particular instant and is independent of the wave forms of the voltage and current. If the network has an impedance of z ohms then, by Ohm's Law, $v = iz$ which implies that p is proportional to v^2. For a purely resistive network with $z = r$, $p = v^2/r = i^2r$.

For reasons that will soon become apparent, it is often necessary, when studying telecommunications systems, to consider the ratio of two powers. Originally the *bel* was defined as a logarithmic way of expressing such a ratio. However it was subsequently decided that the bel was an inconveniently large unit and this led to the introduction of the *decibel* (dB). In order to express the ratio of two powers p_2 and p_1 in decibels one merely computes $10 \log_{10} (p_2/p_1)$. So, for instance, if the ratio of p_2 to p_1 is 2 : 1 then the power ratio is $(10 \log_{10} 2)$ dB $\triangleq$ 3 dB. A positive power ratio is usually referred to as a gain and a negative power ratio as a loss. Thus a ratio of 2 : 1 is a gain of 3 dB but, since $10 \log_{10} \frac{1}{2} \triangleq -3$, a ratio of 1 : 2 is a loss of 3 dB. One of the major advantages of using decibels comes from the fact that they are logarithmic units. Suppose, for example, that a component of a telecommunications system with power ratio $p_2 : p_1$ is connected in cascade following a component with power ratio $p_3 : p_2$ then, obviously, the overall power ratio is $p_3 : p_1$. If we measure the power ratio in decibels then the individual components have ratios $(10 \log_{10} p_2/p_1)$ dB and $(10 \log_{10} p_3/p_2)$ dB while the overall ratio is $(10 \log_{10} p_3/p_1)$ dB. But $\log_{10} p_3/p_1 = \log_{10} p_3/p_2 + \log_{10} p_2/p_1$, i.e., the overall power ratio, when measured in decibels, is obtained by adding the two individual ones. In general, when they are measured in decibels, the power loss or gain of a telecommunications system which has components connected in cascade is the sum of the power gains or losses of the individual components.

We will now return to our simple example and consider what happens, particularly for small signals. Before we can talk sensibly about the system we need to know the capabilities of the microphone and the loudspeaker. First of all we need to know the sensitivity of the microphone, i.e., the electrical power output from the microphone for the minimum required speech input signal level. Then, for the loudspeaker, we must be able to specify the electrical input power it requires to produce an adequately audible output for the minimum required output signal load. Finally, we need to know the power loss due to the transmission channel.

In order to illustrate the calculations involved we will consider a particular example. Suppose that the minimum power output of the microphone is 0.015 mW and that the power which must be delivered to the loudspeaker for minimum signal level is 15 mW. (Note that 1 mW $= 10^{-3}$ W and is called a *milliwatt*.) Suppose also that half the power is lost in the cable, i.e., that there is a power loss of 3 dB. (Recall that we have already shown that a power ratio of 1 : 2 is a loss of 3 dB.) Then, in order to produce a sound at the loudspeaker which corresponds to that at the microphone, we must provide an amplifier which 'recovers' the loss in the cable and 'implements' the gain of 15 : 0.015 which represents the power ratio of loudspeaker to microphone. Thus we must provide an amplifier with a gain of $(10 \log(15/0.015) + 3)$ dB $= 33$ dB.

Now that we know the capacity needed for our amplifier the next question to consider might be where we should place it. One possibility is in the transmitter terminal, a second is in the receiver terminal and we might even wish to consider placing one in each of them. This is not a particularly easy decision and is likely to be influenced by many factors. The amplifier itself will need to be powered and it may be considerably easier to provide the necessary power at one of the terminals rather than at the other. If there is one amplifier and it is placed in the transmitter then, essentially, only the microphone signals will be amplified. But if, on the other hand, it is placed in the receiver then the received signal will be amplified. This received signal is likely to contain unwanted noise which may be acquired by the signal during its transmission and, of course, the noise will also be amplified. Noise may take many forms and, in order to illustrate some of them, we discuss what happens to the signal as it passes through the channel.

The first problem is that some of the signal power may be lost during transmission. As the signal passes through a telecommunications system it suffers attenuation in the passive parts of the system, e.g., lines and radio paths. In addition a certain amount of noise and interference is likely to affect the signal. Although the attenuation can be compensated for by subsequent amplification, in practice the amplifier itself will add further random noise to the signal. Thus each time the signal is boosted it is more heavily contaminated by noise. Clearly, if we are to assess a system, we must have some meaningful way of measuring the noise in a channel and of comparing the levels of noise at different points in the system. In order to do this it is common practice to refer to the *signal-to-noise ratio*, normally abbreviated to S/N, at each point. By convention this is a power ratio and is equal to the signal power divided by the noise power.

When a signal enters the transmission channel it already contains a certain amount of contaminating noise. Then during transmission, whether down a line or over a radio path, both the signal and noise are attenuated. However while this attenuation is taking place extra noise is also being added to the signal. (In the case of a cable system this addition might be 'thermal' noise from its resistive parts while for a radio path it might be 'sky noise'.) Thus the signal-to-noise ratio at the output of the transmission channel is likely to be considerably lower than at the input. Similarly when an amplifier is used, although the signal and noise which are present at its input are amplified by the same factor, the signal-to-noise ratio is lowered still further because the amplifier adds extra noise from both the passive and active components within it. In fact just about every part of a telecommunications system will contribute to the deterioration of the signal-to-noise ratio of the signal passing through it.

Let us now return to the simple telecommunications system of Fig. 2.1. Another important factor to be considered is the ratio of the acoustic power produced by the loudest and quietest inputs to the input terminal. This is normally referred to as the *dynamic range of the message source*. A reasonable quality system should, typically, be able to cope with a dynamic range of about 70 dB. But to achieve this we must ensure that the entire system is able to handle such a range of signals. If any part of the system cannot cope with the highest input then this will probably cause considerable distortion of the signal.

Yet another consideration for a telecommunications system is the bandwidth it can manage. In order to have a meaningful discussion of this we must first review some of the fundamental properties of linear circuits.

Suppose we have a circuit with a set of input signals $X = \{x_1, x_2, \ldots\}$ which produces outputs $Y = \{y_1, y_2, \ldots\}$, where, for each i, y_i is the output

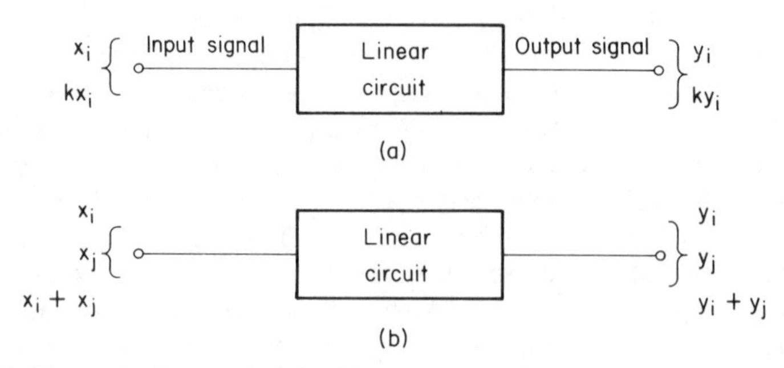

FIG. 2.2. Linear circuit. (a) Principle of homogeneity and (b) principle of superposition.

corresponding to the input x_i. The circuit is said to satisfy the *principle of homogeneity*, if, whenever any x_i is multiplied by a constant and input to the circuit, the output signal is y_i multiplied by the same constant (see Fig. 2.2a). The circuit satisfies the *principle of superposition* if when the input signal is the superposition (or sum) of x_i and x_j (for any two input signals x_i and x_j) the output signal is the sum of y_i and y_j (see Fig. 2.2.b). Any circuit which satisfies both principles is called a *linear circuit*.

Many of the components and circuits of telecommunications systems are either linear or, when restricted to a limited range of values for the input and output, may be considered as such. This range is also usually referred to as the *dynamic range of the appropriate component or circuit*. If our telecommunications system includes components which are not actually linear but we wish it to act as a linear circuit for all messages, then we must ensure that the dynamic range of the entire system is at least as large as that of the message source. Failure to do this will, as we have already seen, probably lead to distortion of the signal output from the receiver. This causes a particular problem for circuits involving scramblers. It means we must make sure that the scrambling technique does not lead to transmitted signals whose dynamic range goes beyond that of the channel, the receiver terminal or, indeed, any part of the transmitter terminal through which it must pass.

So far we have given no justification for our implicit assumption that linear circuits are desirable. We will now see how advantageous linear circuits can be. We know that any circuit modifies the electrical signal at its input to produce an electrical signal at its output. Clearly we would like to be able to analyse the circuit's response to every possible input signal. (We call the set of all possible input signals the *input space*.) However it is almost certainly not practicable or desirable to generate every possible input signal in order to determine the corresponding output. But if the circuit under consideration is linear, then knowledge of the output corresponding to two input signals gives the response to all input signals which are obtained from the original two by either superposition or multiplying by constants. Thus, by determining the actual outputs corresponding to a few input signals, one can use the principles of homogeneity and superposition to deduce the outputs from a much larger number of inputs. A subset of the input space is called a *generating set* if every possible input signal can be obtained by multiplying its elements by suitable constants and/or adding together appropriate combinations of them. Thus if we have a linear circuit and can find a generating set for our input space then, as soon as we know the output corresponding to each of the generating signals, we can use the principles of homogeneity and superposition to deduce the output of any possible input signal.

As we have already observed most telecommunications channels may be regarded as linear circuits, at least for signals within their dynamic range. It is also possible to find a generating set for the input signals and the most popular one is probably the set of sinusoids.

A *sinusoid* is a waveform which is represented by an equation of one of the following two forms: $A\cos(\omega t + \varphi)$ or $A\sin(\omega t + \varphi)$, where A, ω, φ are constants and t represents time. The constant A is called the *amplitude* of the wave and, since both the cosine and sine functions have a maximum value of 1, it is the height of the peaks of the waveform above its average value. (Note that, by convention, A is assumed to be positive.) Since the functions $\sin x$ and $\cos x$ both have period 2π the sinusoids $A\cos(\omega t + \varphi)$ and $A\sin(\omega t + \varphi)$ are also periodic, but have period $2\pi/\omega$. However it is not the usual practice to talk about the period of a sinusoid. Instead it is customary to quote its frequency. The *frequency* is the number of periods (or cycles) which occur in 1 sec. Clearly, for any periodic wave form, if the period is T and the frequency is f then $f = 1/T$ and thus, for a sinusoid, $f = \omega/2\pi$ or $\omega = 2\pi f$. [The unit of frequency is the hertz (Hz) and 1 *hertz* is a frequency of 1 cycle/sec.] Since f is the frequency and $\omega = 2\pi f$, ω is called the *angular frequency* of the sinusoid. (There are other, more convincing, reasons for this terminology but they are not relevant here.) The constant φ determines the initial height of the wave, i.e., the height when $t = 0$, and is called the *phase* of the sinusoid. If two sinusoids have different phases then we say that they are *out-of-phase* and the difference in the two values of φ is called the *phase difference*.

By asserting that the set of sinusoids is a generating set for our input signals we are claiming that the waveform of any input signal can be obtained by adding together an appropriate combination of them. The justification that the sinusoids form a generating set is mathematical and we will postpone it until the next section.

If a signal, or waveform, is written as a sum of sinusoids then the sinusoids which actually occur in this sum are called the *frequency components* of the signal. The *bandwidth of a signal* is then the range of frequencies occupied by the frequency components of the signal and the *bandwidth of a telecommunications system* is the range of frequencies which the system can handle. Thus, as an example, the bandwidth of a typical hi-fi amplifier might be specified as 15 kHz, which would mean that it could handle signals whose frequency components take any value from 0 to 15 kHz. One bandwidth of particular relevance to this book is that of recognisable speech. This, as we shall see in more detail later, is about 3 kHz and extends from approximately 300 Hz to about 3.3 kHz.

If a signal is to be transmitted through a system, then, in order to avoid any distortion, it is clearly necessary to ensure that the range of frequencies which the system can handle includes all the frequency components of the signal. In other words the system bandwidth must be at least as large as that of the signal. It is perhaps not so obvious that it is also desirable that the bandwidth of the system should be no larger than that of the signal. If the system's bandwidth is too large then the system may accept more noise than is necessary and this, of course, will result in a decrease in the signal-to-noise ratio. Obviously noise and interference should be kept to a minimum. Thus, in all telecommunications systems where noise may be significant, it is common practice to ensure that the frequency characteristics of the channel, transmitter terminal and receiver terminal (including amplifiers, etc.) are the same as those of the signal. In particular the bandwidth should be the same for both the system and the message.

As an illustration of this we will consider the tuning of a radio. At any given instant there are numerous signals arriving at the radio's antenna but, nevertheless, it is usually possible to tune the radio so that it only emits the signals of a chosen programme. This is achieved by including, as part of the receiver, an electrical circuit which will only pass frequencies which lie within a small bandwidth, typically about 8 kHz. (Such a circuit is called a *bandpass filter*.) When the radio is tuned, the central frequency of the band passed by this circuit is adjusted so that it corresponds to that of the signal of the chosen programme (see Fig. 2.3).

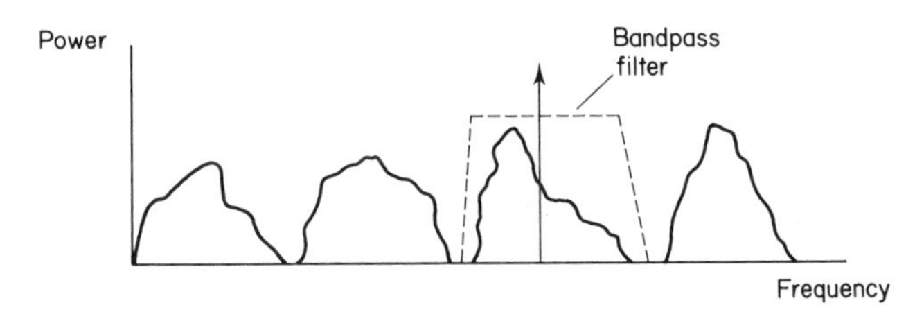

FIG. 2.3. Tuneable receiver.

The bandpass filter is designed so that all signals outside its selected band are attenuated to a negligible level. This careful matching of the bandwidths of the telecommunications system and the message source improves the audio quality of the system. However it causes great problems for the scrambler designer. As we pointed out in Chapter 1, most scramblers are retrofitted to existing telecommunications systems which are likely to operate in narrow bandwidths. But, as we shall see later, most sophisticated forms of scrambling increase the signal bandwidth and so, since the existing bandwidth is likely to be narrow, the user may end up with a system in which the scrambled speech occupies a larger bandwidth than that supported by the rest of the system. This is one of the major reasons for losses in speech quality. The extent of the degradation will, of course, vary from system to system. The degradation may also appear to vary from listener to listener and, for all telecommunications systems, the assessment of the acceptability of the received signal is very subjective.

In any telecommunications system, whether it employs scramblers or not, the listener's perception characteristics are important. When scramblers are included in the system then it is necessary to test the intelligibility of both the received speech and the transmitted speech. Obviously we want the received speech to be understandable while the transmitted speech should have little or no intelligibility to any listener. The 'measure' of the intelligibility in each case is usually nothing more than the reaction of a number of listeners. If a sufficient number of users can understand the received message but not the transmitted message then that aspect of the system is satisfactory.

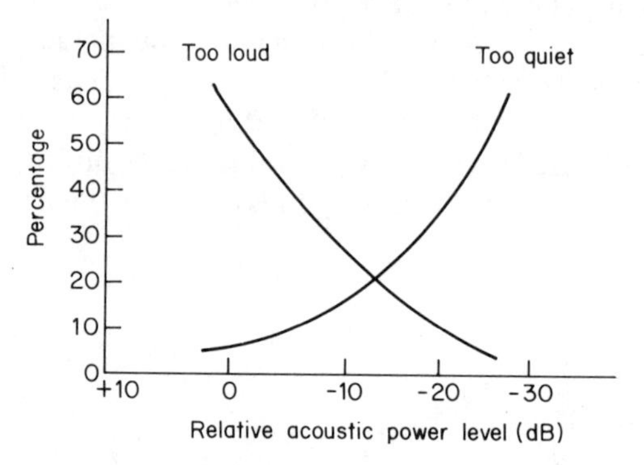

FIG. 2.4. Typical results from user tests for 'loudness'.

Although user trials are the ultimate test for a system, we must never forget that, no matter how good the system may be, it will almost certainly be impossible to please all users. As an illustration consider the graph of Fig. 2.4 which illustrates a number of users' assessment of how loud a system should be. The volume commenced at a particular level, 0 on the horizontal axis, and then the acoustic power was varied. From the graph we can see that, at 5 dB below the original reference level, 10% of the users thought the resulting speech was too quiet while about 40% thought it was too loud. If users can disagree so dramatically in such a simple test then there is clearly no hope of unanimous agreement about levels of intelligibility, etc. The designer can do nothing more than perform sufficient tests to convince himself that he is pleasing most of the people most of the time. At least this is the situation for the received signal. If, during his tests, he finds one solitary listener who can understand his scrambled message he will probably conclude that the system is not secure enough.

B. Examples of Telecommunications Systems

For convenience we shall loosely classify transmission channels under two general headings: (1) bounded, (2) radio. *Bounded channels* will include electrical conduction in wires, cables etc. and optical fibres while *radio channels* include all forms of electromagnetic radiation in space e.g. microwave, satellite, etc.

There is, of course, no reason why a particular telecommunications system should not include both bounded and radio communications. One obvious example of such a system is provided when a telephone conversation takes place between one user in a car while the other is in an office. This is likely to entail a radio link from the car to the local exchange of the second user and then a line from this exchange to the office. However, for the moment, we will consider each of the two categories separately.

1. *Bounded media*

Wire pairs are widely used for telephone communications. They used to be carried overhead on poles but, since this is both unsightly and inconvenient, the normal modern practice is to use buried cables which each carry a large number of twisted wire pairs. The twisting of the pairs is important since it reduces *crosstalk*, i.e., the effect of stray electric and magnetic fields from one pair affecting another.

Although the twisting of the pairs reduces crosstalk, the use of wire pairs is limited. One reason is that crosstalk increases as the frequency increases. Another, even more important, reason is that increasing the frequency also increases the loss (*attenuation*) of the pair. This effect is shown in Fig. 2.5. and Table 2.1 which indicates that the loss will also depend on the metal used as the conductor.

The difficulty of having a frequency-dependent line loss can be overcome, to some extent, by using devices called equalisers and repeaters. An *equaliser* is a device which has the inverse response to that of the line i.e., the attenuation introduced by an equaliser decreases as the frequency increases. Thus

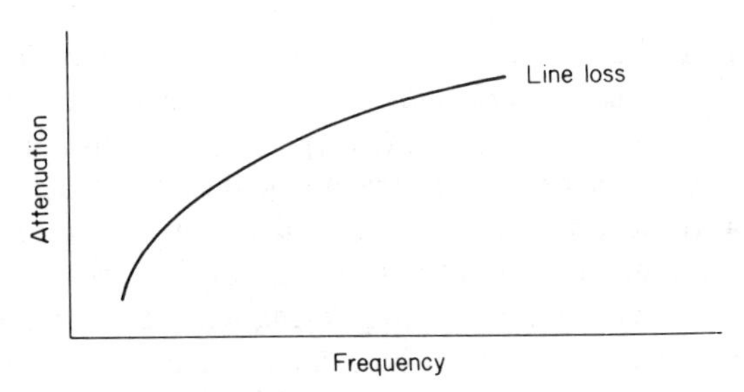

FIG. 2.5. Line loss on a wire pair.

TABLE 2.1

Average Loss for 0.5-mm Diameter Conductor

Conductor	Test frequency (Hz)	Loss (dB/km)
Copper	800	1.2
Copper	3000	2.3
Aluminium	3000	3.4

the idea is to design an equaliser whose response compensates for that of the line. The overall response will then be constant (see Fig. 2.6). Once the loss is constant a *repeater*, which is essentially an amplifier to compensate for the losses, can be added to the line. Thus, by placing equalisers and repeaters at fixed intervals along the cable, it appears that it might be possible to produce a flat response. This spacing of the repeaters and equalisers will clearly depend on the highest frequency to be used; the higher the frequency required the shorter the allowable distance between repeaters and equalisers. Unfortunately, in practice, the attenuation at the higher frequencies is likely to be so bad that too many repeaters and equalisers will be needed, and thus this type of approach can only be used for a very limited frequency range.

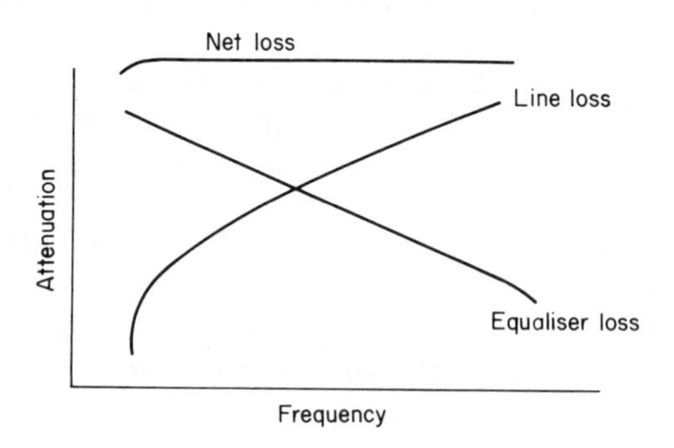

FIG. 2.6. Equaliser and line losses.

There are a number of ways of trying to achieve higher frequency transmissions. One is to use a *coaxial cable* which consists of a pair of concentric cylindrical conductors that are held in position by insulators. The outer conductor is there to act as an electrical shield and, as such, is likely to be less effective at frequencies below 60 kHz. Just as we saw for the twisted wire pair, the usable bandwidth and the repeater spacing are closely connected. For instance, in order to obtain an upper frequency of 61.6 MHz (1 MHz = 10^6 Hz) a coaxial cable with inner and outer diameters of 2.9 and 9.5 mm, respectively, requires a repeater spacing of 1.5 km.

When we discussed bandwidths we pointed out that speech occupies about 3 kHz. In the last few paragraphs we have been discussing channels with frequencies up to 61.6 MHz. In view of the limited range of the human voice, the reader may be wondering why we are so concerned about these very high frequencies. To illustrate the reason we will look at an example. Suppose that we are laying a submarine cable to act as the transmission channel for trans-atlantic telephone calls. Clearly the cost of such an operation is enormous. To use it for one call at a time would make each call very expensive. So the submarine cable is designed so that it can carry thousands of calls simultaneously and this is achieved by sending the various calls within different frequency bands. Clearly the higher the maximum frequency which the cable can carry the larger the number of calls it can carry. Thus our reason for wanting to use high frequencies is to reduce the cost of each transmission. This argument applies not only to submarine cables but to many other types of transmission links including, for example, trunk lines and satellite channels.

It is, of course, not sufficient to say that we transmit the various calls within different frequency bands. We must say how this is achieved. The technique of achieving this multiplicity of calls over a single channel involves the general idea of multiplexing and one particular method is *frequency division multiplexing* (fdm).

The electrical signal generated when speech is directed into a microphone is called the *base-band signal* and normally has a frequency range extending from 300 Hz to 3.3 kHz. In most telecommunications systems the shape and frequency components of this base-band signal are normally modified in some way in order to obtain a form which is more suitable for transmission. This process is called *modulation* and the process of recovering the base-band signal from the modulated signal is called *demodulation*. As we have already observed there are two main reasons for modulation. One is to change the signal into a form and a band where more efficient transmission is possible and the other is to make possible the simultaneous transmission of a number of signals over the same channel. We will return to modulation later and look at the various techniques which are available. For the moment we will merely mention that in frequency division multiplexing many base-band signals are moved to a number of different frequency ranges and that, by combining (*multiplexing*) them to produce a single signal, this then enables the simultaneous transmission of a number of signals (see Fig. 2.7). In any given situation the choice of modulation technique will depend on many factors including, for instance, the environment and the particular telecommunications systems. It may also be influenced by the type of scrambling scheme to be employed.

The system illustrated in Fig. 2.7 is very small and only involves three base-band signals. In practice a coaxial cable with the dimensions described above

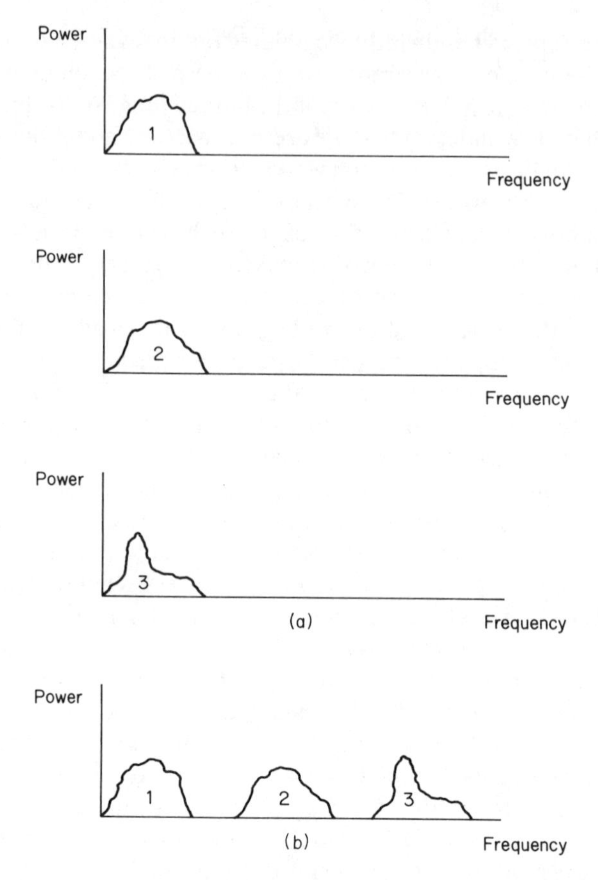

FIG. 2.7. Frequency division multiplexing. (a) The spectra of three different base-band signals and (b) spectrum of the three base-band signals multiplexed together.

is capable of simultaneously transmitting nearly 11,000 different telephone calls. The signals are multiplexed at the transmitter and demultiplexed at the receiver.

It is possible to achieve even wider bandwidths on certain other bounded transmission channels. For instance hollow conducting pipes, known as *waveguides*, can be used for the propagation of radiowaves, (provided that the cross sectional dimensions of the pipe are at least as great as the wavelength of the radio waves; the wavelength is $3 \times 10^8/f$ m, where f is the frequency). Waveguides are used for frequencies in the range of 2 to 11 GHz or, equivalently, for wavelengths in the range 15 to 2.7 cm (1 GHz $= 10^9$ Hz). Radio waves of such high frequencies are called *microwaves*. Although waveguides cannot be used for signals with frequencies below a specific (rather high) value, they have a considerable bandwidth and can therefore transmit many signals simultaneously. A typical 10-GHz system, for instance, will have a bandwidth of more than 200 MHz and be capable of the simultaneous transmission of over half a million telephone messages.

Telephone channels, in common with many other transmission media, exhibit certain amounts of time delay which are likely to vary with the frequency components of the voice signal. This delay can range from 3 to 30 msec and in Fig. 2.8 we show a typical situation relative to a 1-kHz signal. In Chapters 4 and 5, when we consider some particular scramblers, we will discuss the problems which these delays can cause. For the moment we merely remark that these time delays have been the downfall of many scrambling schemes.

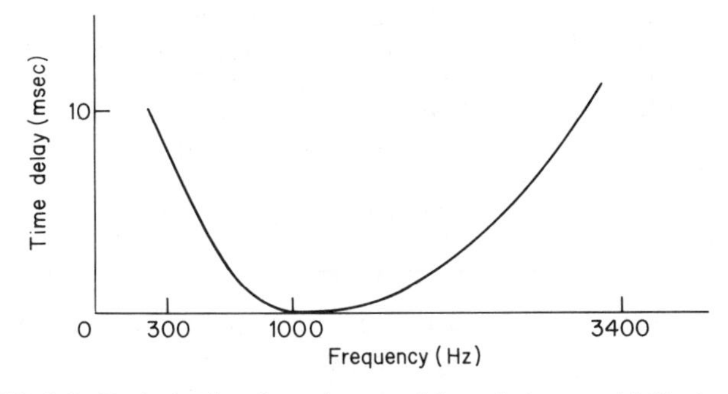

FIG. 2.8. Typical voice channel group delay relative to a 1-kHz signal.

No discussion of bounded media would be complete without mentioning *optical fibres*. This medium uses optical waveguides in the form of glass fibres which carry modulated light signals. Schemes of this type permit vast bandwidths and, as they become more common, are likely to have an important effect on speech security. Among other possible advantages, their use will certainly make the actual interception of the signals considerably harder.

2. *Radio*

Radio transmission channels use radio wave propagation between antennae at the transmitter and receiver. The radio transmitter uses a modulation process to produce a *radio frequency (rf) signal*, i.e., to convert the message signal into a form which is suitable for transmission. Normally the transmitter will also need to contain an amplifier to ensure that the transmitted signal will be strong enough when it reaches the receiver.

Radio waves are unbounded in the sense that they are propagated into the atmosphere. However in practice they will almost certainly be bounded by the earth's surface and ionosphere. (The *ionosphere* is the region, about 50–400 km above the earth's surface, where various conducting layers of ionised gases exist. The different layers tend to reflect different frequency bands.)

When discussing radio it is common practice to assign well-known names to various specific frequency ranges. In Table 2.2 we give a list of these names.

TABLE 2.2

The Various Frequency Bands

Frequency range	Name
0 Hz–3 kHz	Extra low frequency (elf)
3 kHz–30 kHz	Very low frequency (vlf)
30 kHz–300 kHz	Low frequency (lf) or long wave
300 kHz–3 MHz	Medium frequency (mf) or medium wave
3 MHz–30 MHz	High frequency (hf) or short wave
30 MHz–300 MHz	Very high frequency (vhf)
300 MHz–3 GHz	Ultra high frequency (uhf)
3 GHz–30 GHz	Super high frequency (shf)
30 GHz–300 GHz	Extremely high frequency (ehf)

Very-low-frequency waves are used principally for navigational and military purposes. They are bounded by the earth's surface and the ionosphere and are guided by effects which include diffraction at the earth's surface and refraction at the ionosphere.

The lf and mf waves are used mainly for radio broadcasting and rely on propagation over the curvature of the earth's surface. In the mf waveband propagation also takes place by sky waves and this presents a number of problems. For example, sky waves exhibit both regular (i.e., daily and seasonal) and irregular fluctuations with ionospheric conditions. They allow communications over longer distances but this advantage is countered by the fact that they are subject to multipath propagation and selective fading. *Multipath propagation* occurs when the transmitted signal reaches its destination by more than one route. If, for instance, the receiver gets two reflected waves, of which one has been reflected once and the other twice, then the fact that they have travelled paths of different lengths means that the two waves will arrive at the receiver with a relative delay. This, of course, will mean that they probably have different phases. Their phase difference can take any value from 0 to 180°. If it happens to be 0° then they will reinforce each other and the resultant signal may be too large. This will cause distortion. If, at the other extreme, the phase difference is 180° then the signals will cancel each other out. This is known as *selective fading* because, as the conditions fluctuate, certain frequency components seem to fade away. The effect of selective fading can often be heard on the mf band of the radio, especially during the evening. Its effect can be even worse in the hf band.

The hf band is extremely popular and is usually very heavily overcrowded. Its uses include long distance broadcasting plus maritime and aeronautical communications. Unfortunately a consequence of its popularity is that there tends to be considerable interference caused by different stations operating on the same frequency. This tendency for users to concentrate on a few of the frequencies arises from their need to avoid the fading which, as we saw when we discussed the mf waves, results from the sky wave propagation. In this particular band it is common practice to avoid fading by changing frequency to certain 'good' frequencies which are determined by the forecasts of ionospheric conditions and are, as a consequence, known to most users. For short distances hf ground wave propagation also occurs and this tends to be used for land mobile and ship-to-shore communications.

Both vhf and uhf are mainly used over short distances and rely on direct waves. These waves are often a combination of direct and ground reflected waves over distances which, typically, vary from a few kilometers to a few hundred kilometers, depending on both the terrain over which the waves must propagate and the height of the antennae. There is one definite advantage to this type of short range communication and that is the virtual lack of interference from other stations. Both vhf and uhf are used for television broadcasts and, in addition, vhf is also used for high-quality radio.

Most microwave communications are restricted to point-to-point communications. They tend to be transmitted over broad bands and use direct wave propagation. A particular example of this is provided by the so-called *line-of-sight radio relay systems* used in telephone networks. In these systems the stations are mounted on hills or towers in order to achieve a direct, or line-of-sight, path from station to station. Each station consists of a transmitter and receiver for each direction and, by building an appropriate number of stations, links can be established to 'cover' an entire country. There are two advantages to this type of system. The first is the need for only a relatively small transmission power (typically of the order of 10 W) and the second is that highly directional antennae can be employed. This latter remark, of course, applies to all point-to-point systems.

In a radio network both the transmit and receive antennae can be directional or omni-directional. An omni-directional transmitting antennae radiates energy more or less uniformly in all directions. Thus it is likely to be particularly useful when there is a centrally located broadcast antenna transmitting to a number of receivers. Similarly an omni-directional receiving antenna is sensitive to energy from all directions and is advantageous if the receiver is likely to pick-up signals from many different sources.

If, however, a transmitter is to be used only to send signals to one particular receiver then, clearly, energy will be wasted if an omni-directional antenna is used. Figure 2.9 shows a polar diagram for a directional antenna. In this case the antenna is a parabolic reflector and the diagram illustrates how the energy reflected in different directions is likely to vary. (If it were used as a receiving antenna our diagram would should its sensitivity in various directions.) In our particular example the antenna gain is greatest in the reference direction and falls by over 30 dB for a change in direction of only 10°. Directional antennae are less sensitive to interfering signals and this is a great advantage for all directed transmissions. They also have extra advantages for speech security.

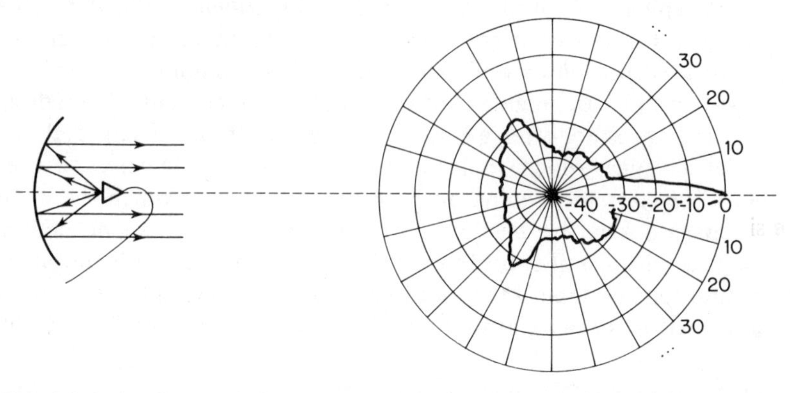

FIG. 2.9. Polar diagram for a parabolic reflector (relative energy radiated in decibels).

The first obvious advantage for speech security is that, since any receiving antenna has to be carefully placed before it will receive the signal, the actual interception of signals is likely to be difficult. The second advantage is concerned with protection against jamming and spoofing rather than against unwanted listeners. A directional antenna is likely to have directions of very low sensitivity as well as its direction of maximum sensitivity. We have already discussed jamming and spoofing so we need not say much about them. In this context, a prospective jammer will set up a powerful transmitting antenna and emit a powerful jamming signal. The aim of this signal is to create such a low signal-to-noise ratio at the receiver's antenna that the communicator's signal will be unretrievable. However, if there is a directional antenna at the receiver the user may be able to position it so that its direction of maximum sensitivity is towards the wanted signal while the direction of minimum sensitivity is towards the jamming signal. If this is achieved then the effect of the jammer will be reduced and the genuine message should be intelligible.

Of course the jamming transmitter may be mobile and, to combat this, we would like to have a directional antenna for which one could change the directions of minimum sensitivity. Another way of phrasing this to say that we would like to be able to change the polar diagram in a controlled way. (Note, incidentally, that the diagram will change if either the direction of the transmitting antenna is changed or if the transmitting frequency is changed). Antennae with this capability are very expensive and have not yet been developed to a sufficiently high level of proficiency. Nevertheless if speech security is an extremely important consideration then this type of antenna may appear extremely high on a user's priority list. The art of antenna design is a fascinating and complex topic. However, it is not directly related to speech scrambling and we shall say no more about it.

Our discussion of the transmission channel led us, quite naturally, into considering various components of the receiver's and transmitter's terminals. The close interaction between the different parts of a telecommunications system make it virtually impossible to discuss one aspect of the system without addressing many others. It is, after all, acceptance of this fact which has persuaded us to include a chapter like this in a book on speech scramblers. We simply could not discuss the scramblers in isolation. Having said that, we will now turn our main attention from the channel to the terminal.

The two most familiar terminals are probably the telephone and the radio receiver. Each of these has characteristics which we have come to accept and, possibly, assume are fundamental properties. For instance, most people take it for granted that a telephone system is always full-duplex and that a broadcast radio is merely simplex. These are merely characteristics of these two terminals when used in their most common environment. When the environment changes then the other properties of the channel may change as well. For instance a mobile radio, as used by police forces, is often a half-duplex device. A more relevant, and in many ways unfortunate, example is that a full-duplex system like the telephone will often be reduced to half-duplex when scrambling is introduced. The reasons for this are complicated and we will not discuss them now. For the moment we will accept it as a fact and look at the consequences. It is important to realise that the fact that a system is half-duplex does not, necessarily, say anything about the channel. Two possibilities are:

(a) the channel allows transmission in either direction, but only one way at a time,

(b) the channel allows full-duplex communications but the terminals are constructed in such a way that transmission is only possible in one direction at any given moment.

When scrambling is added to a telephone system it is usually relatively easy to preserve half-duplex operation. However it is likely to be extremely expensive, and in some cases virtually impossible, to maintain the terminals as full-duplex devices. Once again there are many reasons and some of them are complicated. The fundamental reason is simply that it is difficult to combine or reconcile the properties and characteristics of the scrambler with those of the telephone system. As a simple illustration we will consider the effect of echoes on the system.

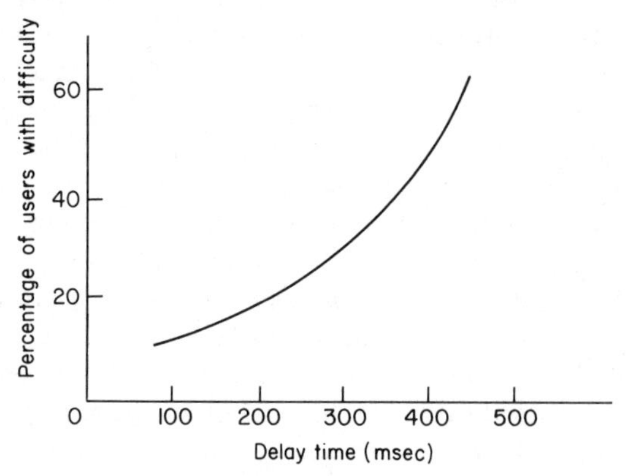

FIG. 2.10. Effect of echo on the message originator.

An *echo* is a delayed version of the message which is produced by reflections in the system. Not surprisingly if these echoes reach the earphone of the message originator they are likely to be very distracting. Furthermore, as Fig. 2.10 illustrates, the degree of distraction will probably increase as the delays get larger. A normal telephone network is designed to ensure that only acceptable delays occur. But if scramblers are introduced to the system they are likely to introduce extra delays which may result in an unacceptable system. Furthermore if the echoes become scrambled the user will be faced with the extra distraction of having unintelligible signals in his earphone.

We can summarize our discussion of voice transmission by saying that we shall, broadly speaking, identify the transmission channel between the terminals by its bandwidth and the impairments which might occur to the signals which it carries. We shall be particularly concerned about the following five principal causes of impairments:

(a) attenuation and its variation with frequency,
(b) noise,
(c) non-linearity of the channel,
(d) changes in propagation time with frequency,
(e) echoes.

Now that we have completed our brief overview of voice message transmission we shall look at some of the methods for analysing signals. Our aim is to establish some of the techniques necessary to examine the properties of speech signals and to tackle the problem of converting the analogue signals to digital ones.

III. Signal Analysis

When we discussed linear circuits we asserted that the waveform of a speech signal could be expressed as the sum of certain sinusoids. Indeed this concept of expressing certain functions of time as the sum of sinusoids is one of the branches of mathematics which has proved most useful to physicists and engineers. We have not, as yet, made any attempt to justify our assertion and have certainly not shown how these sinusoids can be determined. We will now rectify this and begin our study of Fourier analysis.

If $f(t)$ is any periodic function of the variable t then its representation as a sum of sinusoids is called its *Fourier series*, and the process of determining the Fourier series of given functions is called *Fourier analysis*. If the period of $f(t)$ is T and the frequency of repetition is f_1 then, of course, $f_1 = 1/T$. The function $f(t)$ has a Fourier series of the form

$$f(t) = a_0 + \sum_{n=1}^{\infty} a_n \cos(n\omega_1 t) + \sum_{n=1}^{\infty} b_n \sin(n\omega_1 t)$$

where $\omega_1 = 2\pi f_1$. Since f_1 is the frequency of repetition of $f(t)$, f_1 is called the *fundamental frequency* of $f(t)$ and, similarly, ω_1 is the *fundamental angular frequency*. For any positive integer n the terms $a_n \cos(n\omega_1 t)$ and $b_n \sin(n\omega_1 t)$ are called the *harmonics* and occur at angular frequencies $n\omega_1$. To determine the *Fourier coefficients* a_n, b_n we have to integrate $f(t)$ over any complete cycle, i.e., over any interval of length T. Adopting the standard convention that $\oint$ represents integration over one complete cycle we have

$$a_0 = \frac{1}{T} \oint f(t)\, dt$$

$$a_n = \frac{2}{T} \oint f(t) \cos(n\omega_1 t)\, dt$$

$$b_n = \frac{2}{T} \oint f(t) \sin(n\omega_1 t)\, dt$$

We will not attempt to establish these formulae here and any one wishing to see a proof should consult Brown and Glazier (1964). However, we must point out that the function $f(t)$ has to have certain extra properties before these formulae will apply. Fortunately the various signals which we will consider all have these extra properties so we shall ignore them and merely assume that the formulae always hold.

The range of the various frequency components, i.e., the set of integers n for which at least one of a_n or b_n is non-zero, is called the *spectrum* of the function. To illustrate this concept we will determine the spectrum of a square pulse train. The graph of a typical *square pulse train* is shown in Fig. 2.11. In this example $f(t)$ has period T and, during any period of T sec, it takes the value of V for $T/2$ sec and $-V$ for the other $T/2$ sec. In the diagram we have chosen our time interval so that $t = 0$ is at the start of a pulse. In order to determine the Fourier coefficients we must integrate $f(t)$ over any time interval of length T. If we select the interval $t = 0$ to $t = T$, then we have

$$f(t) = \begin{cases} V & \text{for } 0 \leqslant t < T/2 \\ -V & \text{for } T/2 \leqslant t < T \end{cases}$$

Using our formulae for the Fourier coefficients and putting $\omega_1 = 2\pi f_1 = 2\pi/T$ we get

$$a_0 = \frac{1}{T}\int_0^T f(t)\,dt = \frac{1}{T}\left[\int_0^{T/2} V\,dt + \int_{T/2}^T -V\,dt\right] = 0$$

$$a_n = \frac{2}{T}\int_0^T f(t)\cos(n\omega_1 t)\,dt$$

$$= \frac{2}{T}\left[\int_0^{T/2} V\cos(n\omega_1 t)\,dt + \int_{T/2}^T -V\cos(n\omega_1 t)\,dt\right] = 0$$

$$b_n = \frac{2}{T}\int_0^T f(t)\sin(n\omega_1 t)\,dt$$

$$= \frac{2}{T}\left[\int_0^{T/2} V\sin(n\omega_1 t)\,dt + \int_{T/2}^T -V\sin(n\omega_1 t)\,dt\right]$$

$$= \begin{cases} \dfrac{2}{T}\left[\dfrac{VT}{\pi n} + \dfrac{VT}{\pi n}\right] = \dfrac{4V}{\pi n} & \text{if } n \text{ is odd} \quad (\text{Recall that } \omega_1 T = 2\pi) \\ \dfrac{2}{T}[0 + 0] = 0 & \text{if } n \text{ is even} \end{cases}$$

Thus

$$f(t) = \left[\frac{4V}{\pi}\sin(\omega_1 t) + \frac{1}{3}\sin(3\omega_1 t) + \frac{1}{5}\sin(5\omega_1 t) + \cdots\right]$$

$$= \sum_{n=1,\, n\text{odd}}^{\infty} \frac{4V}{n\pi}\sin(n\omega_1 t)$$

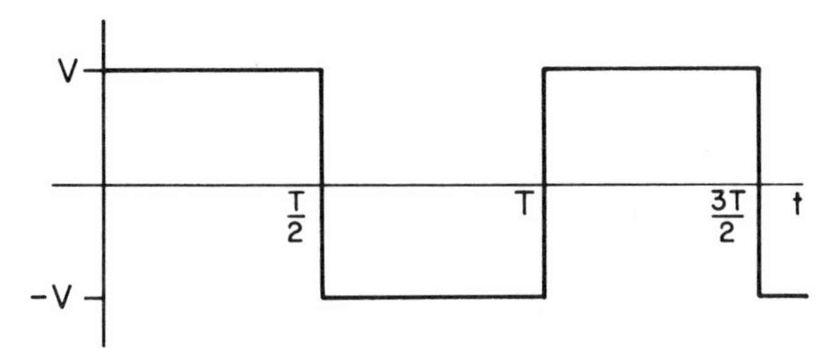

FIG. 2.11. Square pulse train.

For each of the frequency components, i.e., for each odd value of n, $\sin(n\omega_1 t)$ represents the sinusoidal variation at an angular frequency of $n\omega_1$. The corresponding Fourier coefficient, i.e., $4V/n\pi$ is the amplitude corresponding to the harmonic frequency $n\omega_1$. Figure 2.12 shows the amplitude–frequency graph of this periodic square wave. In Fig. 2.13, the four graphs in (a) represent the first four Fourier components of the square wave. Thus the top graph represents $(4V/\pi) \sin \omega_1 t$, the next represents $(4V/3\pi) \sin 3\omega_1 t$ and so on. [Note that since $f_1 = 1/T$ and $\omega_1 = 2\pi f_1$, $\sin \omega_1 t = \sin(2\pi t/T)$ and, hence, $\sin \omega_1 t$ has period T. Similarly $\sin 3\omega_1 t$ has period $T/3$.] The four graphs in (b) then represent the wave obtained by taking only the first one, two, three and four terms of the Fourier series. Thus the top graph of (b) is $(4V/\pi) \sin \omega_1 t$ and the second is $(4V/\pi) \sin \omega_1 t + (4V/3\pi) \sin 3\omega_1 t$. Clearly as the number of the components which are added together increases the waveform obtained will get closer to the square pulse train.

So far our discussion has been restricted to a periodic signal. If $f(t)$ represents a non-periodic signal, then we cannot apply the above formulae to find a Fourier series for it. Heuristically if we try to consider a non-periodic

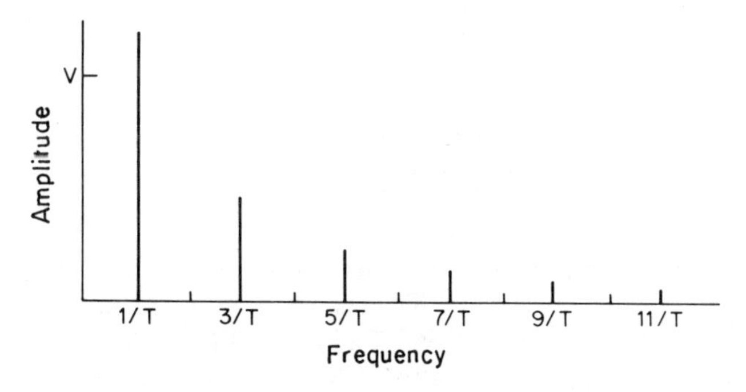

FIG. 2.12. Amplitude–frequency spectrum of the square wave.

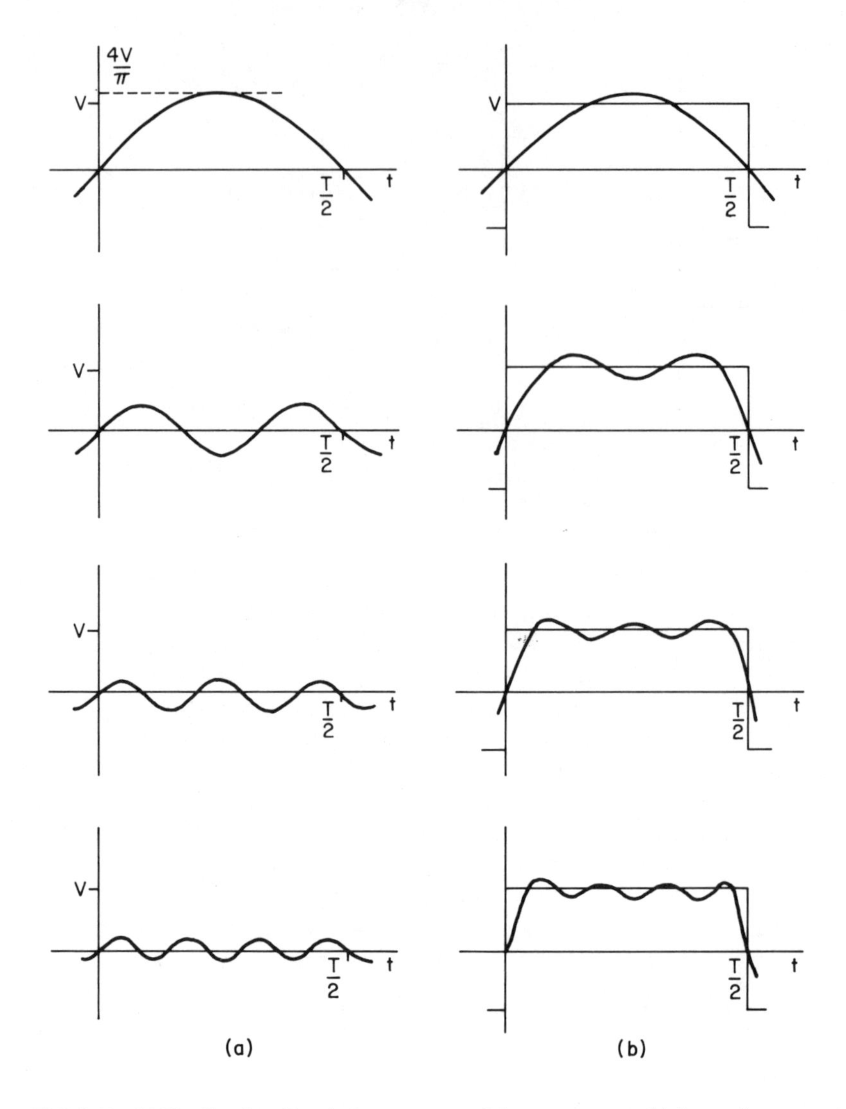

FIG. 2.13. (a) The first four Fourier components of the square wave. (b) Successive approximations obtained by adding the components.

signal as having an infinite period, then it must have an infinitessimally small fundamental frequency. Thus multiples of the fundamental frequency no longer take discrete values. Instead they take all possible values and, if we write $\omega = n\omega_1$, then the summations over n in the Fourier series become integrals over the continuous variable ω. When we introduced the Fourier series of a periodic function $f(t)$ we wrote it as:

$$f(t) = a_0 + \sum_{n=1}^{\infty} a_n \cos(n\omega_1 t) + \sum_{n=1}^{\infty} b_n \sin(n\omega_1 t)$$

But any expression of the form $a \cos x + b \sin x$ can be written in the form $k \cos(x + y)$, where k and y depend on a and b. Hence we have an alternative form of the Fourier series of a periodic function

$$f(t) = \frac{1}{2} k_0 + \sum_{n=1}^{\infty} k_n \cos(n\omega_1 t + \varphi_n)$$

If we now replace our periodic function by a non-periodic one and change the summation to an integral, then we get the Fourier transform

$$f(t) = \frac{1}{\pi} \int_0^{\infty} k(\omega) \cos(\omega t + \varphi(\omega))\, d\omega$$

Thus instead of evaluating constants, as in the periodic case, we now characterise $f(t)$ by determining the functions $k(\omega)$ and $\varphi(\omega)$. (Remember that the variable ω 'corresponds' to $n\omega_1$. This accounts for the $1/\pi$ which appears before the integral.)

If $f(t)$ is non-periodic, then the determination of its spectrum is much harder than for periodic functions. For any given time t the Fourier transform gives the magnitude and phase of each infinitessimal constituent frequency component. Thus, unlike our example of the square pulse train, the graph of the spectrum will not consist of discrete lines but will be continuous.

One method for estimating the frequency spectrum of a non-periodic signal is an analogue technique using an electronic instrument called a *wave analyser* or *spectrum analyser*. The main part of one type of wave analyser consists of a number of band-pass filters. Each filter has a central frequency, f_i, say, and only allows through those frequency components of the signal which lie in a narrow band close to that frequency. Unfortunately in practice it is impossible to construct a filter which can go from no attenuation to full attenuation over a zero frequency range. Consequently, as Fig. 2.14 illustrates, there is always some overlapping between adjacent filters.

The basic idea behind this method is to construct the power density spectrum by attempting to measure the power in each of these small bands, Each filter is attached to a meter which averages the squares of the voltages for those components which pass through it. This enables us to plot the graph of power density against frequency. Clearly the accuracy of this graph depends on the number of these bandpass filters and the size of their bandwidths. (Note that when using this method we are trying to plot a continuous

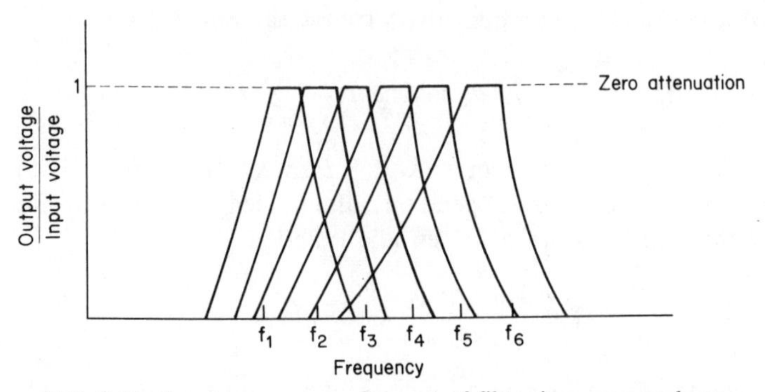

FIG. 2.14. Frequency response for a set of filters in a wave analyser.

graph by determining its values for a number of frequencies. So obviously if we decrease the gap between these frequency values we will obtain a better approximation to the graph.) If we write $\bar{v}_i^2$ for the mean square voltage through the ith filter, then Fig. 2.15 illustrates a wave analyser.

As an alternative to the above method there is a technique which involves digital signal processing. The basic idea is simple. Suppose we have a non-periodic waveform $f(t)$ which we observe for a time interval of T sec. If we assume, quite wrongly of course, that $f(t)$ has period T then we can find the Fourier coefficients to obtain the spectrum of $f(t)$. (This will be a line spectrum and not continuous.) This spectrum will, of course, more or less coincide with the spectrum of $f(t)$ within the chosen time interval but, in general, it is probable that it will be misleading and will not reflect the actual frequency content of $f(t)$. However, if the signal is *band-limited*, i.e., if its

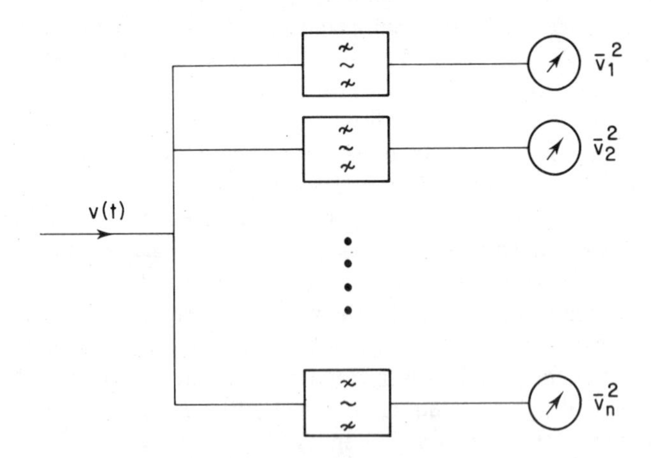

FIG. 2.15. Wave analyser.

range of frequencies is limited, then, by continuously performing Fourier transforms on different samples of length T, we can build up a picture of the spectrum of $f(t)$. So for band-limited signals we can use this technique and, at any given time, obtain an estimate for the spectrum of our signal. In particular if the signal is *stationary*, i.e., if its parameters are independent of the time at which it is measured, then by suitable averaging we can obtain an accurate estimate for the power density of the spectrum.

In order to actually perform a *Fourier transform*, i.e., in order to determine the Fourier coefficients for any one of the observation periods, we need the powerful techniques of modern digital signal processing. The Fourier analysis is usually achieved by sampling the signal, expressing it digitally in terms of these samples and then performing the appropriate arithmetic.

We shall be discussing the arithmetic operations in Chapter 4 and will say more about representing signals digitally when we discuss A/D converters. (The latter discussion occurs later in this chapter.) For the moment we will merely look at two particular power density spectra which might be obtained by using either of the above techniques.

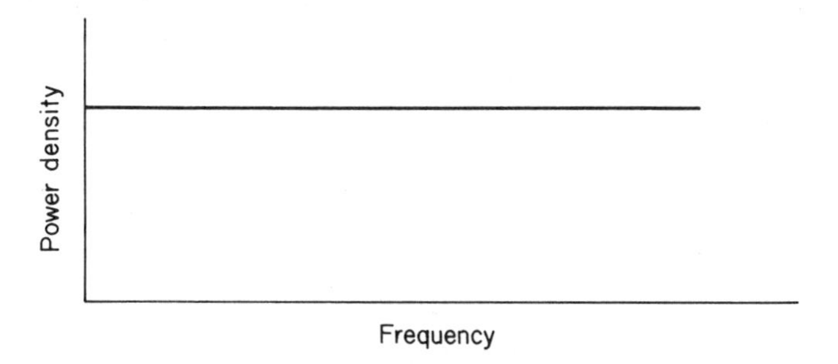

FIG. 2.16. Power density spectrum of white noise.

Figure 2.16 illustrates the power density spectrum of a non-periodic function for which the power density of the signal is independent of the frequency. This is one of the principle characteristics of *white noise*. White noise is important because a white noise source is generally regarded as a source for truly random information. It is particularly relevant for communications because a common technique for testing the robustness of voice transmission is to consider how the introduction of increasing levels of white noise affects the voice quality. The second example, Fig. 2.17, is a 'typical' speech spectrum. In other words, the power density at each part of the spectrum was obtained by averaging a large number of conversations over a long period.

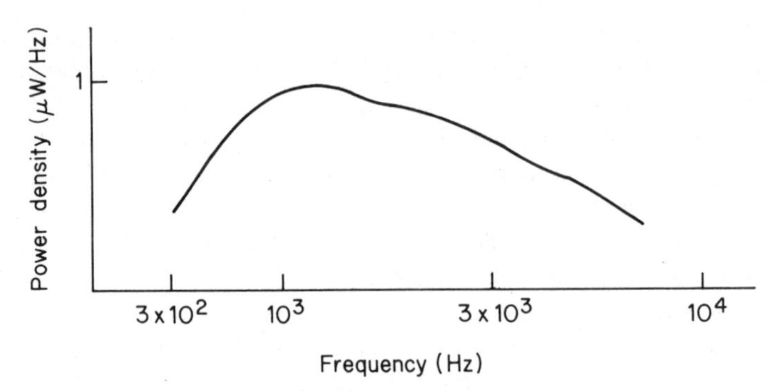

FIG. 2.17. Typical speech spectrum.

IV. Properties of Speech

The familiar sound of the human voice is an extremely complex acoustic signal. It should not be surprising, then, that the electrical signal which results from directing this acoustic signal at a microphone is also very complex. The designer of a scrambler needs to be able to destroy the characteristics of the speech for transmission and yet be able to reconstruct them at the receiver. In order to achieve this goal he needs to have some understanding of the fundamental characteristics of speech. With this in mind we now give a brief discussion on the structure of human speech.

Until very recently most telephones contained a carbon granule microphone. When a user speaks into this microphone his acoustic waves produce a variable pressure on a diaphragm which acts on the carbon granules. Since the conductive properties of the carbon granules alter as the pressure changes, this changing pressure results in a variable resistance in the electrical circuit. As the resistance varies there is a corresponding change in the current flowing through the microphone. This type of microphone has a lower sensitivity to quiet sounds than to loud ones and, as a consequence, exhibits non-linear characteristics. However, this has the advantage that it helps distinguish between the speech and the ambient noise. Such microphones are also cheap and robust. There are, of course, many other types of microphone which are currently being adopted, each with its own merits and demerits.

As we have already observed, Fig. 2.17 shows a typical speech spectrum. There are several observations to make about this graph. The first is that the frequency uses a logarithmic scale and that the power density is measured in microwatts per Hertz, (1 μW/Hz being 10^{-6} W/Hz). The second is that the power density falls rapidly for frequency components which are higher than 3 to 4 kHz. Consequently the very high frequency components make a much smaller contribution to the signal. These observations support our earlier claims that we can consider speech signals as being, essentially, confined to a 3-kHz bandwidth from about 300 to 3300 Hz. It is important to realise that this is by no means a precise evaluation of the range and we will, on occasions, refer to slightly different ranges. Most telephone channels actually allow a bandwidth of 3.1 kHz for speech. (This in fact is the range 300 Hz to 3.4 kHz). Although the lack of the high frequencies does not usually impair the intelligibility of the speech it is, nevertheless, one of the main reasons for the slight difference between someone's normal voice and his 'telephone voice'. When audio quality is crucial, a higher bandwidth must be transmitted and for hi-fi quality a 15–20-kHz band is usually employed.

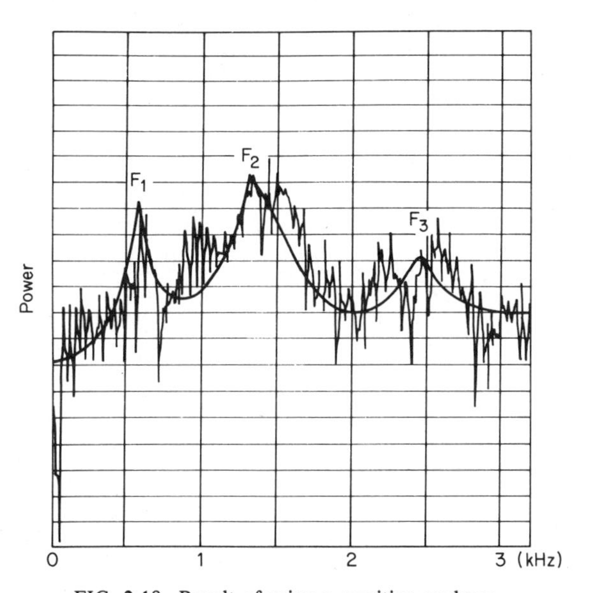

FIG. 2.18. Result of using a sensitive analyser.

If we use a very sensitive analyser and restrict ourselves to frequencies of up to 3 kHz, we should obtain a jagged curve like the one shown in Fig. 2.18. This graph shows the spectrum obtained when a particular sound was made. It shows clearly that there are a number of peaks. These peaks are called *formants* and are produced as a consequence of the way in which speech is formed. The formants are likely to change during a conversation and Fig. 2.19 illustrates how the frequency components change with time. In order to make the comparison between Figs. 2.18 and 2.19 easier we have labelled the formants of Fig. 2.18 F_1, F_2, F_3 and marked Fig. 2.19 in the same way. The change depicted in Fig. 2.19 takes place fairly slowly.

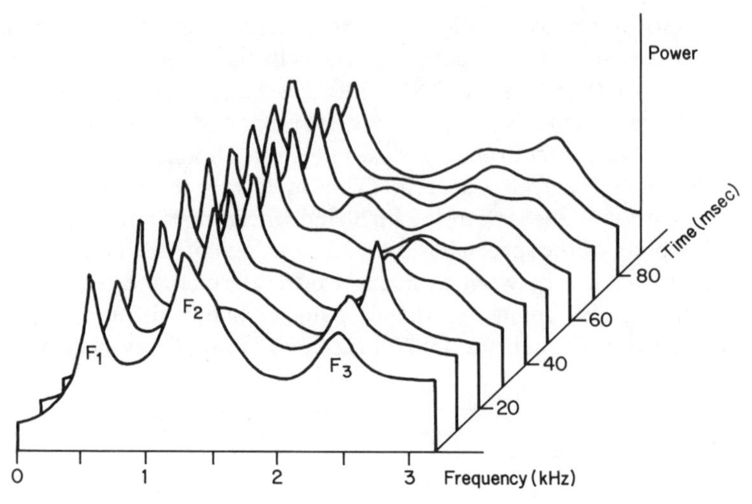

FIG. 2.19. Frequency components changing with time.

In order to describe the properties and characteristics of speech we break it down into its individual component sounds, called *phonemes*. (We will now give a very brief discussion of different phonemes for the English language and how they arise. However an understanding of the details is not necessary. The important fact to realise is that various different letters or sounds give rise to completely different waveforms and that these waveforms are recognisable as different sounds.) Phonemes vary considerably from language to language and we will restrict our attention to English. In the English language there are about forty phonemes which fall into three basic classes: the *vowels* form one complete family while the consonants and some other single syllable phonetic sounds, for instance, ch, form two classes called *plosives* and *fricatives*.

Vowels are produced when the vocal chords convert the stream of air passing through the larynx into a series of pulses. The airstream then passes into a number of cavities of which the most dominant are the nose, mouth and throat. This results in the frequency spectrum of the waveform being modified in a way which is rather similar to the effect that a series of bandpass filters has on a rectangular pulse train. Clearly the sound which emerges depends on the shape and size of these cavities, but it is usually characterised by a large low-frequency content. A vowel sound builds up gradually and, typically, takes about 100 msec to reach its peak amplitude. Figure 2.20 shows typical cavity shapes and amplitude spectra for two vowel sounds.

Plosives are produced by shutting off the airstream and then releasing it with an explosive effect. There are various points at which the airstream may

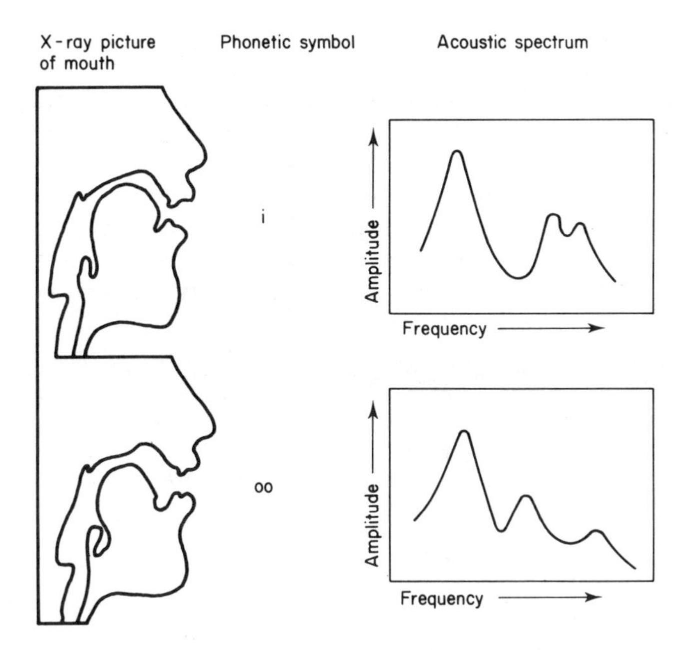

FIG. 2.20. Amplitude spectrum for two vowel sounds.

be blocked, e.g., the palate, tongue or lips. One obvious example of a plosive produced by blocking the airstream with the lips is a 'P'. We will not give a list of plosives but merely note that they tend to be characterised by their high-frequency components and typically reach 90% of their peak amplitude in less than 5 msec.

Fricatives are produced by partially shutting off the airstream to produce a sound like 'white' noise. This sound is then filtered by the vocal tract cavities. A fricative sound typically reaches its peak amplitude in 20 to 50 msec and most of its power density is concentrated between 1 and 3 kHz. One example of a fricative is 'sss . . .'.

We realise that the above discussion is extremely brief and is probably insufficient to enable the reader to distinguish between some of the plosives and fricatives. However, hopefully, it will make the reader realise that his vocal system performs different operations to produce different sounds, and that the difference in these operations is reflected in various distinguishing properties of the resulting signal.

There is yet another characteristic of human speech which needs mentioning. As a human speaks his vocal chords vibrate and the frequency of their oscillation will vary considerably during a conversation. The value of this frequency is called the *pitch frequency*. For a typical male the mean pitch frequency is about 130 Hz while for the average female it is twice as high. Most people have a range of about an octave above and below their mean pitch frequency, i.e., if the mean pitch frequency is f the range will be from about $\frac{1}{2}f$ to $2f$. (An *octave* is a frequency range where the highest frequency is twice the lowest.)

From this discussion the reader should now begin to see what we meant when we said that speech contained information relating to the 'personality' of the speaker. His personality, in this context, is those slight variations of formants, pitch, etc., which enable listeners to recognise him.

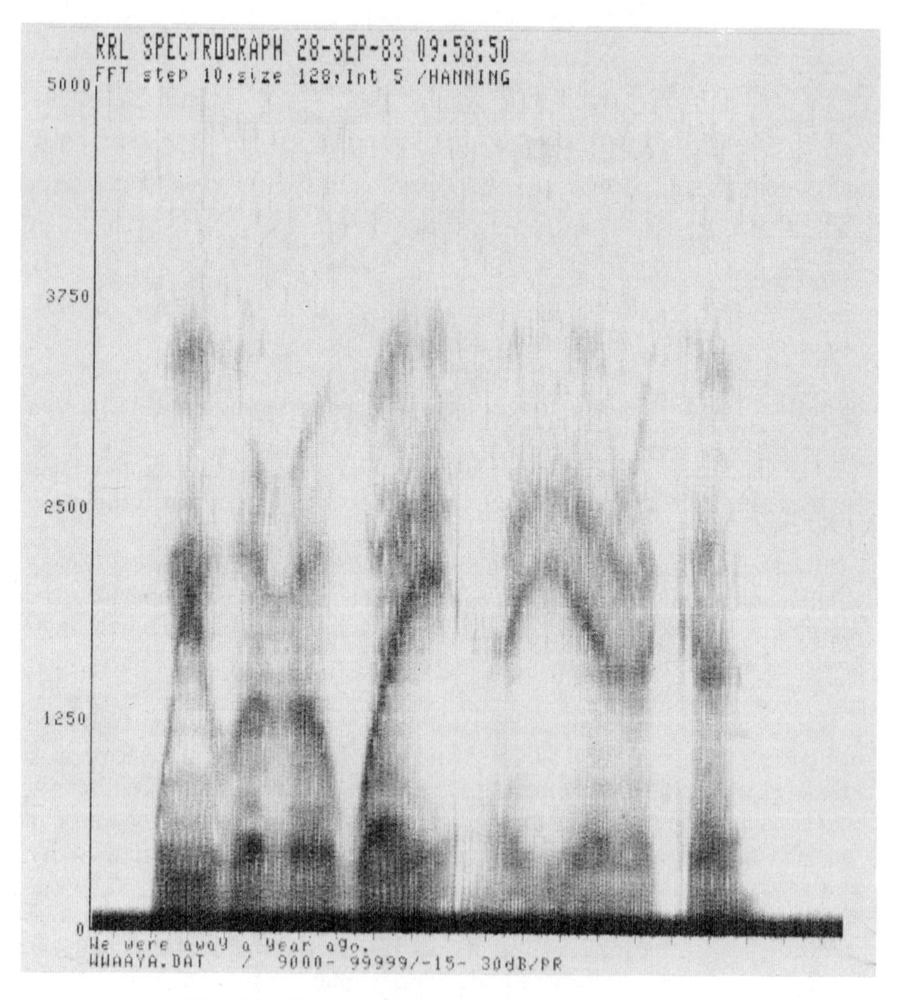

FIG. 2.21. Spectrogram for 'We were away a year ago'.

For any given speech signal we can use the pitch, formants, timing, etc., to form another signal to convey the same spoken message. This reproduction is likely to sound unnatural and some of the speaker's personality will probably be lost. (Exactly how much of this information is lost will depend on the precise parameters used in the formation of the new signal.) This principle of reproduction is the basic idea behind *vocoders*. We shall discuss vocoders later and, for the moment, merely re-emphasize that a scrambled message should conceal the speaker's personality as well as the spoken message.

In Fig. 2.19 we saw a way of inspecting the behaviour of frequency and power with time. These are the three fundamental parameters for speech and we are always interested in knowing how the power in various frequency components varies with time. There is another way of viewing these three parameters simultaneously. This is achieved by using a device called a *spectrograph* to produce a spectrogram. A *spectrogram* is a three-dimensional graph with time on the horizontal axis, frequency on the vertical axis and with the amplitude displayed using a "grey scale". In this scale black represents the maximum amplitude, white represents the minimum and the other amplitudes are represented by various shades of grey; the lighter the shade of grey the smaller the amplitude. Thus a spectrogram is a means of representing a three-dimensional graph in two dimensions (see Fig. 2.21).

V. Analogue to Digital Converters

In Chapter 1 we mentioned digital scrambling methods. Clearly such methods depend on a reliable method to convert analogue signals into digital form. There are many ways of doing this and the particular method chosen is likely to be a significant factor in the choice of scrambling method. It is, therefore, important to have some idea of the various techniques available.

As we saw in Figs. 1.2 and 1.3 a number of scrambling systems make use of A/D converters. In some cases the actual transmission is digital whereas in others the A/D converter is merely used to ease the processing. Thus they are certainly useful devices for scrambler design and implementation. However the reader should not get the impression that speech scrambling is the only, or even the major, application which requires A/D conversion. The whole important concept of digital signal processing relies heavily on A/D converters. Even if we restrict our attention to the digital transmission of speech there are many reasons for desiring this capability which have nothing to do with scramblers. As a consequence there has been a large amount of research into A/D converters and, in particular, the A/D conversion of speech. Although most of this work was not directly concerned with scrambling, the scrambler designer can obviously make use of the modern techniques which have been developed.

Broadly speaking the conversion of speech to a digital signal may be categorised into waveform coders and vocoders. *Waveform coders* attempt to preserve the original waveform without significantly exploiting the characteristics of speech. Consequently this type of conversion is suitable for any band-limited signal and is not restricted to speech. Vocoder methods, on the other hand, use analysis and synthesis techniques to model the vocal tract and attempt to extract the parameters of the assumed speech production model. Of course, as might be expected, there exist a number of systems which attempt to obtain some of the advantages of both methods by using waveform coding in conjunction with speech analysis.

TABLE 2.3

Some of the More Common A/D Conversion Techniques

Class	Technique	Bit rate (kbit/sec)	Quality	Complexity
Waveform	PCM, DM	64	Excellent	Low
		32	Very good	Low
		16	Fairly good	Low
		9.6	Reasonable	Low
		8	Poor	Low
Waveform/vocoder	APC, SBC, ATC	16	Very good	Medium to high
		9.6	Good	
		8	Good	
		4.8	Fairly good	
Vocoder	Channel	1.8–2.4	Fair	High
	LPC	2.4	Fair	High
	formant	0.6–1.2	Poor	Very high

In Table 2.3 we list some of the more common techniques employed today. (Some of the abbreviations may be meaningless to certain readers. We will explain what they mean later.) The bit rate required in each case is extremely important. As we shall see, as the bit rate increases so does the bandwidth needed in the transmission channel. There is one other important observation to make about Table 2.3. This is that the comments about the quality of each technique are subjective; i.e., they are nothing more than our personal opinions. Furthermore they represent our views today. Advances are being made very quickly and they may force us to change our opinions. Another comment, of the same nature, is that the estimates concerning the complexity are all relative. For instance, although a designer may not regard delta modulation (DM) waveform coders as simple, he would certainly admit that it has a much lower complexity than a formant vocoder.

We do not intend to discuss each of these techniques in detail. However we shall want to refer to them later so we will include a brief outline of some of them. We begin with waveform coding.

In *pulse modulation* (PM), the signal is converted into a series of pulses. The message signal is sampled at frequent intervals and the value of each sample is used to determine a property, for example, the amplitude, of a corresponding pulse. In this way the transmitted information corresponds to the values of the message signal at discrete time intervals. This process of sampling is illustrated in Fig. 2.22. In the diagram the vertical lines show the values of the signal at the appropriate time intervals and these values then determine the transmitted information. It is, of course, imperative to transmit sufficiently many samples to ensure that the receiver will be able to recover the original message. The aim is to have as few samples as possible provided that the original message is recoverable and the following theorem gives a precise value for the minimal sampling rate which will guarantee the precise reconstruction of the message.

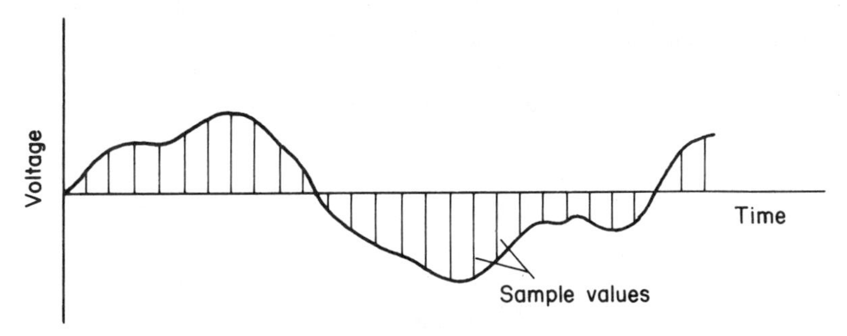

FIG. 2.22. Sample values of a signal.

The Sampling Theorem. Suppose that a function $f(t)$ is limited to a bandwidth of B Hz between frequencies f_1 and f_2, with $f_2 > f_1$. The minimum sampling rate required to characterise the function directly is $2f_2/m$ samples per second, where m is the largest integer not exceeding f_2/B.

This means that, as a rough approximation, a band-limited signal with bandwidth B needs about $2B$ samples per second. In order to obtain some idea of the numbers involved we will work through a small example. Suppose we have a speech signal extending from 300 Hz to 3.4 kHz. Then $B = 3100$ and $(f_2)/B = 3400/3100$. Thus $m = 1$ and $(2f_2)/m = 6800$. Thus, from the sampling theorem the minimum sampling rate which will enable the receiver to recover the signal directly is 6800 samples/sec. In practice when determining the minimum sampling rate for a speech signal it is normally assumed to occupy a 4-kHz bandwidth. This allows the use of simpler filters within the communications systems which form the route of the signal.

In *pulse code modulation* (PCM) the message sample values are sent as a code formed by a pattern of binary pulses. A scheme is used whereby each sample value is transmitted as a sequence of bits. A sequence of bits which represents a sample value is called a *word* and, for speech, a word often consists of 8 bits. If we assume that our words have 8 bits then this means that we can transmit 256 ($= 2^8$) different sample values. However if the difference between the maximum and minimum amplitude values is divided by 256, it is extremely unlikely that each sample will have exactly one of these 256 values. Thus it is customary to transmit the value which is closest to that of the sample. (This approximation, of necessity, introduces an error which is known as the *quantization error*.) To illustrate PCM we will look at an example in which the words have 4 bits. This, of course, implies that there are 16 ($= 2^4$) possible values for the sample. In Fig. 2.23 we illustrate how a word is assigned to a sample value. For this particular example we have used the first of the 4 bits to indicate whether the signal value is above or below the axis. The last three then indicate the distance from this axis. Thus, with this particular encoding rule, 0000 and 1000 both represent the fact that the signal is on the axis and, consequently, coincide. In order to obtain a binary sequence to represent our signal we must look at the sample value for each

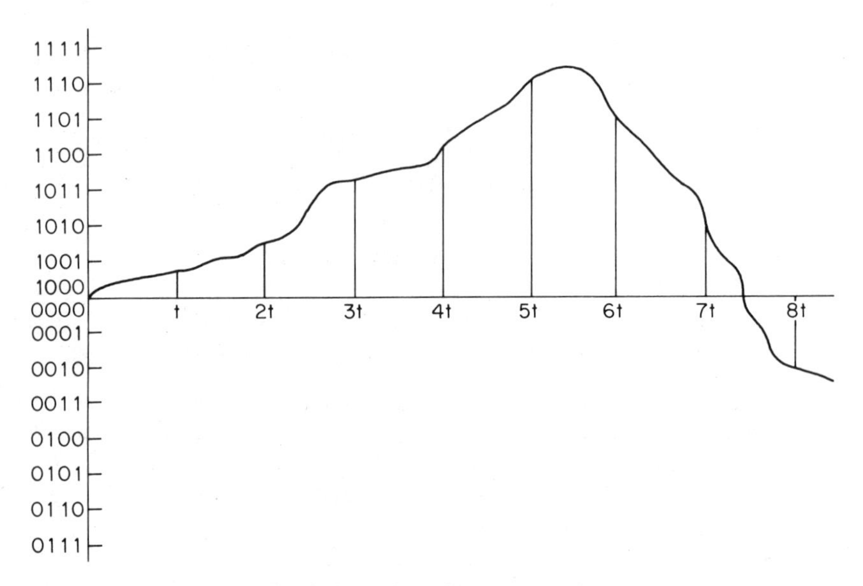

FIG. 2.23. Action of a PCM encoder.

of the prescribed times. At time 0 we have 0000, for time t we have 1001 and for $2t$ the sample value seems marginally nearer to 1001 than 1010 so we get 1001 again. Continuing in this way the PCM signal is 0000 1001 1001 1011 1100 1110 1101 1010 0010. (Note that in many practical systems the codewords may not be evenly spaced. A logarithmic distribution is often used to concentrate them near the axis and provide a uniform signal-to-noise ratio over a wide dynamic range of input signals.)

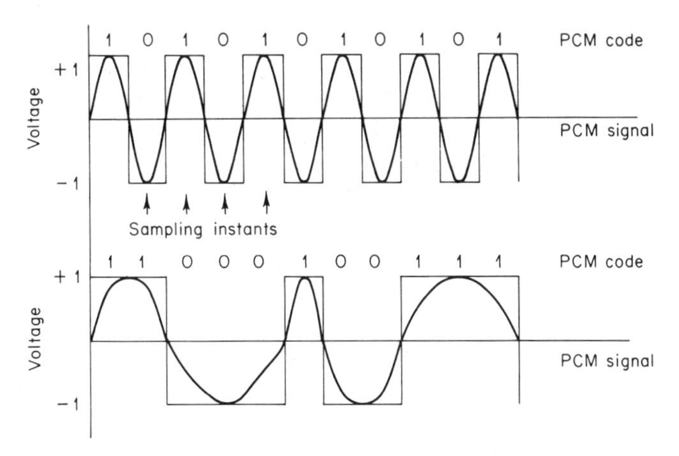

FIG. 2.24. Bandwidth necessary to transmit a PCM signal.

Any PCM signal consists of a sequence of zeros and ones corresponding to the sample values of its message signal. The precise shape of its spectrum will depend on the various patterns of zeros and ones which are transmitted. We can, however, estimate the required bandwidth for a PCM signal. In Fig. 2.24 we illustrate the relation between a PCM code and the corresponding PCM signal. Since the receiver only needs to distinguish between zeros and ones it only needs to be able to decide whether the graph is above or below the horizontal axis. Thus a sequence of all zeros, or all ones, requires a bandwidth just sufficient to pass a sine wave whose frequency is inversely proportional to the length of that sequence. From this it should be clear that a pattern of bits which contains alternate zeros and ones will contain the highest frequency components of the signal. Furthermore it should also be clear that this frequency is half the rate at which the bits are generated by the PCM encoder. In order to quantify what this all means we will work through an example.

Suppose that we have a speech signal with 4-kHz bandwidth. Then, by the sampling theorem, we need to sample 8000 times/sec. If we assume that we have 8-bit codewords then we actually represent the speech signal by 64,000 bits per second. Thus, by our earlier discussion, we need a bandwidth of 32 kHz.

This little example illustrates one of the fundamental problems facing us. If a telecommunications system only allows 4 kHz for a speech channel then we simply cannot transmit our PCM signal over the channel. This is one of the problems we mentioned in Chapter 1 and is one of the reasons for the general interest in low-bit-rate A/D conversion.

The PCM encoder which we have just described measures the height of each sample from the same starting point. However, since in practice speech signals change very slowly, this means that there is unlikely to be a large difference between any two consecutive samples. This suggests that, at least when dealing with speech, it may be better to code the difference between consecutive samples rather than to code each sample. This technique is, in fact, often used and is called *differential PCM* (DPCM). It is used to obtain some of the lower bit rates which are obtainable from PCM (see Table 2.3) and is also used in *delta modulation* (DM).

If a band-limited signal $f(t)$ is the input for a DM then the output, which we denote by $Q(t)$, consists of pulses which are equally spaced and have amplitudes $\pm v$, for some v. We denote the interval between these pulses by T sec, so that the pulses occur with frequency $f_p = 1/T$. One crucial fact is that T must be chosen to make f_p larger than the minimum sampling rate given by the Sampling Theorem. Rather than discuss the relation between $f(t)$

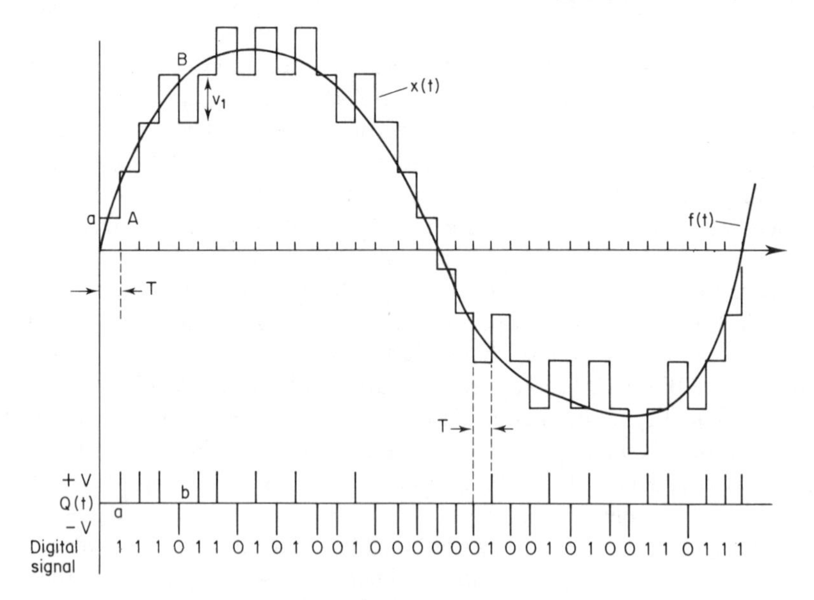

FIG. 2.25. Action of a delta modulator.

and $Q(t)$ in general, we will illustrate it by the example shown in Fig. 2.25. In this diagram the graph of $f(t)$ is drawn. We pick an arbitary point with voltage a and use it as a starting point to determine a function $x(t)$ in the following way. For the first T sec we put $x(t) = a$. At $t = T$ (i.e., at the point A) since $x(t) < f(t)$ we increase $x(t)$ by v_1, (where v_1 is a fixed number chosen by us). For the next T sec $x(t)$ remains constant again, (this time at $a + v_1$), and then when $t = 2T$ we look again at the relative values of $x(t)$ and $f(t)$. In our example we have $x(t) < f(t)$ again, so we add another v_1 to $x(t)$. The shape of $x(t)$ should now be clear. At each multiple of T sec it either increases or decreases by v_1 depending upon whether $x(t) < f(t)$ or $x(t) > f(t)$. In our example we do not have $x(t) > f(t)$ until $4T$ sec, (i.e., at the point marked B), so the first three steps are all upwards. Each time $x(t)$ increases, $Q(t)$ assumes a positive value while $Q(t)$ is negative when $x(t)$ decreases. The pulse $Q(t)$ is shown at the foot of the diagram.

When the input signal is increasing the pulse $Q(t)$ tends to have more ones than zeros while a negative step for $f(t)$ produces the opposite effect. At times when $f(t)$ is more or less constant, for instance near its maxima and minima, $Q(t)$ tends to oscillate between 1 and 0. This is referred to as the *idling state* of $Q(t)$ since it is the condition of $Q(t)$, which in turn defines $x(t)$, for no input signal.

The quality of speech recovered from the digital signal $Q(t)$ is directly related to the efficiency of the A/D converter, the D/A converter of the receiver and the sampling rate of the clear voice input. Voice quality can be improved by using rather more complex delta modulators than the linear system described above. For instance, instead of either adding or subtracting a constant voltage v_1 at each time interval, it is possible to let $x(t)$ follow $f(t)$ more closely. This is achieved by adapting the step height of $x(t)$, in other words to vary the value of v_1, depending on the number of successive ones or zeros in $Q(t)$. Such a scheme is called an *adaptive delta modulation* (ADM). (Similar techniques can be applied to DPCM to obtain *adaptive differential pulse code modulators* (ADPCM).) Recent advances now mean that the bit rate can be reduced to as low as 9.6 kbits/sec, while still preserving a speech quality which some users consider reasonable and even lower, about 8 kbits/sec, with poor quality. However, in practice, 12–18 kbits/sec provides a usable compromise between acceptable speech quality and practical bandwidth limitations. The bandwidth required for this channel can be estimated in a similar way to that used for a PCM encoder. It is about half the maximum rate at which the bits are generated by the delta modulator.

In these last two A/D converters the input signal is sampled at regular time intervals and a digital 'approximation' is then transmitted. Furthermore the minimum possible sampling rate is determined by the sampling theorem. If, for example, our input signal is a sinusoid with frequency f then, instead of sending our digital approximation, we could merely tell the receiver that the input is a sinusoid with frequency *f* and leave him to build up his own signal. This is the principle behind *vocoders*. They are essentially speech synthesis systems which can utilize low-bit-rate output signals. The aim is not to characterize the speech signal but merely to analyse it and then send enough information so that the receiver can build its own signal and reconstruct the message. For instance, in the receiver of a *linear predictive coder* a filter is continuously modified to provide an approximation to the filtering action of the vocal tract. The filter is excited by a pulse or noise sequence corresponding to voiced and unvoiced sounds. The required filter modifying information, together with the excitation (*pitch*) information, is estimated by the analyser in the transmitter.

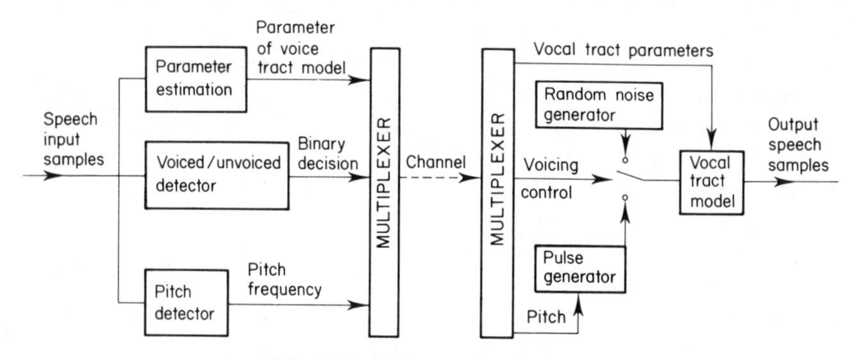

FIG. 2.26. Basic vocoder elements.

In Table 2.3 we listed three types of vocoder. The difference between them is in the vocal tract model. Figure 2.26 shows a block diagram for the basic vocoder elements. In a linear predictive vocoder, the vocal tract is modelled as an electrical analogue of an acoustic tube whose cross-sectional area varies along its length. In contrast, a *channel vocoder* has as its model a bank (16 or more) of parallel filters whose centre frequencies and bandwidths are selected to conform with the perceptual characteristics of the human ear. A *formant vocoder* is in a sense a combination of the above in that there are three or four filters whose centre frequencies are forced to track the resonances of the acoustic model. More details of these and other types of vocoders can be found in Flanagan (1972).

It has been found that the transmitted information in vocoders is sufficient for the receiver to build a signal and reproduce the message. But, depending on the precise parameters of the system being used, some of the characteristics which allow recognition of the speaker may be lost. If too much of the speaker's personality is lost the result may be a rather monotonous single-pitched sound resembling the voice of a 'dalek' or any other voice which film directors tend to attribute to talking computers. To avoid this problem modern vocoders attempt to preserve more of the speaker's identity in the transmitted message.

There are other definite disadvantages of vocoder systems. For instance, since we are dispensing with so much of the redundant information, the system becomes considerably more sensitive to noise on the transmission path. In fact in some vocoder systems it has been found advantageous to make the bit rate as low as possible and then introduce some extra redundancy to allow the receiver to carry out certain error correction methods; the idea being to choose the added redundancy so that, in the receiver, certain error patterns can be discovered and corrected. (We will not discuss error correction systems in this book and the interested reader should consult MacWilliams and Sloane (1978) or Peterson and Weldon (1972)). Another major disadvantage of vocoder systems arises from the physiological differences between various races. Without going into any details, a vocoder designed for a European speaker, for instance, is likely to be much less effective when used by an Oriental. Yet another disadvantage has been that, as a result of their complexity, they have been expensive, large and had a high power consumption. Modern research workers are trying to rectify these drawbacks and this is an area where modern digital signal processing and microelectronics are causing a revolution. The overall complexity of the systems is being reduced and this is resulting in cheaper and smaller devices. This trend is likely to continue for some years.

As well as the waveform analysers and vocoders, Table 2.3 also contains details of three waveform/vocoder systems. For completeness we will give a very brief description of each.

Adaptive predictive coding (APC) is a form of linear predictive coding which incorporates two types of adaptive prediction. The first is a short-term prediction to reduce the correlation due to the vocal tract resonances, and the second is a long-term prediction, over a few tens of milliseconds, to remove the correlation due to pitch periodicities in voiced sound.

A *sub-band coder* (SBC) is a form of channel vocoder which attempts to directly code the speech characteristics in the frequency domain. The speech signal is applied to a bank of bandpass filters, not unlike a spectrum analyser. The output of each filter is then sampled using for instance, a PCM technique.

Adaptive transform coding (ATC) is a technique which is very similar to that of the second form of spectrum analysis estimation which we considered earlier. In this case a spectral representation of speech is obtained using, for example, Fourier transforms, and its parameters are transmitted.

The relative merits of all A/D converters vary according to the circumstances in which they are to be used. In any given situation it is necessary to choose the technique which seems most suited to the telecommunications system. Typical consideratons which may affect the choice include complexity, immunity to errors occurring in the transmission system and the level of speaker recognition which will be accepted. We will discuss these considerations later.

VI. Modulation

We complete this chapter with a brief discussion of some of the more common modulation techniques. As with so many of the other topics in this chapter, we will not attempt to give a comprehensive treatment of the subject. For more details the interested reader should consult Rosie (1973).

There are, as we have already seen, two principal reasons for modulation. One is to facilitate the multiplexing of a number of messages onto a single channel and the other is to transform a message signal into a form which is more suitable for a particular telecommunications system. (Note that we have already discussed certain types of modulation; namely the A/D converters of the last section.) With these two aims in mind we will look at amplitude modulation and frequency modulation. These are, as we shall see, two of the most common modulation techniques and are illustrated in Fig. 2.27.

In Fig. 2.27 the message signal is a sawtooth and the *carrier* is a sinusoid with a much higher fundamental frequency than the message signal. With *amplitude modulation* the instantaneous amplitude of the modulated carrier is made proportional to the instantaneous value of the modulating signal, i.e., the message. Thus as the message signal becomes more positive the amplitude of the modulated carrier increases.

In order to illustrate amplitude modulation we will work through a specific example. Our message signal is, as we know from our discussion of signal analysis, made up of a number of sinusoidal components. For the purpose of this discussion we will concentrate on just one of these components. Let us suppose that one component of our message signal is $v_m \cos(\omega_m t)$ and that the carrier sinusoid is of the form $v_c \cos(\omega_c t)$. Thus the amplitude of our carrier is v_c and we want to obtain a modulated carrier whose amplitude varies with the message signal. This can be achieved by using a device called a *balanced modulator*. In Fig. 2.28 the 'black box' represents a particular type of balanced modulator which is known as a *double-sideband suppressed carrier (dsbsc) amplitude modulator*.

For the particular component of our message signal the output will be $v_m v_c \cos(\omega_m t) \cos(\omega_c t)$. Clearly the amplitude of this output signal varies as the amplitude of our message. If we use the elementary trigonometric identity

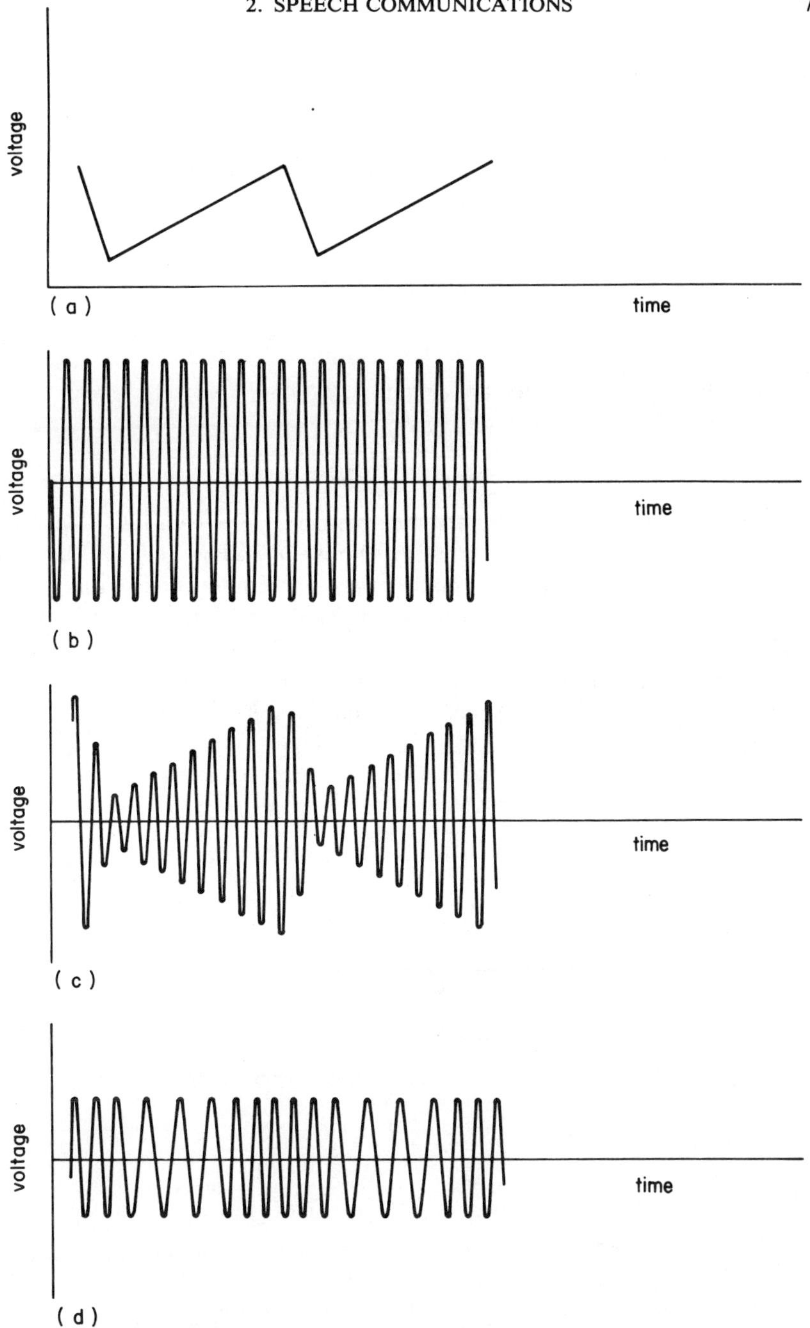

FIG. 2.27. Amplitude and frequency modulation; (a) signal, (b) sinusoidal carrier, (c) amplitude modulation and (d) frequency modulation.

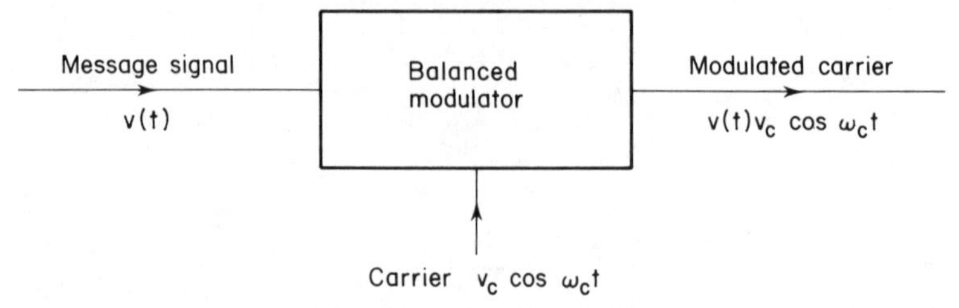

FIG. 2.28. Balanced modulator.

$\cos A \cos B = \frac{1}{2}\cos(A + B) + \frac{1}{2}\cos(A - B)$, then we can express the output of our balanced modulator as

$$\tfrac{1}{2}v_c v_m \cos(\omega_c + \omega_m)t + \tfrac{1}{2}v_c v_m \cos(\omega_c - \omega_m)t$$

When using a balanced modulator the operator is free to choose his carrier signal. In other words the operator can choose v_c and ω_c. We will usually assume that $v_c = 1$ and that ω_c is greater than ω_m. Under these assumptions if the input signal is $v_m \cos(\omega_m t)$ the modulated carrier has an amplitude–angular frequency spectrum as shown in Fig. 2.29. If we were now to consider each sinusoidal component of our speech signal and consider the corresponding output from the balanced modulator, we would obtain a power density spectrum similar to Fig. 2.30. In this diagram the value f_c, which is

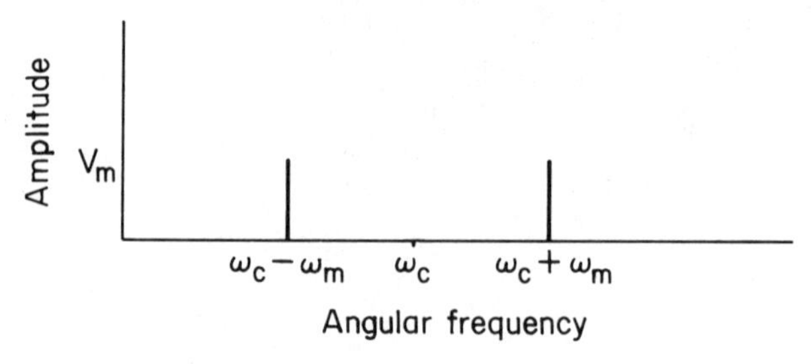

FIG. 2.29. Amplitude–angular frequency spectrum.

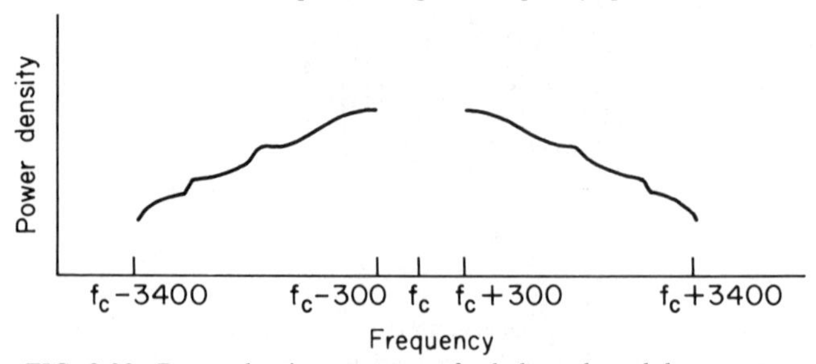

FIG. 2.30. Power density spectrum of a balanced modulator output.

equal to $\omega_c/2\pi$ is called the *carrier frequency*. The two bands of 'side' signals above and below the carrier frequency are called the *upper and lower sidebands* respectively. (Note that in Fig. 2.30 we have assumed that the speech was band limited to 300–3400 Hz and that f_c is greater than 3400.) Under our assumption that $v_c = 1$, the upper sideband is, clearly, similar to the original speech signal except that each frequency component has f_c added to it. The lower sideband is, on the other hand, the mirror image of our original spectrum; i.e., it is similar to the original signal spectrum with the high and low frequencies interchanged. Thus, by a suitable choice of f_c, and by filtering out the lower sideband we can translate the original signal to another band of our choice. This is known as *single-sideband transmission* (SSB). Alternatively we can filter out the upper sideband and obtain the inverted speech signal of Fig. 2.31.

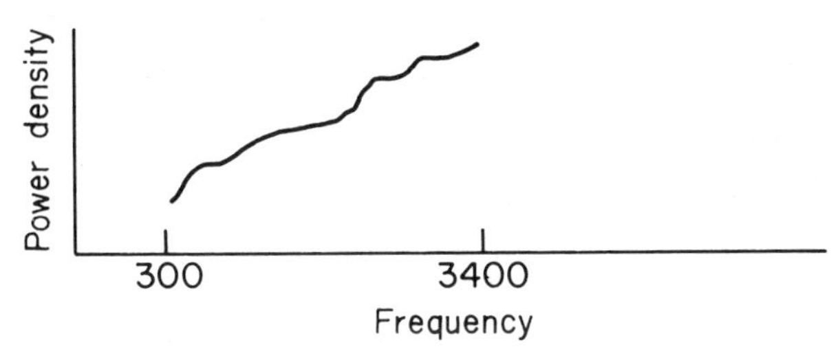

FIG. 2.31. Lower sideband.

In practice the actual filtering may prove difficult and circuits other than the balanced modulator may be used to produce just one of the lower or upper sidebands. It is perhaps worth mentioning that the method described here is very similar to frequency division multiplexing which is used to transmit telephone calls. By choosing suitable carrier frequencies for different signals, each signal can be shifted to a different frequency band and several thousand calls can be carried in a single transmission link. Single-sideband amplitude modulation is also frequently used for speech transmitted over h.f. channels.

In *frequency modulation* (FM) the instantaneous frequency of a carrier is varied in response to the modulating signal. In Fig. 2.27d we showed a sinusoidal carrier modulated by a sawtooth message signal. For this type of modulation it is much harder to estimate the bandwidth of the resulting signal. Clearly, unless it is controlled in some way, it is possible for the frequency modulated signal to have frequency components which extend to infinity on either side. For anyone seeking an approximate guide to the

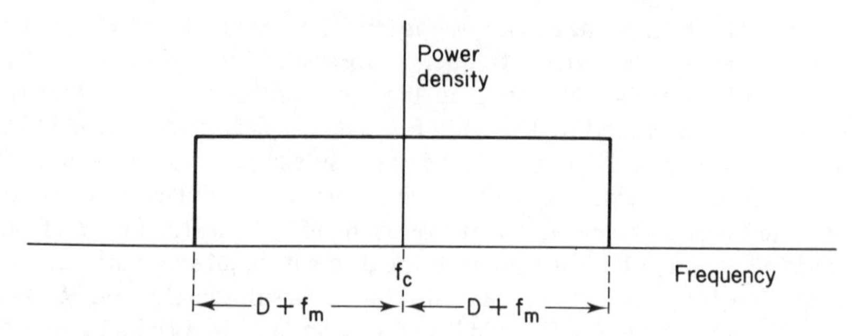

FIG. 2.32. Bandwidth required for a frequency-modulated signal. (D = max[m] deviation; f_m = highest message frequency.)

required bandwidth for a frequency modulated signal, there is a rule-of-thumb called *Carson's rule.* In order to state this rule we first define the deviation to be the difference between the original unmodulated carrier frequency and its frequency at peak modulation. Carson's rule then says that the bandwidth required for the frequency modulated signal is 2× (the maximum deviation + the highest frequency present in the message signal). This is illustrated in Fig. 2.32.

It is important now to emphasize that in practice the choice of a particular modulation scheme will involve many considerations as well as the bandwidth. One of the most important of these is the tolerance to interference and noise during transmission. Furthermore it is not always necessary to restrict oneself to one particular method. Combinations of modulation methods are certainly possible. It is, for instance, common for an analogue signal to be converted into a sequence of two-level (binary) pulses, by, for example, pulse modulation, and for the resulting signal to be regarded as the message signal for frequency modulating a carrier. In this situation the frequency of the modulated carrier will vary between two values which correspond to the two values of the PCM signal. This is often called *frequency shift keying.*

We have already discussed some of the effects of noise on a channel but have not said how it will affect a binary transmission. In fact the relation between the amplitude of the noise and the errors produced in the signal is highly non-linear. There will only be an error if the receiver pulses are excessively affected by the noise. There is, effectively, a threshold where a further small increase in the noise will change a reasonable channel into one which is full of errors. The effectiveness of the channel is usually measured as the proportion of received digits which are in error. This ratio is called the *error rate* and, in Fig. 2.33, we show a typical change in error rate for a PCM signal as additional white noise is introduced to lower the signal to noise ratio.

We shall consider some of the additional effects of noise in later chapters.

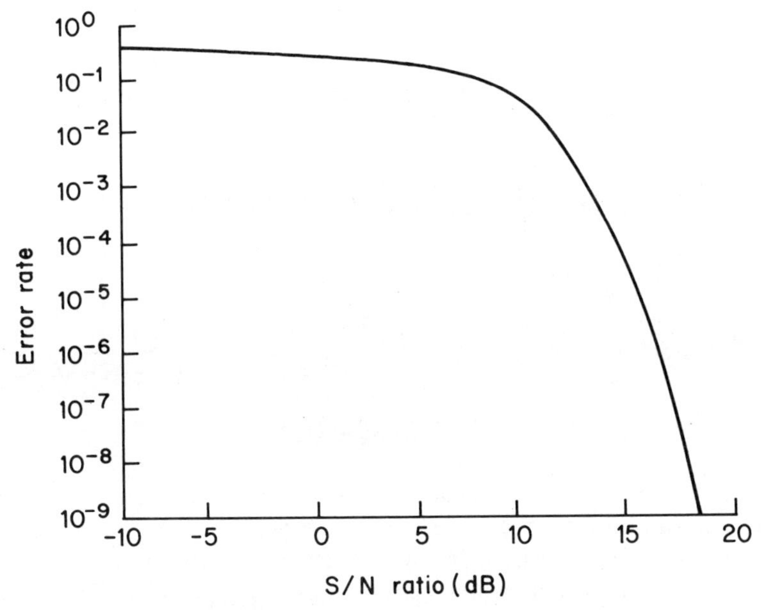

FIG. 2.33. Error rate versus signal-to-noise ratio of PCM.

3. The Principles of Cryptography

I. Introduction

Although, in the two earlier chapters, we have often referred to the security level of a transmission system we have not, as yet, given any idea of how this security might be measured. In this chapter we will introduce some of the basic ideas of cryptography and consider how they can be applied to speech security. From our earlier discussion we know that we can, essentially, characterize speech scramblers as either analogue or digital. With a digital scrambler the analogue message signal is passed through an A/D converter. The resulting digits are then enciphered to obtain a new set of digits which are transmitted to the receiver. The intention is that the encipherment should ensure that anyone who intercepts the transmitted set of digits will be unable to relate them to the original message. Thus the situation is very similar to standard encipherment of data. There are, however, two highly significant differences. The first is that the data will have characteristics which reflect the particular type of A/D converter used and will, of course, also be related to the properties of speech. The second is that we may require certain specific features in our telecommunications system which are normally associated with speech systems but not with data systems. Clearly the design of a digital speech scrambler is likely to be influenced by the considerable advances being made in data cipher systems. The designer has to study the various techniques for data encipherment and see which can be modified to meet his particular requirements.

There is another reason why the scrambler designer should study data cipher systems. There are many occasions, for both analogue and digital scramblers, when we will require a sequence generator for pseudo-random numbers. As we shall see, many of the algorithms employed for data cipher systems can be adapted readily for the generation of sequences of pseudo-random numbers.

In this chapter we will give a brief general introduction to cryptography. In particular we will review some of the data encipherment techniques available and show how they can be adapted to generate sequences of pseudo-random numbers. (It should not be forgotten that much of the chapter will apply to speech as well as to data.) This discussion will, initially, be rather more 'formal' than the earlier ones and we give precise definitions of some of the technical terms which we have used in the earlier chapters. Naturally we will not be able to give an exhaustive treatment of cipher systems and the interested reader is referred to Beker and Piper (1982d).

II. The Basic Properties of Cipher Systems

A system which makes it possible to disguise confidential information in such a way that no unauthorised person will understand it is called a *cipher system*. The information to be concealed is called the *plaintext* (or just the *message*) and the operation of disguising it is known as *enciphering*. The enciphered message is called the *ciphertext* or *cryptogram* and the set of rules used by the encipherer when translating from plaintext to ciphertext is the *algorithm*. In most situations the operation of this algorithm will depend on a *key* which, along with the plaintext, is input to the algorithm. In order that the system may work it is absolutely crucial that the *recipient*, that is the person for whom the cryptogram is intended, should be able to obtain the plaintext from the ciphertext. Thus the recipient must know the key which the encipherer used and this knowledge must enable him to determine the plaintext uniquely. (The process of applying the key to translate the ciphertext back into plaintext is called *deciphering*.) It is generally accepted that, in the type of situation we have just described, the security of a well designed system should not depend on keeping the algorithm secret. There will usually be many keys at the encipherer's disposal and the security of the system will depend on the fact that no one knows, or can deduce, which key has been used. If a system does not depend on a key, or equivalently has only one possibility for the key, then it is often referred to as a *code*. Codes, we must stress, are not necessarily intended to offer any security. An obvious example of a code is an A/D converter where its sole objective is to convert an analogue signal to digital. This is simply a single transformation with no key. Note, by the way, that this explains our use of the term encoding when describing the A/D operation.

Anyone who uses a cipher system must, obviously, feel that there is a risk that someone, known or unknown, might wish to discover the content of his messages. The aim of the cipher is to protect the message if it is intercepted while being transmitted from the encipherer to the recipient. Various authors give different names to this would be interceptor. We have already used the terms interceptor, listener and eavesdropper. Other commonly used terms include bad guy and enemy. We will probably use the term interceptor, but this may change in certain contexts. The important point to stress is that the interceptor will not, in general, know the key and it is this lack of knowledge which, it is hoped, will prevent him from discovering the plaintext.

The art (or science!) of designing cipher systems is known as *cryptography*, while *cryptanalysis* is the name given to the process of deducing the plaintext from the ciphertext without knowing the key. In practice the cryptanalyst may attempt to deduce the key as well as the plaintext. If he is successful he will then have the same information as the recipient and will be able to decipher all further communications until the key is changed.

In order to understand modern cipher systems it is often advantageous to look back at some of the earlier systems and analyse their weaknesses. With this in mind we will begin our discussion by looking at a very simple, and totally insecure, system.

Many young children play games in which they send each other secret messages in code. To do this they usually invent a 'code' by letting each letter of the alphabet represent another one. When they do this they are using a particular example of a *monoalphabetic cipher* or, as it is also known, a *simple substitution cipher*. These ciphers were one of the earliest types used and were certainly employed, for instance, by Julius Caesar. In order to obtain the key, a child will probably write the alphabet on a piece of paper and then, by each letter, put down the letter which will represent it in his ciphered messages. Once the recipient has a copy of this piece of paper he can easily decipher the message, but to anyone without a copy the cryptogram is unintelligible. If, as is usually the case with children, the rule for determining the allocation of letters is arbitrary, then the piece of paper on which the key is written is very important. If it is lost or stolen, then the receiver will not be able to decipher the message. Clearly there are so many possibilities for the key that an interceptor is unlikely to guess the right one. Consequently the mere existence of this piece of paper with the key written on it invites theft by anyone wishing to intercept a message. Although most of these considerations need not bother children, they are of course of concern to the serious cryptographer. The child's system would, undoubtedly, be more secure if both encipherer and decipherer were to remember the key and then destroy the piece of paper. But it is, in general, easier to remember this type of key if, instead of being arbitrary, there is some rule for assigning the ciphertext letters to the plaintext alphabet.

As an example of the type of rule which was used consider the cipher 'machine' of Fig. 3.1. This consists of two concentric rings of which the outer

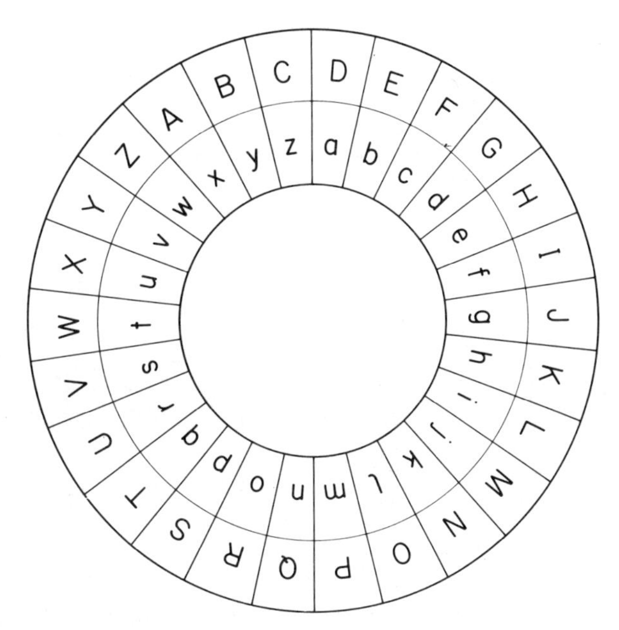

FIG. 3.1. Machine to implement a simple monoalphabetic cipher.

one is free to rotate about the inner. Clearly there are 26 possibilities for their relative positions, and each one may be regarded as a different key with the plaintext alphabet on the inner ring and the corresponding ciphertext letter on the outer. In this case the encipherer and decipherer only need to agree on one letter, for example the letter on the outer ring which corresponds to a, to determine the key. (Thus, for the particular setting in the diagram, the key is the letter D.) For this simple system, often known as a *Caesar cipher system*, remembering the key is easy and the need for the piece of paper has disappeared. However it has been replaced by another, probably worse, snag. Since there are now only 26 possible keys an interceptor might have time to simply try them all.

As we said earlier, simple substitution ciphers offer virtually no security and we will not discuss them in any more detail. However, it is very important to understand why they are so ineffective. The reason is, quite simply, contained in Table 3.1.

Table 3.1 gives the relative frequencies of the alphabetic characters in a sample of more than one hundred thousand characters. Each value listed gives the number of appearances of the appropriate letter as a percentage of the total number of characters. Similar statistics exist for bigrams (pairs of consecutive letters) and trigrams (triples of consecutive letters). A more complete set of these statistics can be found in Beker and Piper (1982d). There

TABLE 3.1

The Relative Frequencies of Letters in English Plaintext

Character	Relative frequency	Character	Relative frequency
A	8.17	N	6.75
B	1.49	O	7.51
C	2.78	P	1.93
D	4.25	Q	0.10
E	12.70	R	5.99
F	2.23	S	6.33
G	2.02	T	9.06
H	6.09	U	2.76
I	6.97	V	0.98
J	0.15	W	2.36
K	0.77	X	0.15
L	4.03	Y	1.97
M	2.41	Z	0.07

have been many other attempts at analysing the statistics of the English language and they are all more or less consistent. Such statistics provide a surprisingly reliable guide for the likely relative frequencies of the characters from most other reasonably long passages of English plaintext. It is this reliability which makes all simple substitution ciphers virtually useless. The reason is fairly easy to see. In any simple substitution cipher system each letter is merely replaced by one other. So, for example, there will be a substitute for E and the frequency of this substitute in the ciphertext will be exactly the same as the frequency of E in the plaintext. Thus, just as E is clearly the most popular letter in the English language, one would expect the substitute for E to be the most popular letter in the cryptogram. Similarly the frequency of each letter in the ciphertext will coincide with that of its equivalent in the plaintext. Thus knowledge of the statistics, plus a certain amount of intelligent guesswork and 'trial and error', will enable a cryptanalyst to break any ciphertext which has resulted from a simple substitution cipher. (This is only true, of course, provided that the ciphertext is long enough for the statistics to be meaningful. So the child's terse rude cryptogram about his teacher may be safe after all!)

Having agreed that simple substitution ciphers are weak, it is now necessary to look for alternatives. One possibility might be to devise a system where, instead of merely substituting one letter for another, something was substituted for each pair of consecutive letters. Or, even more generally, to invent a system where a substitution was made for a set of m consecutive letters. This is precisely the idea behind the ciphering technique known as a *block cipher*. However before we discuss block ciphers we must anticipate a problem which we cannot avoid forever. We have stated, and indeed illustrated, that simple substitution ciphers offer virtually no security. We now intend to look at block ciphers. How can we measure their security? If they are not completely useless what can we say about them? Is it possible that they, or any other system, may be completely unbreakable? Before we begin our discussion of block ciphers we will look at the general problem of assessing the security level of a system. This assessment falls, quite naturally, into two parts. In the first, called *theoretical security*, we look at the security of a system on the assumption that an interceptor has limitless resources and time. Clearly if a system is theoretically unbreakable then we can consider using it! In the second, called *practical security*, we try to be more realistic about the practical limitations on the interceptor's resources and, indeed, on the user's requirements.

A. Theoretical Security

In order to discuss security in any meaningful way we must define all our terms as precisely as possible and be prepared to introduce some mathematical and statistical arguments into the discussion. Anyone who feels uncomfortable with either mathematics or statistics (or both!) need not be put off as we will also give non-technical explanations of the most important details.

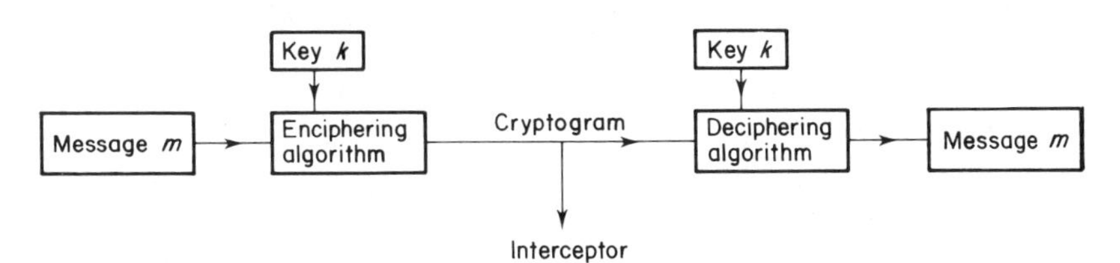

FIG. 3.2. Cipher system.

In Fig. 3.2 we illustrate the type of cipher system that we have been discussing. We must point out that (hopefully!) the interceptor is not really a part of the system. We have included him in the diagram merely to illustrate where the interception is most likely to occur.

Modern cryptography has been greatly influenced by the work of Shannon during the late 1940s. Shannon's approach was to regard the key as determining a transformation from the set of all possible messages to the set of all possible cryptograms. (These two sets are called the *message space* and *cryptogram space*, respectively.) For our discussion we shall actually identify the key and its corresponding transformation. Thus a cipher system is a finite set T of transformations for a (usually) finite message space M onto a cryptogram space C. Each message has associated with it a probability which reflects the chance of it being sent and, similarly, for each transformation there is a probability which reflects the likelihood of it being used. (Messages and cryptograms for which this probability is 0 are not usually included in M or C, respectively.) One fundamental requirement of a cipher system is that knowledge of the cryptogram and transformation should enable the recipient to determine the message uniquely. In mathematical language this means that each of the transformations in T must be reversible, so that if a message m is transformed into the cryptogram c by transformation t, i.e., if $c = t(m)$, then we must have $m = t^{-1}(c)$, where t^{-1} is the inverse of t. Using this terminology then, whereas the receiver will know c and t and thus be able to deduce m, an interceptor will know c and know only the *a priori* probabilities of the various t's. Obviously for a 'good' cipher system we would hope that this information does not help the interceptor to work out, or even guess, the message m. Indeed, ideally we would like it not to enable him to eliminate any possibilities for m. This is the basic objective behind a concept called perfect secrecy which we will now define.

Suppose that we have a cipher system with a message space $M = \{m_1, m_2, \ldots, m_n\}$ and cryptogram space $C = \{c_1, c_2, \ldots, c_u\}$. Suppose also that, for any possible message m_i, the *a priori* probability of m_i being transmitted is $p(m_i)$. When a cryptanalyst intercepts a given cryptogram c_j he can, at least in principle, calculate, for each individual message m_i in the message space, the *a posteriori* probability that m_i was transmitted given that c_j was received. We will denote this new probability by $p_j(m_i)$. If $p_j(m_h)$ were to be much larger than $p_j(m_l)$, for all other messages m_l, then the cryptanalyst would deduce, probably correctly, that m_h was transmitted. Clearly we would like the knowledge of all the *a posteriori* probabilities to give the cryptanalyst no extra information. With this in mind we say that our system has *perfect secrecy* if, for every message m_i and every cryptogram c_j, $p_j(m_i) = p(m_i)$. In order to see that, at least for certain cryptograms c_j, $p_j(m_i)$ need not be the same as $p(m_i)$ consider the following trivial example. Suppose M consists of two messages m_1, m_2 and that C contains three possible cryptograms c_1, c_2 and c_3. Suppose also that $p(m_1) = p(m_2) = \frac{1}{2}$ and that our system has only two possible transformations t_1 and t_2 such that $t_1(m_1) = c_1$ and $t_1(m_2) = c_2$ but that $t_2(m_1) = c_1$ and $t_2(m_2) = c_3$. Then since neither transformation would enable the message m_1 to be represented by the cryptogram c_3, we have $p_3(m_1) = 0$, i.e., $p_3(m_1) \neq p(m_1)$.

If a cipher system has perfect secrecy, i.e., if $p_j(m_i) = p(m_i)$ for all m_i and all j, the fact that a cryptanalyst has intercepted a particular cryptogram gives him no extra information to help him decide which message was sent. Thus no matter how much ciphertext the cryptanalyst obtains he has absolutely no further information to help him determine any of the messages.

Before we investigate whether or not perfect secrecy is achievable we must emphasize two points. The first point is that perfect secrecy is an information theoretic concept which relates solely to the information which the cryptanalyst obtains directly from the intercepted ciphertext. It does not, for instance, allow for the fact that he may have other intelligence sources available or that he might obtain extra information from analysing the traffic on the transmission channel. Thus, in some sense, the term perfect is misleading. The second point is that, in the definition, there is no limitation put on the resources available to the cryptanalyst. If a system has perfect secrecy then, no matter how hard he tries or for how long, the cryptanalyst cannot obtain any information from the intercepted cryptograms.

Clearly perfect secrecy is a highly desirable property. But is it achievable? The simple answer is yes. To show how, suppose that we wish to send at most two messages 'yes' and 'no', and suppose that the probability of transmitting either of them is $\frac{1}{2}$. Suppose, further, that we have two cryptograms c_1 and c_2 and two transformations t_1 and t_2, (both equally likely), such that $t_1(\text{yes}) = c_1$, $t_1(\text{no}) = c_2$ and $t_2(\text{yes}) = c_2$, $t_2(\text{no}) = c_1$. If the cryptanalyst intercepts, for example, c_1 then he knows there are two possibilities; either t_1 was used and the message was yes or t_2 was used and the message was no. But, since each possibility is equally likely, he can only deduce that each message was equally possible. This, of course, he knew before he intercepted the cryptogram, and consequently we have perfect secrecy.

Our example is trivially small. Nevertheless it establishes, without doubt, that perfect secrecy is possible. (The reader might like to mimic our example to construct a system having perfect secrecy with three equally likely messages and three cryptograms. What about n of each?) It is fairly easy to show that for perfect secrecy we need the number of keys, (i.e. transformations), to be at least as large as the total number of possible messages. In fact Shannon showed that if a cipher system has the same number of messages, cryptograms and keys then it has perfect secrecy if, and only if

(a) for any given message m and any given cryptogram c there is exactly one key transforming m into c, i.e. there is a *unique* transformation t with $c = t(m)$ and

(b) all keys are equally likely.

Note that Shannon's result not only tells us how to obtain perfect secrecy but also how to recognize it when we have it!

If a system has perfect secrecy, then, as we have already observed, the cryptanalyst obtains no information whatsoever from the intercepted cryptogram. If this is the case, then we say that the system is unbreakable. From Shannon's work we know that, at least in theory, we can obtain an unbreakable cipher system no matter how large our message space may be.

However in any practical system we are likely to want to transmit a reasonable amount of information. This, of course, requires a large message space which, by Shannon's result, in turn implies a large number of keys. Unfortunately the distribution of a large amount of key material is liable to cause horrendous management problems. In most situations these problems are sufficient to deter communicators from using such systems. Nevertheless there are situations where complete secrecy is of paramount importance and then, despite the obvious problems, such systems are used. If the message space is small then, for instance with our 'yes' and 'no' example, they can even be practical.

There is one particular system which offers perfect secrecy and, because it has had such a great influence on the design of many modern cipher systems, deserves special mention. It is known as the *one-time pad*. Suppose we have a message $m = m_1 m_2 \ldots m_n$ to be enciphered. (Here each m_i might be a character in some appropriate alphabet. So, for instance, if m were an English word, each m_i might be an alphabetic character, whereas if m were a sequence of binary digits then each m_i would be 0 or 1.) In order to encipher m we select a random sequence $k_1 k_2 \ldots k_n$ for which there are the same number of possibilities for each k_i as there are for each m_i. (Here, when saying that we select a random sequence $k_1 k_2 \ldots k_n$, we merely mean that each k_i is chosen at random and is independent of every other k_j.) The enciphering process for a one-time pad is then fully described in Fig. 3.3. In this diagram

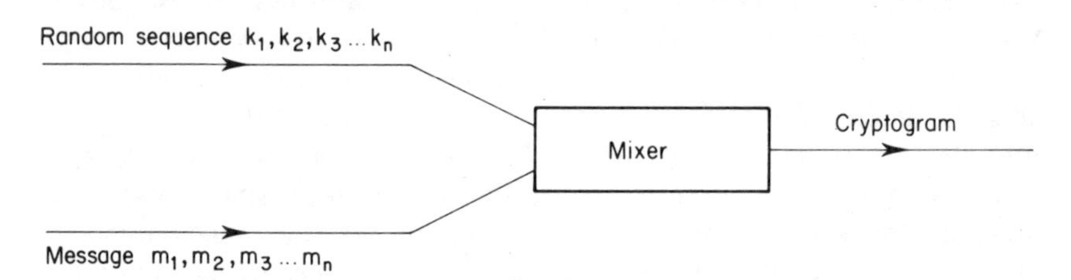

FIG. 3.3. One-time pad.

the mixer acts on each pair k_i and m_i to produce a ciphertext character c_i. One commonly used mixer is a *modulo-26 adder*. In this case, if each m_i is an alphabetic character represented by one of the integers from 0 to 25, each k_i is also an integer from 0 to 25 and the resulting cryptogram is $c = c_1 c_2 \ldots c_n$ where each c_i is the unique integer in the range 0 to 25 given by $c_i \equiv m_i + k_i (\text{mod } 26)$. (Thus if $m_i + k_i$ is less than 26 then $c_i = m_i + k_i$ but if c_i is greater than 25 then $c_i = m_i + k_i - 26$.) A second, possibly even more common, mixer is a *modulo-2 adder* or, to give it its 'engineering name', an *exclusive-or (XOR) gate*. Here the message characters are coded to form a binary sequence $m = m_1 m_2 \ldots m_n$. The sequence $k = k_1 k_2 \ldots k_n$ is then also a sequence of zeros and ones and each c_i of the resulting cryptogram $c = c_1 c_2 \ldots c_n$ is given by $c_i \equiv m_i + k_i (\text{mod } 2)$ or, in engineering notation, $c_i = m_i \oplus k_i$. (Recall that $0 \oplus 0 = 1 \oplus 1 = 0$ and $1 \oplus 0 = 0 \oplus 1 = 1$.)

The name one-time pad is derived from the fact that, when this system was originally proposed, the encipherer and recipient would have identical pads with numbered pages and with a random sequence of characters on each page. The message originator would then precede his message with the appropriate page number to inform the recipient which sequence he was using. As soon as a sequence had been used once its page would be destroyed.

For a point-to-point telecommunications system some version of the one-time pad is certainly feasible. However for a telecommunications network with many terminals the logistics problems associated with key distribution and management (e.g., ensuring that each sequence is used only once) is enormous. Nevertheless the one-time pad is a theoretically unbreakable system and has greatly influenced cryptographers in their attempts to construct secure systems.

B. Practical Security

In our discussion of theoretical security we assumed that the cryptanalyst had unlimited time, facilities and funds. In reality, of course, he is likely to be faced with a totally different situation. He will have to worry about all three of the above resources and, in a number of situations, the time taken to solve a cryptogram will be of the utmost importance to him. As we saw in Chapter 1, it is quite likely that the communicators will only need their messages to be secret for a limited time period, called their required *cover time*. In these situations the message is only of use to the intercepter if he can understand it before the communicators' cover time has lapsed. So if the cover time needed by the encipherer is very short, then time-consuming cryptanalytical techniques may be of little practical value to an interceptor. Thus it is certainly possible for a theoretically insecure system to provide adequate practical security, especially in a tactical environment. On the other hand it is also possible for a theoretically secure system to be highly vulnerable when used in a practical situation. For an example we have only to consider trying to use a one-time pad which, as we have seen, is theoretically unbreakable. It is important to realise that the concepts of perfect secrecy and theoretically unbreakable ciphers ignore many extremely important practical facts. For instance in the discussion of the one-time pad we assumed that the transmission of the key material was not part of the cipher system. This may have been reasonable but it must not be forgotten that the secure transmission of the key material is as crucial as the secure transmission of the messages. (Remember that knowledge of the key gives the interceptor the same information as the intended recipient!) Despite the fact that perfect secrecy is dependent on there being at least as much key material as message, our discussion completely ignored the practical problem of transmitting this large volume of key material to the recipient. Clearly the system can only be practically secure if the encipherer can find a safe way of letting the recipient know the key he has used. There is no doubt that for the one-time pad the actual key management is highly vulnerable and therefore that, although it is theoretically unbreakable, the system may not be practically secure. Once we accept the possibility of using a system which is theoretically breakable, then, when we assess its practical security, we are not asking if the interceptor can break the system but, on the assumption that he can, are asking how long it will take him and how much it is likely to cost. Thus, in order to assess the practical security of a system, we must have some idea of the resources which are likely to be available to a would-be cryptanalyst. In particular we need to know the computer power which he is likely to have at his disposal. We have already discussed this type of problem in Chapter 1 and, as we did then, we stress that it is always advisable to overestimate rather than to underestimate his resources. Thus, if there is any doubt, it is always safest to assume that the cryptanalyst has the best equipment at his disposal. Even under this assumption it may still be possible to have a system which we regard as practically secure. Let us suppose, for example, that we have a system which we know to be breakable but for which a successful attack would require at least 10^{50} storage elements or operations. Donald Davies of the National Physical Laboratory (Davies, 1980) has shown conclusively that if the cryptanalyst needs 10^{50} storage elements to break a system then the cryptographer need not be concerned and can safely regard the system as unbreakable. More specifically he estimated that achieving 10^{50} storage elements would require a memory covering the earth to a height of 10 km. Even if it occupied this volume, the memory bank would have to be so dense that only one atom could be allocated to each memory bit. Of course the details of this estimate are irrelevant. The conclusion, however, is important: if we can set the cryptanalyst a task requiring too much storage then we may regard our system as practically secure. A similar conclusion holds if we set him sufficiently many operations. In neither case would we attempt to specify the lowest 'safe' number for the operations or storage elements. However, given current technology, it is certainly considerably fewer than 10^{50}. Even with as 'few' as 10^{18} necessary operations and on an extremely fast machine capable of executing an operation in 10^{-9} sec, we could feel confident that no one would be able to break the system in less than 30 years. Given this situation we would say that the system has a cover time of over 30 years. (It is worth noting here that there are only 31,536,000 sec in a year!)

When trying to assess the practical security of a system we must estimate the number of operations or storage elements needed to break it and then decide if the cover time is sufficient for our purposes. Having said that we must immediately point out that the number of operations needed will obviously depend on the efficiency of the attack. Thus the cryptanalyst is always seeking ways of reducing the number of operations, and it is the cryptographer's task to be as aware as he can of all the available techniques. In this way the cryptographer will ensure that he does not seriously underestimate the number of operations his 'enemy' may need. Given that there are only a finite number of keys one possible attack is to try each key in turn. Obviously everyone is aware of this and the cryptanalyst is continuously seeking methods which eliminate many possibilities for the key in one go. We can give a simple example of one such technique by looking at simple substitution ciphers. As we saw, one method of attack in this case is to use the statistics and try to identify the ciphertext equivalent for E. Once this has been established, or even once the number of candidates has been narrowed to only a few, all the keys which have different equivalents for E can be eliminated.

Practical cryptology (*cryptology* is the name given to the study of cryptography and cryptanalysis) is a fascinating duel between the cryptographers and the cryptanalysts. On the one hand the cryptanalyst is trying to eliminate large numbers of key possibilities with each single mathematical operation or statistical test. On the other hand the cryptographer is trying to ensure that the amount of work which the cryptanalyst needs to perform does not get too small as the length of the cryptogram increases. It is a battle which the cryptographer dares not lose.

In Chapter 1, when we considered the system from a user's point of view, we recommended that the user should assess his enemy's capabilities. Clearly he is more likely to be able to do this than the system designer. So, if the cryptographer does not know the exact capabilities of the enemy, what assumptions should he make as he begins to design his system? The only safe assumption that the cryptographer can make is that any would-be cryptanalyst has as much knowledge and intelligence information as possible. Once again we emphasize that in practice we are almost always considering theoretically breakable systems (the only exception being the one-time pad). Thus we are accepting that our system is breakable and are merely assessing how long it will take a cryptanalyst to break it. When assessing the security level the cryptographer should assume the following three conditions, called the *worst-case conditions*. He should assume that the cryptanalyst:

(WC1) has a complete knowledge of the cipher system
(WC2) has obtained a considerable amount of ciphertext
(WC3) knows the plaintext equivalent of a certain amount of the ciphertext.

Of course in any given situation the cryptographer must attempt to realistically quantify the terms 'considerable amount' and 'certain amount'. His values will depend on the particular system under consideration.

Condition WC1 implies that we should assume that there is no security in the cipher system itself and accept that all security must come from the interceptor's inability to determine the key. Naturally the cryptanalyst's task is considerably more difficult if he does not know the system and it is now, at least to a certain extent, possible to conceal this information. For instance, with a modern electronic system the function used for enciphering can be 'hidden' in hardware. By using large-scale (or even very large-scale) integration we can 'conceal' the entire function within an extremely small chip. However, although it is a very delicate and time-consuming operation, it is possible to open up one of these chips and we should certainly not assume that the cryptanalyst does not have the ability and patience to do it. Similarly, if a part of the function is included as software within the machine, we can always write a carefully chosen program to disguise it. Once again, provided he has the necessary patience and skill, the cryptanalyst will probably be able to uncover it. Another possibility might be to try tamper-proofing the box containing the essential enciphering and deciphering hardware and software. We have already discussed this problem and, as we saw, for most practical applications only tamper-resistance can, at the present time, be provided without the cost becoming prohibitive. But even if tamper-proofing is used it would still be unwise to assume that the algorithm is not known to the cryptanalyst.

From the manufacturer's or designer's point of view, the acceptance of condition WC1 is welcome. It then removes from him the extremely worrying responsibility involved in keeping a system secret. In fact it is probably true that, in order to keep a system secret with any degree of confidence, one would have to 'shoot' all personnel involved in the design and/or manufacture of the equipment. The scrambler designers' union might find this unacceptable! As an indication that WC1 is widely accepted we point out that a cipher system (DES) has been introduced for which the algorithm has deliberately been made public. We will discuss DES later but clearly the designers and users of DES have accepted WC1.

There is not much to say about WC2. Clearly it is a necessary assumption. If a cryptanalyst can intercept one communication between two parties then he can probably intercept others. Furthermore a number of these communications may have used the same key.

If a cryptanalyst has a complete knowledge of the system plus some plaintext/ciphertext equivalents, then he is able to launch a so-called *known plaintext attack*. This is probably the most important and most commonly used method of breaking ciphers. Any designer is advised to protect himself against such an attack and, as a consequence, he should accept WC3. In a known plaintext attack the cryptanalyst has obtained knowledge of some of the plaintext message, possibly by deduction, intelligent guesswork or even by 'planting' it in some way, i.e., he already knows the plaintext equivalent of part of the cryptogram. He then uses this knowledge to enable him to deduce the rest. For example, for messages in English, he may have deduced the ciphertext equivalent for E. From this knowledge he might then be able to locate the ciphertext equivalent of 'the' and, eventually, break the cryptogram. He might, to take another example, know that the message was a letter and guess that it started 'Dear Sir'. It may not be immediately clear how this type of situation can arise with speech systems. Especially since, in this case, the message is an analogue signal which cannot even be accurately predicted by the message originator. However, as we shall see later, WC3 applies as much, if not more, to many speech systems as it does to data systems.

Once he has accepted WC3 the cryptographer must then decide how much the knowledge of a small proportion of the plaintext/ciphertext equivalent helps the cryptanalyst. Clearly the answer will depend on many things including, obviously, the size of the 'small proportion', i.e., the actual length of known plaintext.

There are, essentially, three main types of modern cipher systems: block ciphers, stream ciphers and public-key ciphers. (This is, of necessity, a very broad classification and the three classes listed are certainly not disjoint.) We will now discuss each of the three types. Naturally our discussion will be brief and for more detail of any of the three types we refer the reader to Beker and Piper (1982d).

III. Block Ciphers

When using a *block cipher* (Fig. 3.4) we first choose an integer s. Then, in order to encipher a message $m = m_1 m_2 \dots m_s m_{s+1} \dots m_{2s} m_{2s+1} \dots$, we split m into 'blocks' of size s. In order to encipher the block $m_1 m_2 \dots m_s$ we use a key k and s functions $f_1, f_2, \dots, f_s$ (usually different) to obtain a

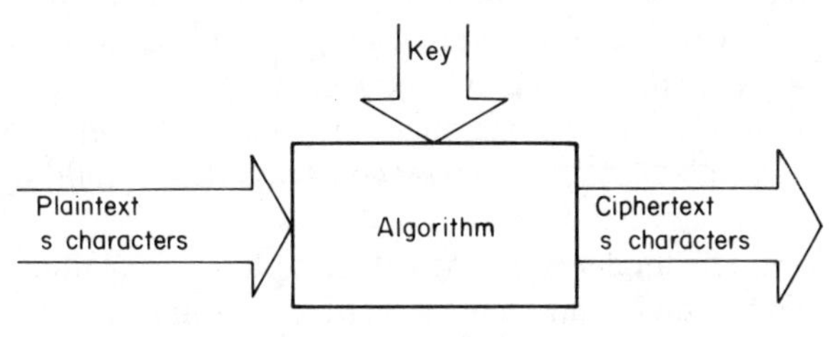

FIG. 3.4. Block cipher.

cryptogram $c_1 c_2 \ldots c_s$. Using the same key and functions we then encipher the next block of s message characters i.e., $m_{s+1} m_{s+2} \ldots m_{2s}$. Thus the message is enciphered s characters at a time, the cryptogram is produced in blocks of s characters and each ciphertext character in a given block usually depends on the complete corresponding plaintext block as well as the key. Since each block of the message is replaced by another block, a block cipher may be regarded as a simple substitution cipher. However, in general, this substitution is likely to be considerably more complex than the monoalphabetic ciphers discussed earlier. In fact a monoalphabetic cipher is merely the special case when each block is identified with a character.

In practice it is desirable to make the functions f_i fairly complicated. The reason for this is that a block cipher tries to utilise confusion and diffusion. These are two of the concepts which were introduced by Shannon and we will say a little about them.

Quite simply, the idea behind *confusion* is to ensure that the relation between a cryptogram and the corresponding key is complex. The objective is to make it difficult for any statistical analysis to indicate properties of the key. To achieve this it is desirable that the encipherment of every single message character should depend on virtually the entire key. If this is so then the cryptanalyst should be unable to determine small parts of the key and, if he is to discover it, will have to find the whole key simultaneously. This will almost certainly involve him in solving considerably more complex equations than would be necessary if he could find the key piece by piece. (Incidentally, this was one of the major defects of the monoalphabetic ciphers which we discussed earlier. In this case the encipherment of one message character involved only a small part of the key, namely the single letter which was substituted for it. Thus the cryptanalyst could break the system by determining small pieces of the key and then using the portion of the key already found to determine others. In fact we have alredy illustrated this type of attack. He could, for example, first find the ciphertext equivalent of E. Then, given this, he could locate the word 'the' etc.)

Whereas confusion ensures a complex relation between the cryptogram and key, *diffusion* ensures the complexity of the relation between the plaintext and ciphertext. It attempts to spread the statistics of the message space over long portions of the cryptogram. The idea is then to ensure that the cryptanalyst needs to intercept a long passage of ciphertext before he can attempt any form of statistical decipherment. This is achieved, in practice, by enciphering large blocks of message characters simultaneously and dependently.

Thus, if we revert to our definition of a block cipher, to introduce the properties of confusion and diffusion each f_i should be a complicated function of as many of the s message characters and as much of the key as possible.

In order to discuss block ciphers we will, for convenience, think of our message and cryptogram characters as binary digits. Then, if our block size is s, the number of possibilities for a block is 2^s and we may regard each message and cryptogram block as one of the integers from 0 to $2^s - 1$ inclusive. Once we have made this identification then each substitution cipher corresponds to a permutation of the set $\{0, 1, \ldots, 2^s - 1\}$. In other words each key k_i determines a permutation α_i on $\{0, 1, \ldots, 2^s - 1\}$.

In case the reader is not familiar with permutations we will give a formal definition and look at a small example. For any positive integer n a *permutation* α on $\{0, 1, \ldots, n - 1\}$ is a transformation which assigns to each integer i in the range 0 to $n - 1$ a unique integer, denoted by $\alpha(i)$, also in the range. Furthermore no two integers have the same value assigned to them. Thus, for example, if we take $n = 8$, one possible permutation α on $\{0, 1, \ldots, 7\}$ is given by $\alpha(0) = 2$, $\alpha(1) = 6$, $\alpha(2) = 1$, $\alpha(3) = 0$, $\alpha(4) = 7$, $\alpha(5) = 4$, $\alpha(6) = 3$, $\alpha(7) = 5$. We often represent α as

$$\begin{bmatrix} 0 & 1 & 2 & 3 & 4 & 5 & 6 & 7 \\ 2 & 6 & 1 & 0 & 7 & 4 & 3 & 5 \end{bmatrix}$$

i.e., we write $\alpha(i)$ underneath i for each i. One fundamental property of permutations is that for any permutation θ on $\{0, 1, \ldots, n - 1\}$ there is a permutation θ^{-1}, called the *inverse* of θ, such that $\theta^{-1}(\theta(i)) = i$ for all i. For our particular example, since $\alpha(0) = 2$ we must have $\alpha^{-1}(2) = 0$. Similarly since $\alpha(1) = 6$ we must have $\alpha^{-1}(6) = 1$. Continuing in this way we get $\alpha^{-1}(0) = 3$, $\alpha^{-1}(1) = 2$, $\alpha^{-1}(2) = 0$, $\alpha^{-1}(3) = 6$, $\alpha^{-1}(4) = 5$, $\alpha^{-1}(5) = 7$, $\alpha^{-1}(6) = 1$, $\alpha^{-1}(7) = 4$ or

$$\alpha^{-1} = \begin{bmatrix} 0 & 1 & 2 & 3 & 4 & 5 & 6 & 7 \\ 3 & 2 & 0 & 6 & 5 & 7 & 1 & 4 \end{bmatrix}$$

(Note that we can obtain α^{-1} from α by simply placing the second row of

$$\begin{bmatrix} 0 & 1 & 2 & 3 & 4 & 5 & 6 & 7 \\ 2 & 6 & 1 & 0 & 7 & 4 & 3 & 5 \end{bmatrix}$$

on top of the first and then altering the order of the columns so that the new top row is in the correct order.)

An alternative way of representing permutations is by giving the associated *permutation matrix*. We will not give a general definition of a permutation matrix but will show what it is for a small example and then for our particular permutation α. Hopefully this will be enough to give the general idea. Suppose that β is the permutation on $\{0, 1, 2\}$ given by $\beta = \left[\begin{smallmatrix} 0 & 1 & 2 \\ 2 & 0 & 1 \end{smallmatrix}\right]$. Then the permutation matrix B of β is the 3×3 matrix with each entry 0 or 1 and exactly one 1 in each row such that

$$B\begin{bmatrix}0\\1\\2\end{bmatrix} = \begin{bmatrix}2\\0\\1\end{bmatrix}$$

Since the first row of

$$B\begin{bmatrix}0\\1\\2\end{bmatrix}$$

is 2, the first row of B must have a 1 in the position which will involve 2 when we work out the product. Since 2 is in the third row this means that the first row of B must be 001. similar considerations give

$$B = \begin{bmatrix}0 & 0 & 1\\1 & 0 & 0\\0 & 1 & 0\end{bmatrix}$$

Clearly $\beta^{-1} = \left[\begin{smallmatrix}0 & 1 & 2\\1 & 2 & 0\end{smallmatrix}\right]$and the permutation matrix of β^{-1} is

$$\begin{bmatrix}0 & 1 & 0\\0 & 0 & 1\\1 & 0 & 0\end{bmatrix}$$

By direct calculation we can check that this is the matrix B^{-1} and in fact, for any permutation γ, if C is the permutation matrix of γ, then the permutation matrix of γ^{-1} is C^{-1}. However we can actually obtain the permutation matrix of γ^{-1} from C without going through the somewhat lengthy process of finding its inverse. Every permutation matrix has exactly one 1 in each row and exactly one 1 in each column. Furthermore if P is a permutation matrix then P is orthogonal which means that $P^{T} = P^{-1}$, where P^{T} denotes the *transpose* of P. Thus, in our small example, we could have found the permutation matrix of β^{-1} by merely writing down the transpose of B, i.e., by writing the matrix whose rows are the corresponding columns of B. For our earlier example where

$$\alpha = \begin{bmatrix}0 & 1 & 2 & 3 & 4 & 5 & 6 & 7\\2 & 6 & 1 & 0 & 7 & 4 & 3 & 5\end{bmatrix}$$

then since, for example, $\alpha(0) = 2$ and 2 is in the third position, the first row of its permutation matrix must have its 1 in the third position. This argument applied to the other seven rows gives the following 8×8 permutation matrix

$$\begin{bmatrix} 0 & 0 & 1 & 0 & 0 & 0 & 0 & 0 \\ 0 & 0 & 0 & 0 & 0 & 0 & 1 & 0 \\ 0 & 1 & 0 & 0 & 0 & 0 & 0 & 0 \\ 1 & 0 & 0 & 0 & 0 & 0 & 0 & 0 \\ 0 & 0 & 0 & 0 & 0 & 0 & 0 & 1 \\ 0 & 0 & 0 & 0 & 1 & 0 & 0 & 0 \\ 0 & 0 & 0 & 1 & 0 & 0 & 0 & 0 \\ 0 & 0 & 0 & 0 & 0 & 1 & 0 & 0 \end{bmatrix}$$

Clearly the transpose of this matrix is

$$\begin{bmatrix} 0 & 0 & 0 & 1 & 0 & 0 & 0 & 0 \\ 0 & 0 & 1 & 0 & 0 & 0 & 0 & 0 \\ 1 & 0 & 0 & 0 & 0 & 0 & 0 & 0 \\ 0 & 0 & 0 & 0 & 0 & 0 & 1 & 0 \\ 0 & 0 & 0 & 0 & 0 & 1 & 0 & 0 \\ 0 & 0 & 0 & 0 & 0 & 0 & 0 & 1 \\ 0 & 1 & 0 & 0 & 0 & 0 & 0 & 0 \\ 0 & 0 & 0 & 0 & 1 & 0 & 0 & 0 \end{bmatrix}$$

The reader should now convince himself that this second matrix is indeed the permutation matrix of α^{-1}.

Let us now revert back to our discussion of block ciphers and illustrate how using permutations can help us to write down the keys. We will consider an example with $s = 3$. Thus we have eight possible messages and eight possible cryptograms. If, for example, the input is 101 then, since 101 is the binary representation of 5, we will represent it as 5. In this way each message and cryptogram can be represented as one of $\{0, 1, \ldots, 7\}$. Each key now determines one of the permutations on this set $\{0, 1, \ldots, 7\}$. In Fig 3.5 we illustrate one possibility. (Note that we have used the permutation which we discussed earlier.) From Fig. 3.5 we can work out the output for any given input. Suppose for example the input is 011. Then, since 011 corresponds to 3 and

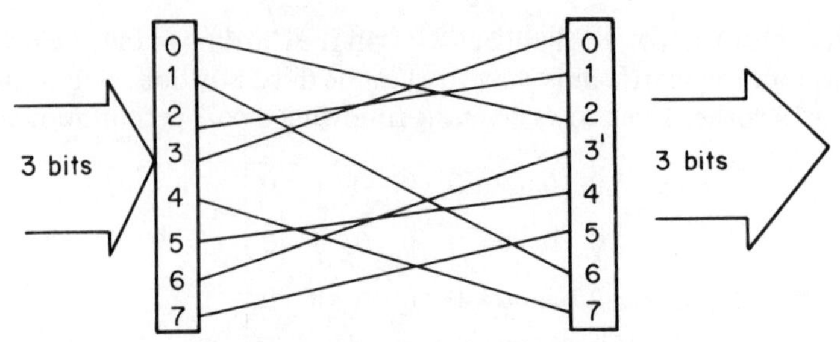

FIG. 3.5. Possible permutation when $s = 3$.

3 is mapped onto 0, the output will be 000. Similarly, since 110 corresponds to 6 and 6 is mapped onto 3, if the input is 110 the output will be 011.

Before we continue to discuss arbitrary block ciphers we must point out yet further ways of describing the cipher represented by Fig. 3.5. We can write down a *look-up table* or a *truth table.* In Table 3.2 we have given the look-up table for the permutation of Fig. 3.5. Table 3.3, although it contains

TABLE 3.2

A Look-up Table for Fig. 3.5

m_1	m_2	m_3	c
0	0	0	010
0	0	1	110
0	1	0	001
0	1	1	000
1	0	0	111
1	0	1	100
1	1	0	011
1	1	1	101

TABLE 3.3

The Truth Table for Fig. 3.5

m_1	m_2	m_3	c_1	m_1	m_2	m_3	c_2	m_1	m_2	m_3	c_3
0	0	0	0	0	0	0	1	0	0	0	0
0	0	1	1	0	0	1	1	0	0	1	0
0	1	0	0	0	1	0	0	0	1	0	1
0	1	1	0	0	1	1	0	0	1	1	0
1	0	0	1	1	0	0	1	1	0	0	1
1	0	1	1	1	0	1	0	1	0	1	0
1	1	0	0	1	1	0	1	1	1	0	1
1	1	1	1	1	1	1	0	1	1	1	1

the same information, is slightly different. This second table shows the truth tables for each of the functions f_1, f_2, f_3 which define the block cipher for the key exhibited in Fig. 3.5. (So, for example, $f_1(010) = 0$, $f_2(010) = 0$, $f_3(010) = 1$.)

For a block cipher with block size s there are 2^s possible message blocks and, consequently, $(2^s)!$ possible permutations. (For any positive integer n, $n! = 1 \times 2 \times \cdots \times (n-1) \times n$ and is equal to the total number of permutation on n symbols.) Obviously it would be useful if, for each one of them, we had a key which enabled us to use that particular permutation. As we shall see, this is not usually the situation and there will normally only be a comparatively small number available to us.

Since a block cipher is a substitution cipher it is likely to be vulnerable to statistical attacks involving the analysis of the cipher blocks. These attacks are likely to be similar to those in which the statistics of the English language can be used to break monoalphabetic ciphers. Another problem with a block cipher is that an interceptor is often able to compile a directory of corresponding blocks of plaintext and ciphertext. Clearly the size of such a directory is likely to depend on the number of possibilities for the plaintext blocks, i.e., on the block size. Both these methods of attack can be thwarted by choosing a sufficiently large value for s. With this in mind Meyer (1974) suggests that the minimum block size should be equivalent to four characters. If this is accepted, then if, for instance, an 8-bit character code is used, s should be at least 32. But if we choose $s = 32$ and want to be able to use all the possible permutations on 0 to $2^{32} - 1$ then we require a key space capable of producing $(2^{32})!$ permutations. Clearly $(2^{32})!$ is so large that we cannot manage it and we can only choose $s = 32$ if we are prepared to accept a severe restriction on the available permutations. Even if s is less than 32, $(2^s)!$ may still be too large. For instance if s is as small as 6 then, since $(2^6)! \cong 2^{296}$, we still need a 296-bit key to be able to obtain all permutations.

One feasible and attractive way to restrict our permutations is to use only those which are defined by certain simple, mathematical functions. When we do this we arrange for each key to determine a mathematical function which, in turn, gives an appropriate permutation. There will be many occasions when we will need to generate 'random' permutations or, alternatively, to make a random selection from a carefully chosen set of 'good' permutations. There are many algorithms for generating random permutations and an interesting discussion of them is contained in Sloane (1982). One particularly fast and simple algorithm is the following. Let $x_1 = 1$, $x_2 = 2$, ..., $x_n = n$. Then for $i = n, n-1, ..., 2$ we generate a random number U, uniformly distributed between 0 and 1, put $k = [iU] + 1$ and then exchange the values assigned to x_i and x_k. (Here, for any real number y, $[y]$ denotes the largest integer which is less than or equal to y.) Our random permutation is then

$$\begin{bmatrix} 1 & 2 & 3 & \cdots & n \\ x_1 & x_2 & x_3 & \cdots & x_n \end{bmatrix}$$

In order to work through a simple example of this algorithm we let $n = 5$. So we start with $x_1 = 1$, $x_2 = 2$, $x_3 = 3$, $x_4 = 4$, $x_5 = 5$. If our first value for $U = 0.40369$ then $[5U] + 1 = 3$ so we have $x_1 = 1$, $x_2 = 2$, $x_3 = 5$, $x_4 = 4$, $x_5 = 3$. If the next value for $U = 0.55563$ then $[4U] + 1 = 3$ so we get $x_1 = 1$, $x_2 = 2$, $x_3 = 4$, $x_4 = 5$, $x_5 = 3$. If the third value for $U = 0.63700$ then $[3U] + 1 = 2$ which gives $x_1 = 1$, $x_2 = 4$, $x_3 = 2$, $x_4 = 5$, $x_5 = 3$. Finally if the fourth value is $U = 0.63207$ then $[2U] + 1 = 2$, so our final values are $x_1 = 1$, $x_2 = 4$, $x_3 = 2$, $x_4 = 5$, $x_5 = 3$ and the permutation is $\left[\begin{smallmatrix} 1 & 2 & 3 & 4 & 5 \\ 1 & 4 & 2 & 5 & 3 \end{smallmatrix}\right]$.

Of course we have, in a sense, 'fudged' the issue by assuming that we can generate random numbers. However this is a topic we shall repeatedly discuss, (see for example our discussion of shift registers in Section IV of this chapter), so we are happy to avoid it here. There will also be instances when we shall discuss methods for choosing good permutations from which to make random selections. Since the definition of good will change according to the discussion we will postpone a discussion of this type of process until Chapter 4 when we will have specific examples.

When we were discussing our worst case conditions we mentioned the existence of a cipher system for which the entire enciphering algorithm has been made public. This system is a block cipher and is called the *Data Encryption Standard* (or DES). Although we will look at a little of the history and some of the general problems which arise from cryptographic standards, we will not discuss the operational details of DES. Instead we merely observe that it is based on the principle of a Feistel cipher system. This is an interesting, and particularly important, example of a block cipher system. For a *Feistel cipher system* the block size has to be even and, if the block size is $2n$, each message block is divided into two halves and written as $m = (m_0, m_1)$. In this system each key k defines a set of subkeys $\{k_1, k_2, \ldots, k_h\}$ and each subkey k_i determines a transformation f_{k_i} which maps each block of size n onto another one. The message μ is then enciphered in h 'rounds' using the following rules:

$$\begin{aligned} &\text{At round } 1: \quad \mu_0 = (m_0, m_1) \to \mu_1 = (m_1, m_2) \\ &\quad\vdots \\ &\text{At round } i: \quad \mu_{i-1} = (m_{i-1}, m_i) \to \mu_i = (m_i, m_{i+i}) \\ &\quad\vdots \\ &\text{At round } h: \quad \mu_{h-1} = (m_{h-1}, m_h) \to \mu_h = (m_h, m_{h+1}) \end{aligned}$$

where $m_{i+1} = m_{i-1} + f_{k_i}(m_i)$ for each $i \geqslant 1$. The ciphertext is then the $2n$-bit block $m_h m_{h+1}$.

To decipher we note that, since all additions are modulo 2, the equation $m_{i+1} = m_{i-1} + f_{k_i}(m_i)$ may also be written as $m_{i-1} = m_{i+1} + f_{k_i}(m_i)$. Thus if we reverse the two halves of the ciphertext block and apply the encipherment procedure in the reverse order we have

$$\bar{\mu}_h = (m_{h+1}, m_h) \rightarrow \bar{\mu}_{h-1} = (m_h, m_{h-1}) \qquad \text{at round } 1$$
$$\vdots$$
$$\bar{\mu}_i = (m_{i+1}, m_i) \rightarrow \bar{\mu}_{i-1} = (m_i, m_{i-1}) \qquad \text{at round } h + 1 - i$$
$$\vdots$$
$$\bar{\mu}_1 = (m_2, m_1) \rightarrow \bar{\mu}_0 = (m_1, m_0) \qquad \text{at round } h$$

Thus we can decipher provided that we can reproduce each f_{k_j} at the appropriate moment. It is important to note that we do not require that the functions have any special properties. In particular, they do not need to be reversible. Examples of Feistel ciphers utilising different functions and some of the effects of this on their security level are given in Beker and Piper (1982d).

The search for a standard encryption algorithm was initiated in 1973 by the United States National Bureau of Standards (NBS). Their stated intention was that the method of encryption selected as a standard should be amenable to the various types of equipment built by many manufacturers of computer and terminal equipment. They also wanted all information relating to this project to be publicly available. Although their first search was unsuccessful the second, begun in August 1974, produced an algorithm which showed sufficient merit to justify further examination. After undergoing U.S. Government review for acceptability as a federal standard the algorithm was published for public comment in March 1975. There was a wide variety of public opinion and, after considering the various reactions to their proposals, the NBS held two workshops to consider DES. In 1978, according to Ruth Davis (Davis, 1978), both workshops expressed the view that DES was satisfactory as a standard for the next 10–15 years.

The Data Encryption Standard has had a very mixed reception. Since it is the first system with a publicly known algorithm, any discussion of DES is likely to raise the thorny question of whether there should be a standard. Another question, of more direct relevance, is whether or not DES should be the standard. This of course relates to the security level attained by DES. There are a number of recent publications which describe the DES algorithm, (see for example Beker and Piper, 1982d; Konheim, 1981) and discuss its merits. We refer the reader to these. We must, however, say a little about the general question of whether or not a standard should exist.

When we discussed our worst-case conditions we stated that the system designer should accept WC1. It might, at first sight, seem that publication of the algorithm is a logical consequence of this. However, prior to DES, we know of no publication which contained a complete algorithm for practical useage. Thus DES is the first example where an algorithm has actually been published and the world's cryptanalysts have been challenged to break it. With any system like DES there is always a danger, hopefully very small, that someone will find a way to break it. When a system is published as a standard this focuses the attention of all cryptanalysts on the same system and must therefore increase the chances of it being broken. Furthermore if a standard is widely used then the cryptanalyst knows that, by breaking it, he will gain access to many users' messages. Thus if he finds an attack which works it will be worth his while to implement it even if it is likely to be expensive and time consuming. If someone does manage to break a standard which has been adopted on a nationwide, or even worldwide, basis then, of course, that standard will have to be changed. This is likely to be a colossal, extremely expensive task.

To counterbalance the above disadvantages there are, fortunately, a number of advantages to having a standard. One of the main ones relates to the cost and 'peace of mind' for the user. If a chip, or set of chips, is designed to implement the standard, then they can be produced in sufficient quantity that the cost to the user will be low. However, we must point out that, in practice, the algorithm is only a comparatively small part of a system, and so the overall savings will not be as significant as it might appear. Despite this, the existence of a standard might considerably increase the number of users of cipher systems. The reason is simple. There have been many examples of custom-built systems which have been very insecure. Thus people who do not have the resources and/or ability to assess systems may be reluctant to use them. Unless they have a great deal of confidence in the designers of their systems, these people may feel much more inclined to use a standard which many people have both used and studied. Another obvious advantage of using the standard is the compatibility which can be attained between various systems. However, as we have said before, the risk remains that if one network is broken, then they all are.

Given that a standard is to be used then the versatility of a block cipher system makes it a very strong 'candidate' for that standard. As we shall see, block ciphers can be configured in many different ways and thus facilitate various types of application.

One fundamental characteristic of the block cipher is that, since the message is enciphered in blocks, a number of message characters will be enciphered simultaneously and dependently. Thus each character of the ciphertext depends on a number of message characters and, at the receiver, each part of the message depends on many ciphertext characters. Thus if there is one single error in the transmission of the ciphertext there are likely to be many errors in the received message. (This effect, where one error causes many more, is called *error propagation*.) There are occasions when error propagation might appear to be a boon. In any situation where complete accuracy is essential then any single error in the data must be detected. With a block cipher this single error is likely to 'blow up' into many and the recipient will then be aware that something is wrong. However, when complete accuracy is essential the receiver will almost certainly contain some automated procedure for error detection.

Consequently the advantage of an error-propagating system is not as necessary as it might have appeared and furthermore error propagation might actually lower the success rate of the automated error detection. In practice the propagation of errors is often considered a major disadvantage and there are many situations where the occasional error is of no consequence. For instance if the message is a passage of English text then the redundancy of the English language is so great that a few errors are unlikely to prevent the receiver from deciphering correctly. For a second example where error propagation may be undesirable we consider the encipherment of digital speech. Here, to take a typical situation, 16-kbit/sec delta-modulated speech may withstand error rates of up to 10% in the transmission path. So if an error-propagating cipher system is added to a bad, but usable, transmission channel the result is likely to be totally unusable. When we consider radio applications, the effect of this is a significant drop in the range of the radio. Yet another consequence of error propagation is that properties such as information formats are likely to be lost.

IV. Stream Ciphers

A *stream cipher* is one in which errors are not propagated. It is characterised by the fact that the encipherment of each bit of data is independent of the rest of the message.

Apart from Shannon's work, the most significant factors in the development of the design of cipher systems were the advent of the computer and then, in the 1960s, the expanding use of microelectronics. (It is worth noting that it was the need to break a cipher system during the Second World War that led to the development of Colossus, one of the first dedicated calculating machines that we now know simply as computers.) They meant that a whole new range of functions was available to the cryptographer; but they also compelled him to increase his mathematical knowledge. Many of these new functions can only be expressed in terms of a mathematical language which is considerably more advanced than any of the mathematical knowledge previously required in this book.

The development of the stream cipher was greatly influenced by the fact that Shannon had proved the one-time pad to be unbreakable. Many cryptographers felt that if they could emulate the one-time-pad system in some way then they would have a system with a guaranteed high security level. They were also encouraged by the fact that since the 1920s many of the mechanical and electromechanical machines had operated in a way similar to the one-time pad, in the sense that they produced long sequences of displacements which were applied, character by character, to the plaintext message. However, there was one fundamental difference. The sequence produced by one of these machines was completely determined by the key and was not random. Nevertheless, by choosing the algorithm carefully, it was possible to generate a sequence which appeared to be random (in the sense that there was no obvious relation between the elements). Many cryptographers believed that such systems were highly secure but, as we shall see, this is not necessarily so.

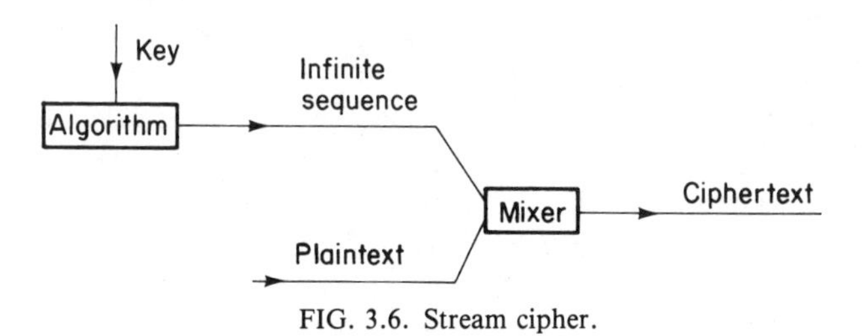

FIG. 3.6. Stream cipher.

A typical stream cipher is shown in Fig. 3.6. In this system the key is fed into an algorithm which uses this key to generate an infinite sequence. The algorithm is usually referred to as the *sequence generator* or *keystream generator*. We re-emphasize that a stream cipher is not error propagating. Error propagation is usually considered a disadvantage and the stream cipher is undoubtedly the most common system used in current cipher equipment. It is also possibly the most important. Consequently we will consider in some detail the various properties which such a system must exhibit to be secure against the worst-case conditions. At times the discussion will be highly mathematical. Although the reader does not need to understand the details of all the arguments he must realise that mathematics plays a fundamental role in this type of analysis. Some of the most complicated looking systems may have extremely elementary mathematical flaws in them. Since the implementation of the majority of stream cipher systems employs electronic techniques, both the plaintext and the infinite sequence usually use a binary character set.

There is another reason for studying stream ciphers in detail. Their keystream generators are also very important for the production of pseudo-random sequences of digits. (A *pseudo-random sequence* of digits is a sequence of digits which appears to be random, in the sense that there is no obvious relation between the various numbers, but is in fact totally deterministic and reproducible from a relatively short 'seed' sequence. In practice this seed is the key.) In the later chapters we shall frequently need sequence generators of this type.

As we said before we began our discussion of block ciphers, it would be a mistake to think of block ciphers and stream ciphers as being totally independent of each other. As an illustration of this we now observe that there are many ways in which a block cipher can be used as a sequence generator for a stream cipher. We illustrate one such technique in Fig. 3.7.

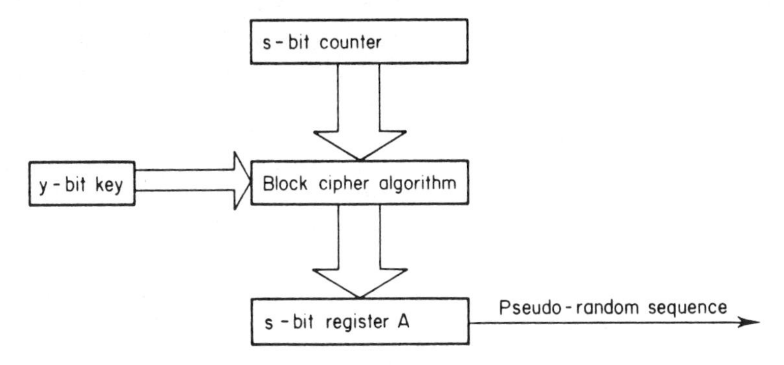

FIG. 3.7. Block cipher used to produce a pseudo-random sequence.

In this example the data input to the algorithm are replaced by a counter which increments every time the block cipher and register are clocked. (This counter could be replaced by almost any deterministic circuit of our choice.) After the y-bit key has also been input, the block cipher algorithm then produces an s-bit block which it holds in register A. Thus each time the counter is incremented we obtain a new s-bit block in A. For any i of our choice, provided of course that i is not greater than s, we can output i of these bits each time, and in this way we obtain our binary sequence. Clearly the properties of the output sequence depend on the block cipher algorithm and on the choice of i, but with a suitably well-designed algorithm the sequence should appear random. The choice of i is likely to depend on our speed requirements and on the time necessary for the block cipher algorithm to produce an output. If, for instance, $s = 100$ and the algorithm has a maximum speed of 100 times/sec, then if we require 10 kbit/sec we must put $i = 100$ and take all 100 bits which the block cipher produces. If, on the other hand, we only require 2 kbit/sec we might choose to put $i = 20$.

If, in the system depicted in Fig. 3.7, the counter counts from 0 to $2^s - 1$ in increments of 1 then, if the key is not changed, after 2^s clocks the situation will revert back to the initial state. Consequently it will begin to reproduce the original sequence. This, of course, means that, if we use the system of Fig. 3.7 and do not change the key, the sequence produced will have the property that it repeats itself after 2^s rounds. Any sequence which consists of repetitions of a fixed shorter sequence is said to be *periodic* and the shortest part of the sequence which is repeated is called a *cycle*. Furthermore the length of a cycle is called the *period* of the sequence. If we let (s_t) represent the sequence $s_0 s_1 s_2 s_3 \ldots$ then if (s_t) has period p we know that (s_t) starts to repeat itself after p terms. Thus $s_p = s_0$, $s_{p+1} = s_1$ and, for any m, $s_{m+p} = s_m$.

Any sequence generated by a practicable sequence generator will be periodic. Once we have used a length of sequence which is longer than the period then the rest of the sequence is completely predictable. Thus if we use a sequence with a small period then, since there is a danger that we will use part of the sequence more than once, our security level may drop. For this reason it is absolutely crucial that, whenever we use a sequence generator, we know the period of the sequence we are using. Or, if we do not know it precisely, that we have a lower bound for its value. There are a number of theorems which guarantee a minimum period for any sequence when using a particular type of sequence generator in a certain way. The importance of these results should be clear and we will discuss them later.

Although it is necessary to use a sequence with a large period it is important to remember that we also need our sequence to appear random. We are relying on this sequence to 'destroy' the statistical properties of the transmitted message so that the cryptanalyst cannot use a statistical analysis to attack our system. Since any periodic sequence is obviously not truly random we must try to decide what we mean by 'appear random'. We must attempt to answer questions like: 'when is a periodic system random enough that we can use it?' Thus, before we look at other possible sequence generators, we will discuss the concept of randomness.

A. Randomness

Our first problem is to decide what we mean by randomness. Before attempting to give a formal definition we will try to decide what we want our randomness properties to indicate. Clearly, as we have already observed, no periodic sequence is truly random. In cryptography it is unpredictability rather than randomness which is normally required. We want to know that if a cryptanalyst intercepts part of the sequence he will have no information on how to predict what comes next. Again this is, strictly speaking, impossible for any periodic sequence, since as soon as he knows a complete cycle the cryptanalyst knows the entire sequence. Nevertheless, it is not unreasonable to try to ensure that, if a segment of ciphertext which is considerably shorter than the period is intercepted, no further information is imparted. A sequence satisfying these general properties is normally called a pseudo-random sequence. We emphasize that this concept is as important for block ciphers as stream ciphers.

To attempt a definition of randomness we need to introduce more terminology and define the statistical concepts of runs and autocorrelation functions. If (s_t) is any binary sequence, then a *run* is a string of consecutive identical sequence elements which is neither preceded nor succeeded by the same symbol. Thus, for example, 0111001 begins with a run of 1 zero, contains a run of 3 ones, a run of 2 zeros and then ends with a run of 1 one. A run of zeros is called a *gap* while a run of ones is a *block*.

Suppose that (s_t) is a binary sequence of period p. For any fixed a, we compare the first p terms of (s_t) with its *translate* (s_{t+a}). (For every i the ith entry of (s_{t+a}) is s_{i+a}. For a fuller discussion see Section IV.B.) If A is the number of positions in which these two sequences agree, and $D(=p - A)$ is the number of positions in which they disagree, then the *autocorrelation function* $C(a)$ is defined by

$$C(a) = (A - D)/p.$$

Clearly $C(a+p) = C(a)$ for all a, and so it suffices to consider those a satisfying $0 \leqslant a < p$. When $a = 0$ we have *in-phase autocorrelation*. In this case, clearly, $A = p$ and $D = 0$, so that $C(0) = 1$. For $a \neq 0$ we have *out-of-phase autocorrelation*.

The following three randomness postulates for a binary sequence of period p were proposed by Golomb (1967).

(R1) If p is even then the cycle of length p shall contain an equal number of zeros and ones. If p is odd then the number of zeros shall be one more or one less than the number of ones.

(R2) In the cycle of length p, half the runs have length 1, a quarter have length 2, an eighth have length 3 and, in general, for each i for which there are at least 2^{i+1} runs, $1/2^i$ of the runs have length i. Moreover, for each of these lengths which are greater than one, there are equally many gaps and blocks.

(R3) The out-of-phase autocorrelation is a constant.

The 'classical' way of attempting to obtain a truly random sequence is to flip a 'perfect coin', and record whether it comes down heads or tails. In this context, Golomb gave the following interpretation of his postulates: "In flipping a 'perfect coin', R1 is the postulate that heads and tails occur about equally often, and R2 is the assertion that after a run of n heads (tails) there is a fifty–fifty chance that it will end with the next coin flip. Finally R3 is the notion of independent trials—knowing how the toss came out on a previous trial gives no information for the current trial''.

Any sequence which satisfies these three axioms is called a *PN-sequence*, where the *PN* stands for *pseudo-noise*. We do not want to enter into a discussion about the merits or demerits of Golomb's postulates. We will, for the purposes of this discussion, accept that a set of properties of this type is a reasonable requirement for a binary keystream sequence. We are not prepared to use a sequence merely because it satisfies R1, R2 and R3. Neither shall we reject a sequence because it fails to satisfy them. We shall require something similar to R1, R2, R3 and then apply a number of other restrictions before accepting the sequence. From our earlier discussions we know that, if they are to be used as enciphering sequences in a stream cipher system, our sequences must resemble random sequences. In practice the sequences used in cipher systems have large periods. A period of less than 10^{10} is rarely used, and periods as long as 10^{50} are not uncommon. Although knowledge of properties of the entire sequence is crucial, and gives us confidence in the system, it tells us little about small sections of the sequence; but if an interceptor does obtain some of our ciphertext it will almost certainly be a relatively small section. Thus it is important to apply statistical tests to sections of our sequence, and to check that they also appear to be random. This type of randomness is often referred to as '*local randomness*'. There are many popular tests for local randomness; we will list five. These types of tests are also used for testing true random number generators for use in key generation.

Our aim is now merely to describe five particular tests, and give an indication of their usefulness. In practice the five tests might be combined to form part of a computer package, and we would expect our sequence to pass all five. But we must decide what we mean by 'pass'. To do this we establish statistical values corresponding to truly random sequences, and then set a pass mark. As an illustration, suppose our pass mark is to be 95%. This means that a given sequence passes the test if its value lies in the range in which we would expect 95% of all truly random sequences. It is usual to denote the pass mark as $(100 - \alpha)\%$, where α is called the *significance level* of the test.

Throughout the following discussion we will assume that a sample of n bits of our sequence contains n_0 zeros and n_1 ones.

1. The Frequency Test

This is perhaps the most obvious of the tests, and is applied to ensure that there is roughly the same number of zeros and ones. For this we merely compute

$$\chi^2 = (n_0 - n_1)^2/n$$

Clearly, if $n_o = n_1$ then $\chi^2 = 0$, and the larger the value of χ^2 the greater the discrepancy between the observed and the expected frequencies. To decide if the value obtained is good enough for the sequence to pass, we merely have to compare our value with a table of the χ^2 distribution, for one degree of freedom. (Such tables are commonly available and give the values for χ^2 corresponding to the various significance levels.) For instance if we have decided on a 5% significance level we find from standard tables that the values of χ^2 is 3.84. So, quite simply, if our value is no greater than 3.84 the sequence passes. Otherwise we must reject it.

2. The Serial Test

The serial test is used to ensure that the transition probabilities are reasonable, i.e., that the probability of consecutive entries being equal or different is about the same. This will then give us some level of confidence that each bit is independent of its predecessor. Suppose 01 occurs n_{01} times, 10 occurs n_{10} times, 00 occurs n_{00} times and 11 occurs n_{11} times. Then $n_{01} + n_{00} = n_0$ or $n_0 - 1$, $n_{10} + n_{11} = n_1$ or $n_1 - 1$ and $n_{10} + n_{01} + n_{00} + n_{11} = n - 1$. (Note the -1 occurs because in a section of length m there are only $m - 1$ transitions.) Ideally we want $n_{01} = n_{10} = n_{00} = n_{11} \cong (n - 1)/4$. Good (1957) has shown that

$$\frac{4}{n-1} \sum_{i=0}^{1} \sum_{j=0}^{1} (n_{ij})^2 - \frac{2}{n} \sum_{i=0}^{1} (n_i)^2 + 1$$

is approximately distributed as χ^2 with two degrees of freedom.

3. The Poker Test

For any integer m the number of possibilities for a section of length m of a binary sequence is 2^m. In this test the sequence of length n bits is partitioned into blocks of size m, called 'hands', and we then count the frequency of each type of hand in our sequence. If these frequencies are $f_0, f_1, f_2, \ldots, f_{2^m-1}$, and if $\sum_{i=0}^{2^m-1} f_i = F$ then $F = [n/m]$, where, as before, $[n/m]$ denotes the largest integer which is not greater than n/m. Next, as before, we evaluate

$$\chi^2 = \frac{2^m}{F} \sum_{i=0}^{2^m-1} (f_i)^2 - F$$

and then compare our value with the value for χ^2 having $2^m - 1$ degrees of freedom.

We can apply this test many times for different values of m. There are, however, situations where certain values of m may be more relevant than others. Suppose, for example, that if our sequence 'passes' this test then we will want to use it to encipher data which has been converted to binary using a specific code. Then we are likely to be particularly interested in applying the poker test when m takes the value which is equal to the number of bits representing a character in that particular code. (This might typically be 5 or 7.)

There is a variation of the poker test which is occasionally useful. In this variation we evaluate the numbers $x_0, x_1, \ldots, x_m$ where, if m is the block length, x_i is the number of m-bit blocks having i ones and $m - i$ zeros. We may then apply the χ^2 test with m degrees of freedom, where

$$\chi^2 = \frac{2^m}{F} \sum_{i=0}^{m} \frac{(x_i)^2}{\binom{m}{i}} - F$$

4. The Autocorrelation Test

Suppose the sequence of n bits which we wish to test for randomness properties is $a_1, \ldots, a_n$. Then set

$$A(d) = \sum_{i=1}^{n-d} a_i a_{i+d} \qquad 0 \leqslant d \leqslant n - 1$$

Clearly

$$A(0) = \sum_{i=1}^{n} (a_i)^2 = \sum_{i=1}^{n} a_i = n_1$$

If the sequence has n_0 zeros and n_1 ones which are randomly distributed, the expected value of $A(d)\,(d \neq 0)$ is

$$\mu = n_1^2(n - d)/n^2$$

This enables us to use standard hypothesis testing techniques to decide whether or not we believe our sequence has a 'random' distribution.

5. The Runs Test

For the runs test we divide the sequence into blocks and gaps. We let r_{0i} be the number of gaps of length i, and r_{1i} be the number of blocks of length i. If r_0 and r_1 are the number of gaps and blocks, respectively, then

$$r_0 = \sum_{i=1}^{n} r_{0i} \qquad \text{and} \qquad r_1 = \sum_{i=1}^{n} r_{1i}$$

Using the notation of the serial test, it is easy to see $n_{01} = r_0$ or $r_0 - 1$, $n_{10} = r_1$ or $r_1 - 1$, $n_{00} = n_0 - r_0$ and $n_{11} = n_1 - r_1$.

We would not be applying this test if the sequence had not already passed the serial test, and so we know that the total numbers of gaps and blocks are within acceptable limits. We now expect about half the gaps (or blocks) to have length 1, one quarter to have length 2 and so on (see Golomb's postulate R2). We will not worry about the precise statistical test which should now be used, but refer the interested reader to Mood (1940).

Now that we have given some idea of what we mean by a random sequence we are happy to list two specific requirements for a sequence generator as:

(A1) the sequence produced must have a guaranteed minimum length for its period.

(A2) the sequence must appear to be random.

In case it is not clear we must emphasize that we are not saying that A1 and A2 together make a sequence generator acceptable. They do not. We are merely asserting that they are necessary properties and that any sequence generator which does not have them should be rejected. We will soon be adding extra requirements.

B. Shift Registers

Now that we have some idea of the type of sequence which we need, we can begin to investigate some of the possibilities for the enciphering algorithm and to look at their implementation. Most of the current cipher systems which are commercially available either employ DES or are based on stream ciphers. Although the keystream sequence is generated in various ways, nearly all the methods involve the use of a shift register. There are a number of reasons for this. One is that they are easily obtainable and comparatively inexpensive. Another reason is that, when they are used in certain ways, there are a number of mathematical and statistical techniques for analysing the sequences which they generate and, as a consequence, of assessing the security level of the system. Because of their importance we devote an entire section to shift registers and the sequences which they generate.

An *n-stage shift register* consists of n binary storage elements $S_0, S_1, \ldots, S_{n-1}$, called *stages*, connected in series. The contents of the stages change in time with a clock pulse according to the following rule: If $s_i(t)$ denotes the content of S_i after the tth time pulse, then $s_i(t+1) = s_{i+1}(t)$ for $i = 0, \ldots, n-2$ and $s_{n-1}(t+1) = f(s_0(t), s_1(t), \ldots, s_{n-1}(t))$. The function f is called the *feedback function* of the register. If, for any t, we write $s_t = s_0(t)$, then we say that the register *generates* the sequence (s_t). Clearly $s_i = s_0(i)$ for all i satisfying $0 \leqslant i \leqslant n-1$, and the sequence (s_t) is completely determined by $s_0, s_1, \ldots, s_{n-1}$ and the feedback function f.

If $f(s_0(t), s_1(t), \ldots, s_{n-1}(t)) = \sum_{i=0}^{n-1} c_i s_i(t) \pmod 2$ with each c_i equal to 0 or 1, then the shift register is said to have *linear feedback*. The constants $c_0, c_1, \ldots, c_{n-1}$ are called the *feedback coefficients*. This can be represented by the diagram in Fig. 3.8, where $c_i = 1$ stands for a closed connection and $c_i = 0$ for an open one.

The content of the shift register at any given time is called its *state* and we may regard the state as either an n-bit binary vector or as a binary number

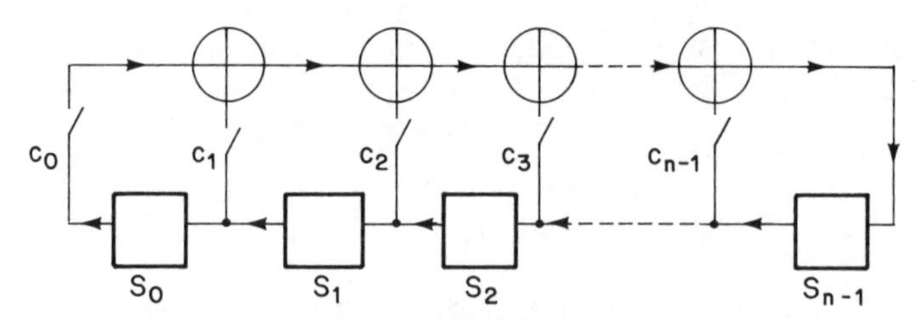

FIG. 3.8. Linear-feedback shift register.

in the range 0 to $2^n - 1$. Clearly every state has a unique successor. If the feedback function is linear with each $c_i = 0$, then, no matter which initial state we use, after the nth clock pulse each stage S_i will contain 0 and will remain 0 from then on. Thus, to keep the shift register alive, we must always ensure that at least one of the c_i is non-zero, i.e., that at least one switch is closed. If $c_o \neq 1$ then the content of S_0 contributes nothing to the feedback into S_{n-1} so, after the first clock pulse, the state of the register will be independent of $s_0(0)$. In this case we are not really using the full capacity of the register and so, to eliminate this defect, we will always assume that $c_0 = 1$.

If we let $s(t)$ denote the binary column vector $(s_0(t), s_1(t), \ldots, s_{n-1}(t))^T$, then the action of the linear shift register may be described by the matrix equation $s(t + 1) = Ms(t)$ where

$$M = \begin{bmatrix} 0 & 1 & 0 & \cdots & 0 \\ 0 & 0 & 1 & \cdots & 0 \\ \vdots & \vdots & \vdots & & \vdots \\ 0 & 0 & 0 & \cdots & 1 \\ c_0 & c_1 & c_2 & \cdots & c_{n-1} \end{bmatrix}$$

Since we are assuming $c_0 = 1$, the matrix M is nonsingular. This means, of course, that we can now always deduce $s(t)$ from $s(t + 1)$, and that, apart from the initial state, each state now has a unique predecessor as well as a unique successor. Since there are only 2^n possible states, a repetition must occur among the first $2^n + 1$ states. As soon as this repetition occurs the sequence of state vectors will continue to repeat itself. Although there are 2^n possible states, the nonsingularity of M guarantees that, provided the initial state is not all zeros, the all-zero vector will never occur as a state. Thus, no matter which values are assigned to the feedback coefficients, the succession of states of an n-stage shift register with linear feedback is periodic with $p \leqslant 2^n - 1$. The value of p will, of course, vary and will depend on both the initial state and the values of the feedback coefficient. Before looking at how p can vary we will show, by giving a small example, that, at least in some cases, a period of $2^n - 1$ can be achieved.

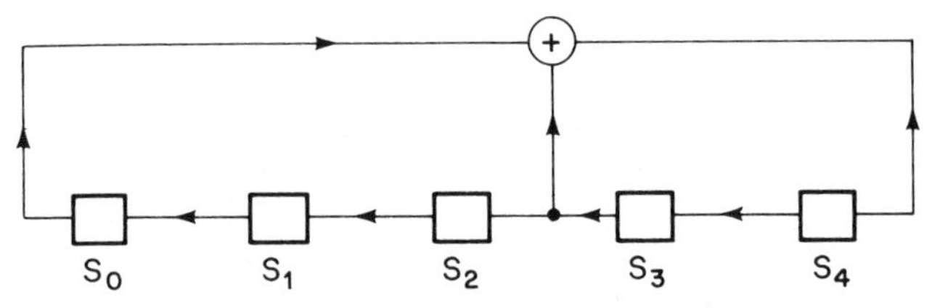

FIG. 3.9. Shift register for our example.

For our example we will consider a five-stage shift register with feedback function $s_0 + s_3$. The situation is illustrated in Fig. 3.9. (Note we have adopted the common convention of not drawing the open switches.) If we take 01010 as our initial set then, when $t = 1$, the state will be $1010f(0, 1, 0, 1, 0)$. However, $f(0, 1, 0, 1, 0) = 0 + 1 = 1$ and so when $t = 1$ the state is 10101. The sequence of states is given in Table 3.4. An inspection of the table shows

TABLE 3.4

The Sequence of States for Our Example

t		t		t		t	
0	01010	8	01100	16	11100	24	10010
1	10101	9	11000	17	11001	25	00100
2	01011	10	10001	18	10011	26	01000
3	10111	11	00011	19	00110	27	10000
4	01110	12	00111	20	01101	28	00001
5	11101	13	01111	21	11010	29	00010
6	11011	14	11111	22	10100	30	00101
7	10110	15	11110	23	01001	31	01010

that the first repetition of a state occurs when $t = 31$ and thus for our example the succession of states has period $31(= 2^5 - 1)$.

From our discussion before this example it is clear that the sequence obtained by outputting the content of S_0 at each clock is an infinite sequence with the property $s_{t+n} = \sum_{i=0}^{n-1} c_i s_{t+i}$. Such an equation is called a *linear recurrence relation* of order n and the binary sequence (s_t) is called a *linear recurring sequence.* At any given time t the state of the register represents a section of the sequence, i.e., the next n entries. Thus, since the succession of states has period $p \leqslant 2^n - 1$, the sequence (s_t) is periodic with period $p \leqslant 2^n - 1$. For an n-stage shift register, there are 2^n different initial states which, of course, give rise to 2^n different periodic binary sequences. If (s_t) is one such sequence and if its period is p then $s_0 s_1 \dots s_{p-1}$ will form a cycle. But if we start at any one of the p elements in this cycle we would get another cycle. Thus for instance $s_2 s_3 \ldots s_{p-1} s_0 s_1$ is also a cycle of (s_t). But if we start with $s_2 s_3 \ldots s_n s_{n+1}$ then the sequence we get will not be (s_t) but (u_t) where, for example, $u_t = s_{t+2}$. Thus (u_t) is essentially (s_t) with the first two terms deleted. When this occurs we say that (u_t) is a *translate* of (s_t) and the number by which each term is translated is called the *shift*. So, in our particular example, the shift is 2. Clearly by starting at any element of the cycle $s_0 s_1 \ldots s_{p-1}$ we can obtain p different translates of (s_t) (where the translate with shift 0 is (s_t) itself). It should also be clear that each of these p translates can be generated by the same register using exactly the same feedback coefficients.

The initial state 00...0 corresponds to a cycle of length 1 and the resulting sequence is called the *null sequence*, or *zero sequence*, denoted by (0). The remaining $2^n - 1$ sequences will be distributed among cycles of various lengths. If these $2^n - 1$ sequences all lie on one cycle of length $2^n - 1$, then we have a maximum length cycle and each of these sequences of maximum period is called an *m-sequence*. Clearly all possible state vectors except 00...0 will occur once among the first $2^n - 1$ states of the shift register during the generation of an m-sequence.

If, as is the case when discussing sequences generated by shift registers with linear feedback, we have a linear recurrence $s_{t+n} = \sum_{i=0}^{n-1} c_i s_{t+i}$, then we associate with it a polynomial $f(x)$, called its *characteristic polynomial*, defined by

$$f(x) = 1 + c_1 x + c_2 x^2 + \cdots + c_{n-1} x^{n-1} + x^n$$

(The characteristic polynomial has constant term 1 because we are always assuming that $c_0 = 1$.) Once we have chosen the feedback coefficients, or equivalently once we have set the switches, we may identify the shift register with its characteristic polynomial $f(x)$ and shall talk about the sequences *generated by* $f(x)$. Of course, as before, different initial states will give rise to different periodic polynomials which are generated by the same polynomial.

The aggregate of all infinite binary recurring sequences (s_t) generated by a given $f(x)$ is called the *solution space* of $f(x)$, and is denoted by $\Omega(f)$. Thus $\Omega(f)$ consists of 2^n sequences corresponding to all 2^n initial states. With the obvious definitions of addition and scalar multiplication, $\Omega(f)$ is an n-dimensional vector space over Z_2. (Note Z_2 is merely the set consisting of 0 and 1 with the two operations of addition and multiplication modulo 2. Thus, in Z_2, $1 + 1 = 0 + 0 = 0$, $0 + 1 = 1 + 0 = 1$, $1 \cdot 1 = 1$, $1 \cdot 0 = 0 \cdot 1 = 0 \cdot 0 = 0$. With these rules for addition and multiplication all the 'normal' rules of arithmetic 'work'.)

There are a number of very useful results relating properties of the characteristic polynomial with the period of the sequence. If the reader is not familiar with the terminology, then he should not concern himself too much with the precise results stated below. The important point to appreciate, given in Result 3, is that we have a means of ensuring that the sequence our shift register produces has period $2^n - 1$. There exist comprehensive lists of primitive polynomials that may be used for the feedback function. In order to state these results we have to introduce the exponent of a polynomial. A binary polynomial $f(x)$ has *exponent* e if $f(x)$ divides $x^e + 1$ but does not divide $x^r + 1$ for any $r < e$. We note that any binary polynomial $f(x)$ with constant term 1 has an exponent e and that, if $f(x)$ has degree n, $e \leqslant 2^n - 1$. A *primitive polynomial* of degree n is one with exponent $2^n - 1$. [Any reader interested in seeing proofs of these assertions should see, for example, Beker and Piper (1982d).] The exponent of a characteristic polynomial is particularly relevant when trying to determine the possible periods of sequences which can be generated by it. The following three results show why.

Result 1: Suppose $f(x)$ is a polynomial over Z_2 with exponent e. Then the period of any sequence (s_t) in $\Omega(f)$ divides e.

Result 2: Suppose $f(x)$ is an irreducible polynomial over Z_2 with exponent e. Then the period of any non-null sequence (s_t) in $\Omega(f)$ is e.

Result 3: Suppose $f(x)$ is a polynomial over Z_2. Then $\Omega(f)$ contains an m-sequence if and only if $f(x)$ is primitive.

As a consequence of these results we know that, by taking any primitive polynomial as our characteristic polynomial, we will obtain an m-sequence by choosing any nonzero initial state.

If we have any m-sequence (with period $2^n - 1$) then it can be shown that any cycle, i.e., any $2^n - 1$ consecutive entries, contains precisely 2^{n-1} ones and $2^{n-1} - 1$ zeros. Furthermore its out-of-phase autocorrelation is always $-1/(2^n - 1)$. These facts, plus other simple statistical tests, suggest that an m-sequence is reasonably 'pattern-free' and suitable for use as a foundation for generating the 'random sequence' referred to earlier. In fact it can be shown that an m-sequence is a PN-sequence. Thus sequences generated by primitive polynomials will, for suitably large values of n, satisfy the conditions A1 and A2 which we require for our keystream sequence.

Despite the fact that it may have period $2^n - 1$, any sequence generated by an n-stage shift register with linear feedback is completely determined by its characteristic polynomial $f(x)$ and any one of its state vectors. Thus the entire sequence is known once we know the n feedback coefficients and any n consecutive entries of the sequence. But, as we have already seen, the feedback coefficients are the coefficients of a linear relation of order n which is satisfied by the sequence (s_t). Unfortunately, at least from the cryptographer's point of view, a great deal is known about the solution of linear recurrence relations. As a consequence of this knowledge, an m-sequence of period $2^n - 1$ can be completely determined by any $2n$ consecutive entries.

If the known entries are $s_r, s_{r+1}, \ldots, s_{r+2n-1}$, then all that is involved in determining the feedback constants (and hence the entire sequence) is the inversion of the nonsingular $n \times n$ matrix

$$\begin{bmatrix} s_r & \cdots & s_{r+n-1} \\ s_{r+1} & \cdots & s_{r+n} \\ \vdots & & \vdots \\ s_{r+n-1} & \cdots & s_{r+2n-1} \end{bmatrix}$$

This is a routine operation unless n is very large; but there are many practical snags (not to mention the cost) in trying to use very large shift registers. So, for our particular problem, despite the fact that the sequences satisfy our conditions A1 and A2, the use of a shift register with linear feedback is not satisfactory. Our problems arose, basically, because once the cryptanalyst has obtained $2n$ consecutive bits of our sequence he only has to solve n linear equations in n unknowns to obtain the entire sequence. If we wish to use shift registers in the generation of our sequence then we must try to remove the 'linearity' from the system.

We must be quite sure what we mean by this. In order to see why, it is important to make one crucial, and at first sight confusing, observation. If (u_t) is any binary sequence of period p, then (u_t) can be generated on a p-stage register with initial state $u_0 u_1 \ldots u_{p-1}$ and characteristic polynomial $x^p + 1$. In other words any periodic binary sequence is a linear shift register sequence. Thus for any periodic binary sequence, no matter how it is generated, there is an integer v such that knowledge of $2v$ consecutive entries determines the entire sequence. Furthermore the work involved will consist, essentially, of inverting a $v \times v$ matrix. Clearly it is this value v which the cryptographer must ensure is large. With this in mind we define the *linear equivalence* of a periodic binary sequence to be the size of the smallest shift register which can generate it with a linear feedback function. (Note that this is the value v which we have just discussed!) What the cryptographer wants is to use one, or many, 'small' registers, probably in some non-linear way, to obtain a sequence with a large enough linear equivalence, v say, so that the possibility of a cryptanalyst being able to deduce $2v$ consecutive bits of the sequence and then to invert a $v \times v$ matrix does not bother him.

We now wish to add an extra condition to our earlier requirements for a sequence generator. We now require:

(A1) the sequence produced must have a guaranteed minimum length for its period.

(A2) the sequence must appear to be random.
(A3) the sequence must have a large linear equivalence.

It must be stressed, as always, that having a sequence with a large linear equivalence is necessary, but not sufficient, for a good sequence generator. There are many examples of weak sequences which have high linear equivalences. There are so many ways of attempting to generate sequences with the right properties that we cannot possibly discuss them all. Instead we refer the reader to Beker and Piper (1982d), which contains a discussion of many different techniques.

We will give an example of just one possibility. This is a method, called multiplexing, which combines two shift registers which each have linear feedback. We must emphasize that, in practice, any system used would be far more complex than anything we can exhibit here. However our example will serve as an illustration of the type of results which are available.

Let SR1 and SR2 be two shift registers with m and n stages, respectively ($m > 1$, $n > 1$), such that each has a linear feedback function. We denote the stages of SR1 by A_0, .., A_{m-1} and those of SR2 by $B_0, \ldots, B_{n-1}$. Furthermore we let $a_i(t)$ and $b_j(t)$ denote the contents of A_i and B_j at time t. To define a multiplexed sequence we assume that both shift registers have primitive characteristic polynomials, i.e., that SR1 generates a binary sequence (a_t) of period $2^m - 1$ and SR2 generates a binary sequence (b_t) of period $2^n - 1$. A *multiplexer* is a device used to produce a sequence, which we call a *multiplexed sequence*, related to the states of SR1 and SR2 in the following way. We first choose an integer k in the range $1 \leqslant k \leqslant m$. We can only choose $k = m$ if $2^m - 1 \leqslant n$, and if $k \neq m$ then k must also satisfy $2^k \leqslant n$. Having chosen k, we now choose k stages $a_{x_1}, a_{x_2}, \ldots, a_{x_k}$ of SR1 and, for convenience, we assume $0 \leqslant x_1 < x_2 < \cdots < x_k \leqslant m - 1$. At any time t, the binary k-tuple $(a_{x_1}(t), a_{x_2}(t), \ldots, a_{x_k}(t))$ is interpreted as the binary representation of a natural number which we denote by N_t. For each value of t the

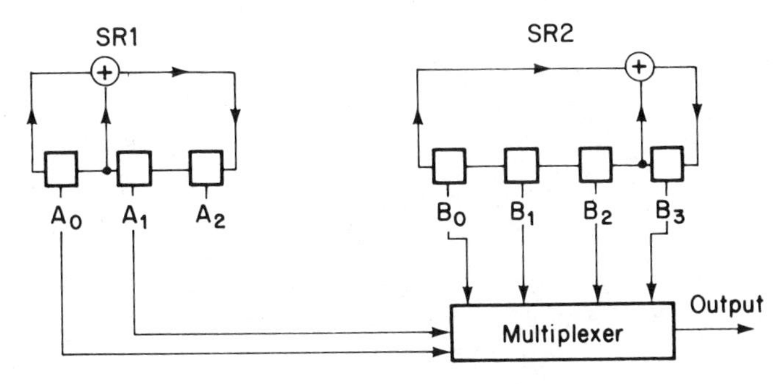

FIG. 3.10. Example of multiplexing.

number N_t then determines an address in SR2 which we denote by $\theta(N_t)$. Our multiplexed sequence (u_t) is now defined by $u_t = b_{\theta(N_t)}$. (Thus u_t is the entry in the stage $B_{\theta(N_t)}$ at time t.)

Since multiplexing is such an important concept we will work through a small example. We will take $m = 3$ and $n = 4$ and the switch settings as shown in Fig. 3.10. We will assume that the initial state of SR1 is 100 and that of SR2 is 1000. For this example we take $k = 2$, $x_1 = 0$, $x_2 = 1$ and let the addresses determined by the numbers 0, 1, 2, 3 by given by $\theta(0) = 2$, $\theta(1) = 3$, $\theta(2) = 0$, $\theta(3) = 1$. The first seven states of each register are

SR1	SR2
100	1000
001	0001
010	0011
101	0111
011	1111
111	1110
110	1101

From this we see that $N_0 = 2$, $N_1 = 0$, $N_2 = 1$, $N_3 = 2$, $N_4 = 1$, $N_5 = 3$ and $N_6 = 3$. Thus $\theta(N_0) = 0$, $\theta(N_1) = 2$, $\theta(N_2) = 3$, $\theta(N_3) = 0$, $\theta(N_4) = 3$, $\theta(N_5) = 1$, $\theta(N_6) = 1$ and, finally, $u_0 = b_0(0) = 1$, $u_1 = b_2(1) = 0$, $u_2 = b_3(2) = 1$, $u_3 = b_0(3) = 0$, $u_4 = b_3(4) = 1$, $u_5 = b_1(5) = 1$ and $u_6 = b_1(6) = 1$.

Straightforward computation gives the first 120 terms of (u_t) as 10101111 01000000101111111101000000111100011111011011111110110000000010101000 100000111101110101001110100101101101011110100000. In any multiplexed sequence each entry depends on the previous states of both registers. So as soon as the two states repeat simultaneously the multiplexed sequence must begin to repeat itself. Thus, in general, a multiplexed sequence will be periodic with period $p \leqslant (2^m - 1)(2^n - 1)$. (Note that in our example $p = 105 = (2^3 - 1)(2^4 - 1)$, so it is certainly possible to have $p = (2^m - 1)(2^n - 1)$.)

A great deal is known about the period of multiplexed sequences and, more importantly, about their linear equivalence. Most of the 'good' results, i.e., ones which say that the multiplexed sequence might be suitable for use as a keystream sequence, depend on some limitations being placed on the permitted values of m and n. However the cryptographer is free to choose the values of m and n, so restrictions of this type need not worry him. As an illustration of this type of result we mention that if $(m, n) = 1$, (i.e., if m and n have no common factor other than 1), the period of a multiplexed sequence is $(2^m - 1)(2^n - 1)$. This is a powerful and rather surprising result. It does not depend on either characteristic polynomial (recall that they are primitive, by definition), the value of k or the way in which the addresses are allocated. From this result we can certainly obtain sequences satisfying A1.

What about A2? If $(m, n) = 1$ then it can be shown that the mean value of the out-of-phase autocorrelation is $(p - e)/e(pe - 1) \cong 1/e^2 - 1/pe$ (where $p = 2^m - 1$ and $e = 2^n - 1$ are the periods of the two original sequences). Since $1/e^2 - 1/pe$ is small this is encouraging but, of course, the mean itself gives no specific information about specific values of the autocorrelation $C(a)$. It is desirable to have $C(a) \cong 0$ for all a with $1 \leqslant a \leqslant pe - 1$. Fortunately, if n is fairly large in comparison with m, it is straightforward to show $C(a) \cong -1/(2^n - 1)$ for most values of a.

What about A3? An example of the type of result about the linear equivalence is the following: If $(m, n) = 1$ the linear equivalence d of a multiplexed sequence is related to the k stages selected from SR1 in the following way:

(a) $d \leqslant n(\sum_{i=0}^{k}\binom{m}{i})$ if $1 \leqslant k \leqslant m - 1$, with equality if $k = 1, 2, m - 1$ or if the k stages are spaced at equal intervals

(b) $d = n(2^m - 1)$ if $k = m$.

It should be noted that if the k stages are unevenly distributed then equality need not occur in (a). Although this result does not tell us d for all possible situations it does mean that, by suitable choice of m, n and k, we can use two linear shift registers to obtain a sequence of controllable linear equivalence.

For a more detailed discussion of multiplexing and a proof of the above results see Jennings (1980). All that we have done here is indicated that it is possible to generate, in a controlled way, sequences satisfying our conditions A1, A2 and A3. Of course, in practice, these sequences need to be examined in much more detail before they can be employed in a cipher system.

V. Public-Key Systems

The security of the early 'pencil and paper' cipher systems was, as we have seen, minimal and relied on the secrecy of both the key and the enciphering algorithm. As systems improved it became feasible to allow the cryptographer to accept our worst-case conditions WC1, WC2 and WC3. In particular this meant that the designer assumed that his algorithm was known, and that all security lay within the key. Any system discussed so far, whether good or bad, has had the requirements that, prior to the transmission of each message, the sender and receiver must have agreed on the key, and that this key must remain secret. These requirements pose many problems. For instance, as we saw for the one-time pad, if the key is too large then transmitting it and keeping it secret is just as great a problem as disguising a message. As we have already stressed, the problems of key management must not be underestimated.

As recently as 1976, Diffie and Hellman (1976c) suggested a way of overcoming some of these problems. They observed that the key is essentially in two (not, of course, unrelated) 'halves'; the encipherment key and decipherment key. Although the decipherer needs to know the key used by the encipherer, there is no reason whatsoever why the encipherer needs to know the decipherment key. In the systems which they proposed, called *public-key cryptosystems*, they suggested that, as well as the enciphering algorithm, the encipherment key should also be made public. In the systems which we have discussed so far, knowledge of the encipherment key and procedure would enable a cryptanalyst to deduce the decipherment key. For a public-key system we require a situation where given the encipherment procedure and key, and, perhaps, even the decipherment procedure, it is impossible, or at least computationally infeasible, to deduce the decipherment key. Once we have such a system, anyone wishing to use it can be assigned an encipherment key which may be published in a public directory. Anyone wishing to send a message to one of the users will merely consult the directory to see which encipherment key he should use. In this way any user, who will of course have his own secret decipherment key, will be able to decipher any cryptogram without even needing to know the identity of the sender.

The idea of a public-key system is ingenious and such systems are just beginning to be adopted in practice. A number of suggestions for possible systems have been published and the most feasible appears to be the RSA system named after its creators Ron Rivest, Adi Shamir and Len Adleman (1978). Our description of it will be brief and, for more details, we refer the reader to Beker and Piper (1982d).

For the *RSA system* the public encipherment key is a pair of positive integers h and n. Before encipherment each message must be divided into blocks which can be encoded as an integer between 0 and $n - 1$. Each block m_i of the message is then enciphered by raising it to the hth power (modulo n). Thus, if c_i is the corresponding ciphertext block, c_i is the integer between 0 and $n - 1$ satisfying $c_i \equiv m_i^h (\text{mod } n)$. To decipher we raise c_i to another power d such that $m_i \equiv c_i^d (\text{mod } n)$. Thus in order to obtain an RSA system we must be able to generate triples of integers h, d and n such that h and d have the required properties modulo n; namely if $y \equiv x^h (\text{mod } n)$ then $x \equiv y^d (\text{mod } n)$. The security relies on the fact that knowledge of h and n will not enable a cryptanalyst to determine d. One obvious requirement then is that the integers must be large.

In the proposed system n is the product of two large primes p and q. We will not discuss the problem of finding large primes but stress that, although n is made public, p and q must be kept secret. For reasons which we will not explain, h is chosen to satisfy $(h, (p - 1)(q - 1)) = 1$ and d is then computed so that $dh \equiv 1(\text{mod}(p - 1)(q - 1))$. Any values for n, h and d chosen in this way will work, and it should be clear that there are many choices for n and, for any given n, many choices for h. However, for any given h and n, d is unique. It is also true, although again we offer no justification, that the implementation of the encipherment and decipherment procedures is reasonably straightforward, but does require a great deal of processing power.

From the last paragraph it is clear that knowledge of p, q and h would enable a cryptanalyst to determine d, and so to break the system. However, it is extremely unlikely that a cryptanalyst will be able to determine p and q from n. It is not, unfortunately, certain that it is necessary for him to factor n before he can break the system. There are a number of papers which discuss the security of the RSA system and further research is continuing to determine the level of security offered by both this and other possible public-key systems. It certainly appears promising and highly likely that public-key systems will be adopted and that their use will increase.

Finally it is worth stressing that public-key algorithms, the RSA system for instance, are block ciphers and as such can also be used as pseudo-random sequence generators. Although this has not occurred very much to date it is likely to increase in the future as the processing required becomes less of a problem.

As we now go on to discuss particular scrambling algorithms the reader will become aware of the importance of sequence generators and data encipherment techniques in this context. Our review of such systems has, of necessity, been brief. It has however been our intention to give some insight into the construction of such algorithms so that when, in future chapters, we make comments like "suppose we have a sequence generator satisfying conditions A1, A2 and A3" or "suppose we have a block cipher with an s-bit data input and y-bit key input", the reader should appreciate the difficulties which might be encountered in constructing such a device!

4. Frequency Domain Scrambling

I. Introduction

In the earlier chapters we discussed some of the general problems involved with speech transmission and with attempting to secure a telecommunications system. For the remainder of the book we will look at various specific scrambling schemes and ways in which they might be implemented. We shall simply consider a succession of possibilities, analyse their effectiveness and discuss their relative merits. In doing this we will, of course, use many of the ideas which we have introduced earlier. As was probably apparent in those earlier chapters, it is usually impossible to consider any one aspect of speech security without involving many others. Thus, whenever we discuss a particular scrambling technique, we will have to consider how it might be affected by the characteristics of the transmission channel. Similarly, when we consider security we will have to consider the residual intelligibility as well as any sophisticated attack which a cryptanalyst might mount. There is no obvious way to divide the subject into disjoint topics and, no matter how one attempts to 'break it up', there is bound to be some overlap between the different chapters.

Our approach is, first of all, to divide all scramblers into one of the two general, broad classifications of analogue or digital. The next three chapters are devoted to analogue scramblers and we sub-divide our discussion of the topic into three parts. In this chapter we shall, essentially, restrict ourselves to scrambling in the frequency domain. Chapter 5 will address time domain scrambling and then, in Chapter 6, we shall consider scrambling schemes which do not fit neatly into either of these two categories. We shall also look at the so called two-dimensional scramblers, i.e., those that operate in both the frequency and time domain. Chapter 6 also contains some general implementation techniques including, for instance, synchronization. The final chapter is devoted to the specific problems of handling digitized speech.

In this chapter we shall, as we indicated in Chapter 3, use many of the concepts related to data encipherment.

As we have already observed, our classification is slightly artificial since there will be a certain amount of overlap between the chapters. For instance, there exist methods of scrambling in the frequency domain which produce an identical effect to certain time domain scrambling techniques. Clearly such techniques could be classified under either frequency or time domain scrambling. Nevertheless the above subdivision is reasonably convenient and does at least make sense historically. Most of the earliest devices utilised frequency domain scrambling and the majority of the time domain techniques were developed later.

When David Kahn wrote his excellent book 'The Codebreakers' (Kahn, 1967), he discussed one of the earliest scrambling schemes and then said

> Later methods operate more directly on the speech itself, often in ways that resemble transposition, substitution and null ciphers. In most of the substitution systems, ciphering selects one component out of the many that make up the complex phenomenon of speech and alter it. It usually chooses frequency, though some scramblers distort volume.

This was written in 1967. Today, just 17 years later, many other techniques exist. Nevertheless a large proportion of them still use the frequency domain. The importance of frequency domain scrambling cannot be overemphasised.

II. Frequency Inverters

Frequency inverters have existed for many years but offer a very low level of security. Nevertheless we shall discuss them in considerable detail. There are two main reasons for this. The first is that a frequency inverter is easily understood and, consequently, we can use it to introduce a number of analysis techniques which we will then apply to more sophisticated systems. The second is that many modern scramblers employ frequency inversion in addition to their other techniques.

The action of a *frequency inverter* is described quite accurately by its name. It literally moves the frequency components of the signal so that the lower frequencies are moved to the upper part of the band while the higher frequencies are moved to the lower band. If we assume that our signal is in the range 300–3000 Hz, then Fig. 4.1 shows the signal before and after scrambling. For anyone who is not too happy with diagrams, a more informative representation of frequency inversion is given by the two spectrograms of Fig. 4.2. Spectrograms are very useful to the scrambler designer because, as can be seen from our example, they show him what is happening to his signal. This then enables him to identify any imperfections being caused by his system. Unfortunately, from the designer's point of view, it can also give the interceptor considerable insight into how the signal has been transformed.

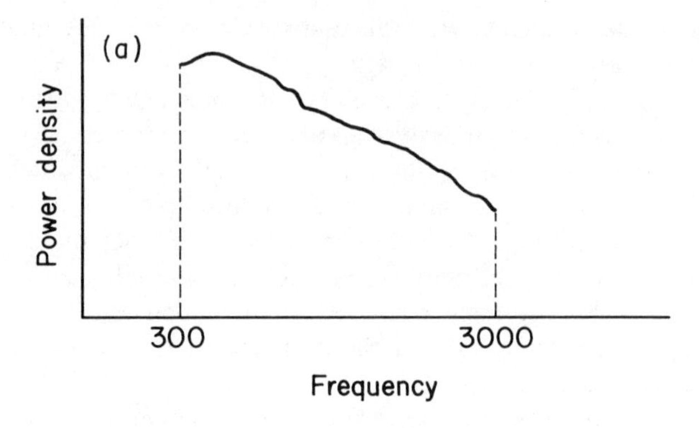

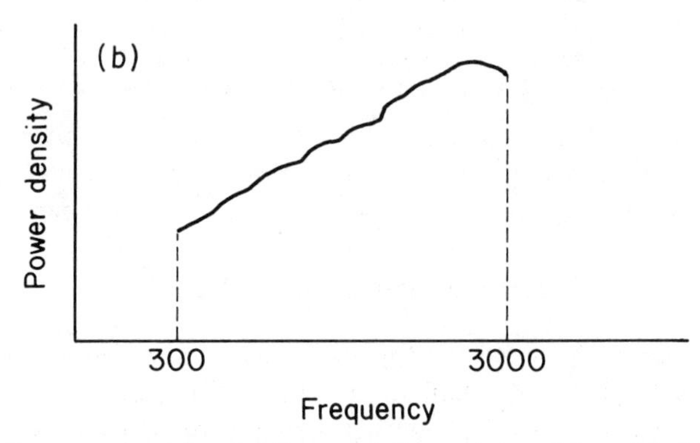

FIG. 4.1. Frequency inversion. (a) Power density spectrum of the original signal and (b) power density spectrum of the inverted speech.

If we refer back to Chapter 2 then we will see that Fig. 2.31 is almost identical to Fig. 4.1(b). Thus, if we use a balanced modulator, or some similar device, and then remove the upper sideband, we achieve frequency inversion. When we do this then, in order to ensure that the lower sideband, i.e., the inverted speech, occupies the correct waveband, we must choose our carrier frequency carefully. As an illustration if we suppose that our signal is originally in the 300–3000-Hz band then reference to Fig. 2.30 shows that we require $f_c = 3300$ Hz. As we saw in Chapter 2, balanced modulators are used for frequency division multiplexing of telephone channels. Consequently there are some readily available devices for frequency inversion.

As an alternative to these devices we will look, in considerable detail, at a method which is particularly suitable for processing a digitized signal. In this discussion we will take the opportunity to acquaint the reader with the extremely important concept of the *discrete Fourier transform* (DFT).

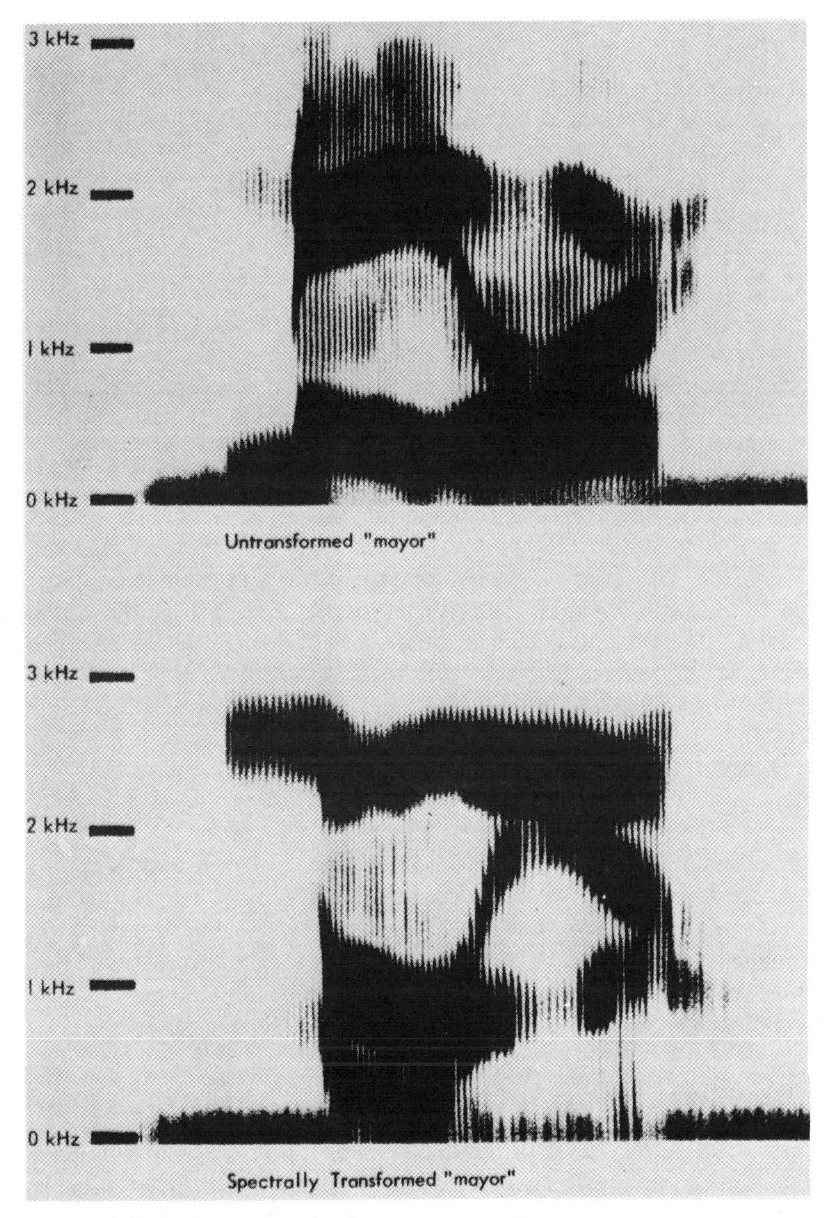

FIG. 4.2. Spectrographic recordings of the word 'mayor' before and after frequency inversion. [From Blesser (1972).]

Suppose that we have a band-limited system which has already been digitized ready for processing. Suppose, also, that the input speech is being sampled using pulse code modulation (PCM) and that, for each integer n with $n \geqslant 0, x(n)$ denotes the nth sample. If we now change the sign on each alternate sample value, i.e., if we replace $x(n)$ by $-x(n)$ for all odd values of n, then this has the effect of inverting the frequency components of the signal. (We will prove this assertion later in this section. For the moment we will accept it and discuss some of its consequences.) If, for example, we were using the sign-magnitude PCM system described in Section V of Chapter 2, the frequency inversion would be achieved by simply changing the most significant bit of each alternate sample. So, if we take the example of Fig. 2.23, an original signal of 0000 1001 1001 1011 1100 1110 1101 1010 0010 is frequency inverted by changing it to 0000 0001 1001 0011 1100 0110 1101 0010 0010.

Before giving our formal proof, we will give some credence to our assertion by discussing an extreme situation. Suppose that we have a *constant signal*, i.e. one with a frequency of 0 Hz, and that its amplitude is A. If we sample at a rate of n per second then the first n samples of the new signal will be $A, -A, A, -A, \ldots, A, -A$. (For convenience we have assumed that n is even). This signal has a frequency of $\frac{1}{2}n$ which, according to the sampling theorem, is the highest we could obtain for this sampling rate.

As in the analogue case, the effect of inverting samples can be seen by studying spectrograms before and after the operation. As an illustration, in Fig. 4.3 we show spectrograms of the original speech and the resultant speech after *alternate sample inversion* of a PCM signal. These show quite clearly that the frequency spectrum has been inverted and give more realistic support to our claim.

The simplicity of alternate sample inversion is very attractive, provided that the signal has to be digitized for other reasons. However, it is important to re-emphasise that it is the alternate samples which we are inverting and not alternate bits. It is far less easy to see the effect of sign changes on coding techniques such as ADM or ADPCM. This situation has been studied by Kak and Jayant (1977). It is more complicated than the simple frequency inversion which we have just introduced, and we will not discuss it in detail.

A. The Discrete Fourier Transform

When we introduced the Fourier transform and the concept of sampling, we stated that it was possible to perform a Fourier transform on a block of samples. This is a very important idea and is achieved by performing a discrete Fourier transform (DFT). In this section we will discuss the DFT in general and then use it to establish our claim that inverting the sign of alternate samples results in frequency inversion.

Suppose that we have a block of n samples for a given waveform. If

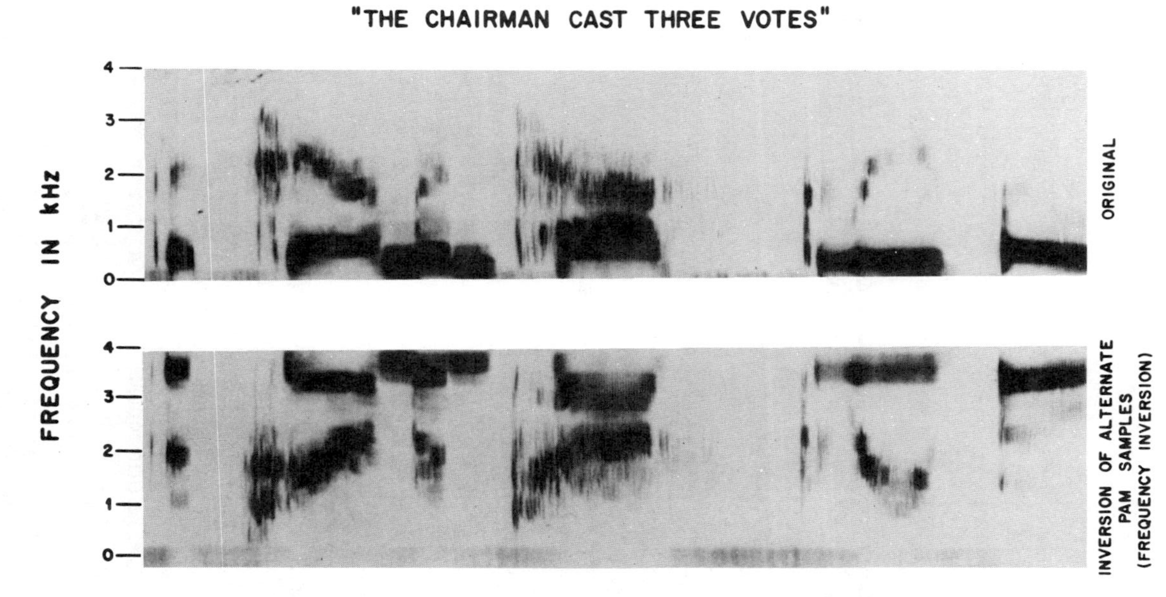

FIG. 4.3. Spectrogram to illustrate alternate sample inversion of a PCM. [From Kak and Jayant (1977). Reprinted from The Bell System Technical Journal. Copyright 1977, AT&T.]

these samples are $x(0), x(1), \ldots, x(n-1)$ and if we denote the *spectral coefficients*, (i.e., *the DFT samples*), by $X(0), X(1), \ldots, X(n-1)$, then the transform is given by:

$$\begin{bmatrix} X(0) \\ X(1) \\ X(2) \\ \vdots \\ X(n-1) \end{bmatrix} = \begin{bmatrix} 1 & 1 & 1 & \cdots & 1 \\ 1 & \omega & \omega^2 & \cdots & \omega^{n-1} \\ 1 & \omega^2 & \omega^4 & \cdots & \omega^{2(n-1)} \\ \vdots & \vdots & \vdots & \ddots & \vdots \\ 1 & \omega^{n-1} & \omega^{2(n-1)} & \cdots & \omega^{(n-1)^2} \end{bmatrix} \begin{bmatrix} x(0) \\ x(1) \\ x(2) \\ \vdots \\ x(n-1) \end{bmatrix} \quad (1)$$

where $\omega = \exp(-j(2T/n))$. Two important, but easily established, properties of ω are $\omega^n = 1$ and $\sum_{i=0}^{n-1} \omega^i = 0$. From the matrix equation [Eq. (1)] we see that, for any r,

$$X(r) = \sum_{s=0}^{n-1} \omega^{rs} x(s)$$

If we write X for the column vector with $X(r)$ in the rth position, x for the corresponding column vector with $x(r)$ in its rth position and F for the transform matrix of Eq. (1) then, clearly, $X = Fx$. Straightforward verification shows that F is invertible and that its inverse is given by

$$F^{-1} = \frac{1}{n} \begin{bmatrix} 1 & 1 & 1 & \cdots & 1 \\ 1 & \omega^{-1} & \omega^{-2} & \cdots & \omega^{-(n-1)} \\ 1 & \omega^{-2} & \omega^{-4} & \cdots & \omega^{-2(n-1)} \\ \vdots & \vdots & \vdots & \ddots & \vdots \\ 1 & \omega^{-(n-1)} & \omega^{-2(n-1)} & \cdots & \omega^{-(n-1)^2} \end{bmatrix}$$

From the equation $X = Fx$ we see that $x = F^{-1}Fx = F^{-1}X$ and thus we can also obtain the sample values from the spectral coefficients.

It is important to realise that in order to utilise our DFT we have to assume that the waveform is repeating every n samples. Thus, if our sampling rate is n_s samples/sec, then, since we take one sample every $1/n_s$ sec, we are assuming that the waveform repeats every n/n_s sec; but this implies that the fundamental frequency must be at least n_s/n Hz and the line spectrum we obtain will be harmonics of n_s/n. Since our sampling rate is n_s samples/sec we know, from the sampling theorem, that we can only obtain the frequency spectrum for a bandwidth of $\frac{1}{2}n_s$ Hz. If we assume this band is from 0 to $\frac{1}{2}n_s$ Hz then the highest frequency component of the DFT corresponds to that harmonic of n_s/n which occurs at $\frac{1}{2}n_s$ Hz. Thus, since $n_s/2$ divided by n_s/n is $\frac{1}{2}n$, the highest frequency component is the $(\frac{1}{2}n)$th harmonic.

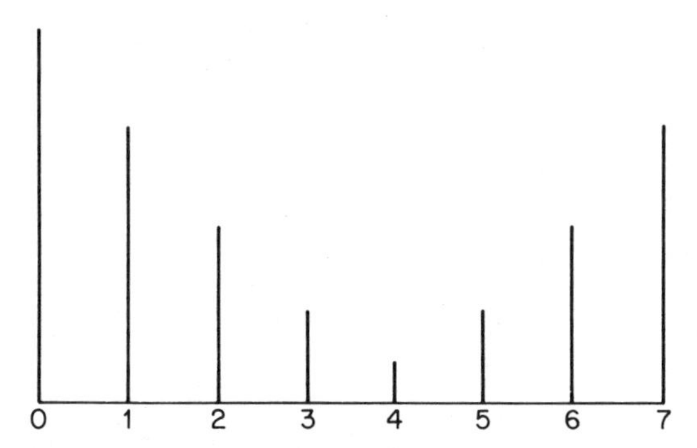

FIG. 4.4. Typical DFT line spectrum for $n = 8$.

From this discussion we see that $X(0)$ corresponds to the spectral component at a frequency of 0 Hz and $X(1)$ corresponds to the spectral component at a frequency of (n_s/n) Hz. If, for convenience, we assume that n is even, then we can state the frequencies associated with $X(2)$, $X(3)$, etc. until we get to $X(\frac{1}{2}n)$ which is the spectral coefficient corresponding to the maximum frequency of $\frac{1}{2}n_s$ Hz. The remaining spectral coefficients from $X(\frac{1}{2}n + 1)$ up to $X(n - 1)$ essentially mirror image the spectrum obtained so far. To be precise $X(\frac{1}{2}n + i) = X^*(\frac{1}{2}n - i)$ for $i = 1, 2, \ldots, \frac{1}{2}n - 1$. However in this particular context it is sufficient to ignore the complex conjugation. This means we can, for example, treat $X(\frac{1}{2}n + i)$ as equal to $X(\frac{1}{2}n - i)$. As an illustration, we include a typical spectrum with $n = 8$ (see Fig. 4.4).

Before we discuss frequency inversion in general we will see what it means for our small sample in Fig. 4.4. From the diagram it is clear that this can be achieved by cyclically permuting each frequency coefficient four positions to the 'right'. In other words if the new spectrum is X' with $X'(r)$ in the rth position, then X' is given by $X'(4) = X(0)$, $X'(5) = X(1)$, $X'(6) = X(2)$, $X'(7) = X(3)$, $X'(0) = X(4)$, $X'(1) = X(5)$, $X'(2) = X(6)$ and $X'(3) = X(7)$. The result is illustrated in Fig. 4.5.

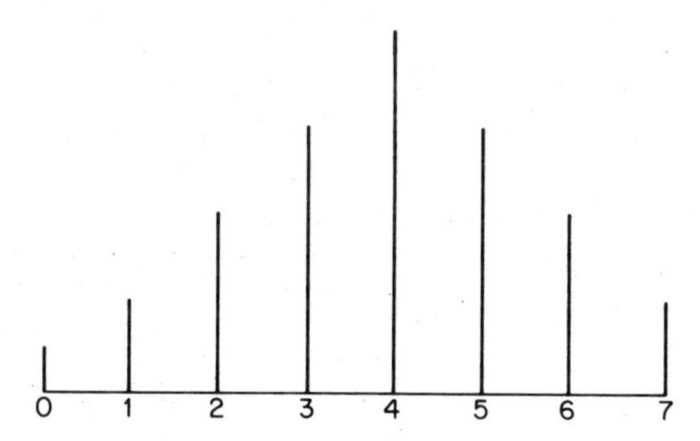

FIG. 4.5. Frequency inverted DFT spectrum of Fig. 4.4.

In general frequency inversion can be achieved by a cyclic permutation which shifts all the coefficients $\frac{1}{2}n$ to the right. Thus if X' represents the new spectrum and has $X'(r)$ in its rth position then $X'(\frac{1}{2}n) = X(0)$, $X'(\frac{1}{2}n + 1) = X(1), \ldots, X'(0) = X(\frac{1}{2}n), \ldots, X'(\frac{1}{2}n - 1) = X(n - 1)$.

For our small example we can represent this frequency inversion by the matrix equation

$$\begin{bmatrix} X'(0) \\ X'(1) \\ X'(2) \\ X'(3) \\ X'(4) \\ X'(5) \\ X'(6) \\ X'(7) \end{bmatrix} = \begin{bmatrix} 0 & 0 & 0 & 0 & 1 & 0 & 0 & 0 \\ 0 & 0 & 0 & 0 & 0 & 1 & 0 & 0 \\ 0 & 0 & 0 & 0 & 0 & 0 & 1 & 0 \\ 0 & 0 & 0 & 0 & 0 & 0 & 0 & 1 \\ 1 & 0 & 0 & 0 & 0 & 0 & 0 & 0 \\ 0 & 1 & 0 & 0 & 0 & 0 & 0 & 0 \\ 0 & 0 & 1 & 0 & 0 & 0 & 0 & 0 \\ 0 & 0 & 0 & 1 & 0 & 0 & 0 & 0 \end{bmatrix} \begin{bmatrix} X(0) \\ X(1) \\ X(2) \\ X(3) \\ X(4) \\ X(5) \\ X(6) \\ X(7) \end{bmatrix}$$

Clearly the matrix in this equation is the permutation matrix which represents the cyclic permutation moving all values four positions to the right. In general frequency inversion will correspond to a permutation $X' = PX$ where P is given by

$$P = \left[\begin{array}{ccccc|ccccc} \multicolumn{5}{c|}{\overbrace{\qquad\qquad}^{\frac{1}{2}n}} & \multicolumn{5}{c}{\overbrace{\qquad\qquad}^{\frac{1}{2}n}} \\ 0 & 0 & 0 & \cdots & 0 & 1 & 0 & 0 & \cdots & 0 \\ 0 & 0 & 0 & \cdots & 0 & 0 & 1 & 0 & \cdots & 0 \\ 0 & 0 & 0 & \cdots & 0 & 0 & 0 & 1 & \cdots & 0 \\ \vdots & \vdots & \vdots & \ddots & \vdots & \vdots & \vdots & \vdots & \ddots & \vdots \\ 0 & 0 & 0 & \cdots & 0 & 0 & 0 & 0 & \cdots & 1 \\ \hline 1 & 0 & 0 & \cdots & 0 & 0 & 0 & 0 & \cdots & 0 \\ 0 & 1 & 0 & \cdots & 0 & 0 & 0 & 0 & \cdots & 0 \\ 0 & 0 & 1 & \cdots & 0 & 0 & 0 & 0 & \cdots & 0 \\ \vdots & \vdots & \vdots & \ddots & \vdots & \vdots & \vdots & \vdots & \ddots & \vdots \\ 0 & 0 & 0 & \cdots & 1 & 0 & 0 & 0 & \cdots & 0 \end{array}\right] \begin{array}{l} \\ \left.\begin{array}{c} \\ \\ \\ \\ \\ \end{array}\right\} \frac{1}{2}n \\ \left.\begin{array}{c} \\ \\ \\ \\ \\ \end{array}\right\} \frac{1}{2}n \end{array}$$

But if x is our original signal and y is the final signal then $X = Fx$ and $y = F^{-1}X'$. Thus $y = F^{-1}X' = F^{-1}PX = F^{-1}PFx$. So if we evaluate $F^{-1}PF$ we will know precisely how to obtain our frequency inverted signal directly from the sample values. But doing this gives

$$F^{-1}PF = \begin{bmatrix} 1 & 0 & 0 & 0 & 0 & \cdots & 0 \\ 0 & -1 & 0 & 0 & 0 & \cdots & 0 \\ 0 & 0 & 1 & 0 & 0 & \cdots & 0 \\ 0 & 0 & 0 & -1 & 0 & \cdots & 0 \\ 0 & 0 & 0 & 0 & 1 & \cdots & 0 \\ \vdots & \vdots & \vdots & \vdots & \vdots & \ddots & \vdots \end{bmatrix}$$

In other words

$$\begin{bmatrix} y_0 \\ y_1 \\ y_2 \\ y_3 \\ y_4 \\ \vdots \end{bmatrix} = \begin{bmatrix} x_0 \\ -x_1 \\ x_2 \\ -x_3 \\ x_4 \\ \vdots \end{bmatrix}$$

Thus, we have established our claim that inverting the sign of each alternate sample inverts the frequency spectrum.

The discrete Fourier transform is an exceptionally useful tool in many aspects of speech processing and it is important to understand its function and to be able to manipulate it.

B. The Security Level

We have now seen an analogue technique and a digital technique for accomplishing frequency inversion. But when we first introduced the idea of frequency inversion we said that it provided a very low level of security. We will now explain why this is so. Our explanation is, to a large extent, based on the paper by Barry Blesser (Blesser, 1972). This paper describes a series of experiments designed to estimate whether or not a person could learn to understand the frequency inverted speech. We begin by quoting a paragraph from Blesser.

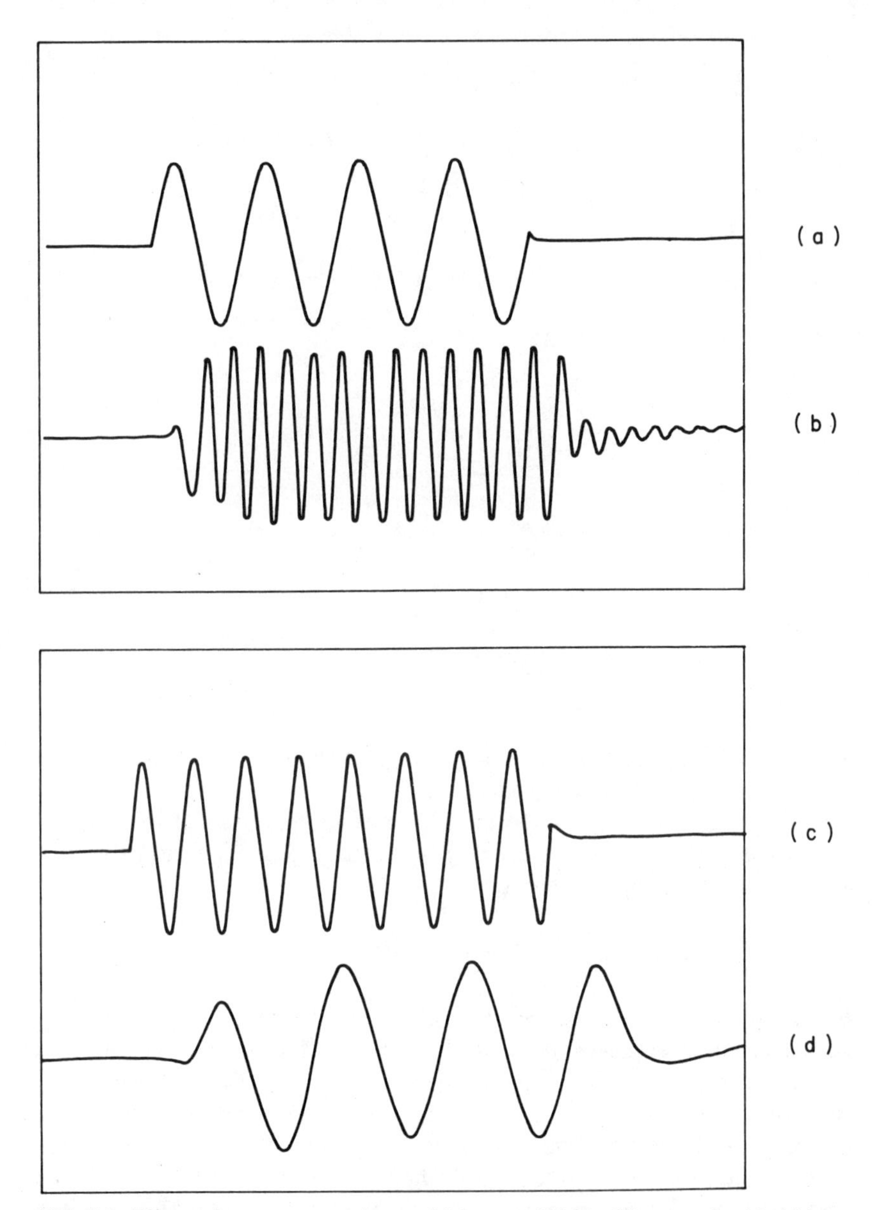

FIG. 4.6. Effects of system on tone bursts. (a) Input at 700 Hz, (b) output for (a), (c) input at 2200 Hz, (d) output for (c). [From Blesser (1972).]

This kind of transformation, in contrast to additive noise, amplitude distortion and filtering, does not obscure or remove the information contained in the frequency spectrum. Rather, it rearranges the information to create a new signal that bears a one-to-one correspondence to the old signal. In one sense, spectrally transformed English speech is a new language that happens to have the same vocabulary, semantics, and syntactic structure as English, but the actual sounds in the 'language' are alien or foreign. One might imagine that spectrally transformed speech could be produced by a 'being' whose mouth is so distorted that his articulators give rise to a speech signal with a spectrum that would be the rotation of normal English.

Blesser considered the frequency inversion of a band-limited speech signal ranging from 200–3000 Hz. Thus, from Fig. 2.30, every frequency f is transformed into one at $3200 - f$. The effect of this is shown in Fig. 4.6. Before we describe Blesser's experiments and discuss their results, we will use our knowledge of speech and try to predict certain properties which we might expect our transformed waveform to exhibit.

The pitch of a speech signal is believed to be related to the fundamental frequency of the waveform in the sense that the apparent pitch of a harmonic series corresponds to the repetition time of the envelope. Figure 4.7 shows the time waveform of the two vowels 'a' and 'u' before and after transformation. In each case the original vowel sounds have a distinctive pitch which is retained in the frequency inverted speech. This is usually the case and the perceived pitch contour of a transformed sound will be the same as that for the original speech signal. So, for instance, if the pitch rises at the end of an utterance, which is a characteristic of most questions, then the pitch will also increase at the end of the corresponding inverted passage. Thus questions in the original speech remain questions after inversions. Another consequence of the same phenomenon is that any higher pitch for emphasised words or syllables will be unaffected and, as a consequence, any accent which the speaker may have will be apparent in the inverted speech.

If we look back at Fig. 4.1 we can see that the overall power of an inverted signal is the same as that for the original one. This does not, however, imply that the loudness is unaffected. In fact there is a very dramatic effect on the loudness. The reason for this is that the human ear responds differently at various frequencies. The ear is normally far more sensitive to the frequencies at the top of the speech waveband than it is to the low frequency components. Thus, after inversion, any low frequency noise becomes a high frequency whine at about 3 kHz. Since this low frequency noise is very common, it has a significant effect on the inverted signal. Another consequence is that low-intensity, low-frequency formants are likely to be moved to a part of the band for which the ear is more sensitive and, hence, have their importance increased.

Measurement of noise in terms of its effect on a user, as opposed to measuring its absolute power, is a very important topic and is the motivation behind psophometry. *Psophometry* attempts to measure the extent to which

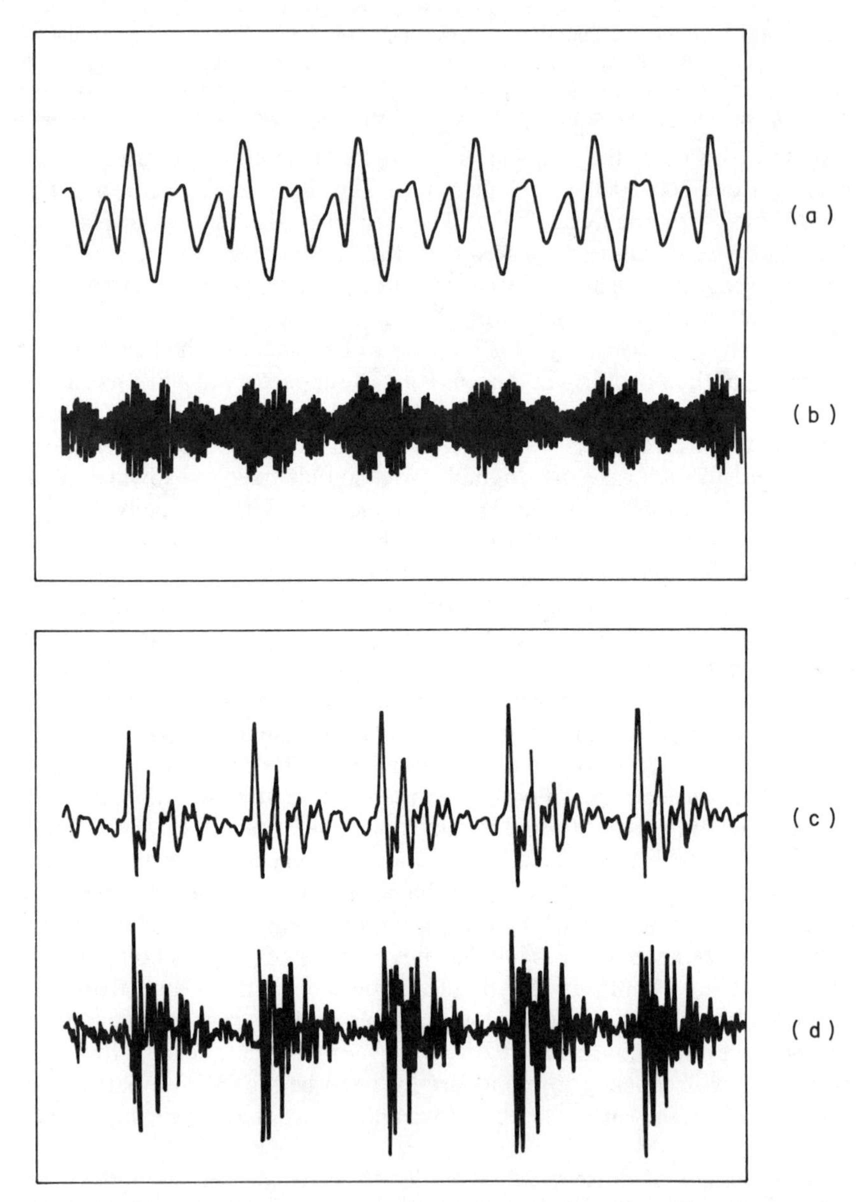

FIG. 4.7. Time waveforms for vowels; (a) u before transformation, (b) u after transformation, (c) a before transformation, (d) a after transformation. [From Blesser (1972).]

noise interferes with communications. Different frequencies of noise are likely to cause various levels of interference with, for a narrow band voice channel, the most disturbing ones being around 1 kHz. The idea behind psophometry is to weight the noise power at each frequency according to a weighting function which is shown in Fig. 4.8. From this graph it can be deduced that white noise over the entire waveband is, when weighted appropriately, about 2.4 dB lower than the same basic power at 1 kHz. Although this type of information is helpful to the scrambler designer we must not forget that it may also assist an enemy who might wish to disrupt communications at the least power cost.

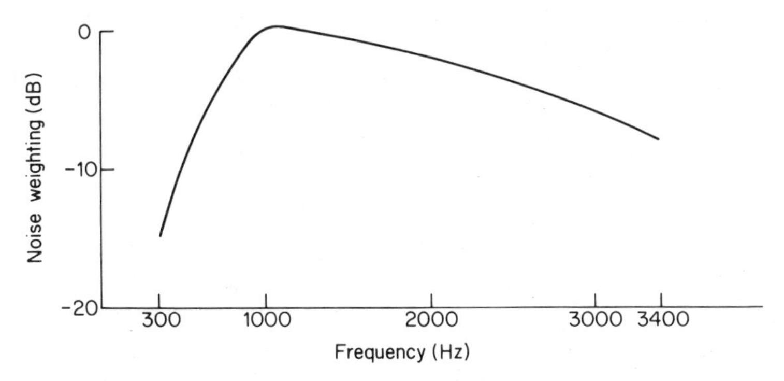

FIG. 4.8. Psophometric weighting function.

So far we have discussed the relation between pitch and loudness for a speech signal before and after frequency inversion. Another common property of the new signal is that the temporal order of the sound pattern is completely unchanged by the transformation. Thus, to give one important example, a pause in the original speech remains a pause after the inversion. Similarly the sequential order of the phonemes remains as it was originally. Another, equally important, fact is that many of the phoneme 'cues' are unchanged. These cues, which may be either spectral or non spectral, are the various characteristics which enable us to identify a particular phoneme or type of phoneme without necessarily hearing it. For instance, the sudden release of energy following the stop interval, which is characteristic of plosives, remains unchanged by frequency inversion. Similarly, since noise is transformed into noise, the noise component of a fricative is also unaltered.

No matter how many predictions and/or deductions we make regarding the likely sound of the inverted speech signals, there is no substitute for actually listening to it; hence the need for experiments like those conducted by Blesser. For his experiment Blesser used six pairs of male subjects. The intention was that each pair should undergo 20 sessions of 45 minutes each but, in practice, only two of the pairs completed all the sessions. In each session, apart from the first and last, each pair spent 30 minutes trying to converse using frequency inverted speech and the remaining 15 minutes were taken up by a series of pretaped tests. The conversation time provided the necessary exposure to the frequency inverted speech for the subjects to learn, while the pretaped tests were designed to attempt to provide an objective measure of their learning and progress. The testing series was also used to try to identify which variables were responsible for the subject's ability to learn to communicate with their partner. The achievements were decided by using the first session to set a base-line level and the last session then measured their final level.

For the details of the tests used and of the results we refer the reader to Blesser's original paper (Blesser, 1972). The results can be fairly summarised by saying that initially the subjects were completely unable to communicate but that, after several hours of practice, they were able to converse reasonably well. In other words the subjects learnt how to understand frequency-inverted speech. It is perhaps worth pointing out that, according to Blesser, there was no obvious improvement in the subjects' learning after the first few sessions. In fact, each subject seemed to have reached the limit of his learning by the fourth or fifth lesson. Nevertheless the conclusion to be drawn from Blesser's work is clear. His subjects were able to understand frequency-inverted speech and, as a consequence, the security offered by systems which rely on speech inverters is low. In Chapter 6 we shall look at the results of further tests on the intelligibility of scrambled frequency-inverted speech.

Blesser's results refer to speech inversion, which is an example of a fixed spectral transformation. In fact if the spectral transformation is fixed then, no matter which system is adopted, a listener has the inherent ability to learn to understand just as if he were learning a new language. Using a fixed transformation means that we have only one key, i.e., that we have a code and not a cipher. It is the lack of choice for the key which causes this practical weakness. A second disadvantage of using a code is that, once an interceptor knows the type of transformation which has taken place, he is able to retransform the signal to its original form just as easily as the receiver. In fact, either by building his own descrambler or by obtaining one of the user's descramblers, he can listen directly to any communication.

These types of attack can only be thwarted by a scrambler which is able to use more than one transformation and is able to change the transformation it is using. Once this facility is introduced the interceptor who is trying to 'understand' the scrambled speech is, essentially, faced with trying to learn a language for which the rules are changing. This change of transformation can be effected by the introduction of a key which controls the precise parameters of the transformation being used. Clearly an interceptor's descrambler is useless without knowledge of the current key. The frequency with which the parameters need to be changed will vary according to the system. They might be changed only occasionally, possibly every few hours, or on a message to message basis. It might even be desirable to change them several times per message. We shall see examples of situations of each type.

III. Band-Shift Inverters

Although a *band-shift inverter* is based on the frequency inverter, a key is introduced in an attempt to secure the system from any interceptor who happens to possess an appropriate descrambler and to make it harder for him to learn the 'language'. Since the user is able to vary his key the band-shift inverter is our first example of a scrambler which is a genuine cipher system.

When we discussed inversion we began with a signal band limited to 300–3000 Hz. We showed that, if our inverted signal is to be in the same band, our carrier frequency must be 3300 Hz. If instead we let our carrier frequency

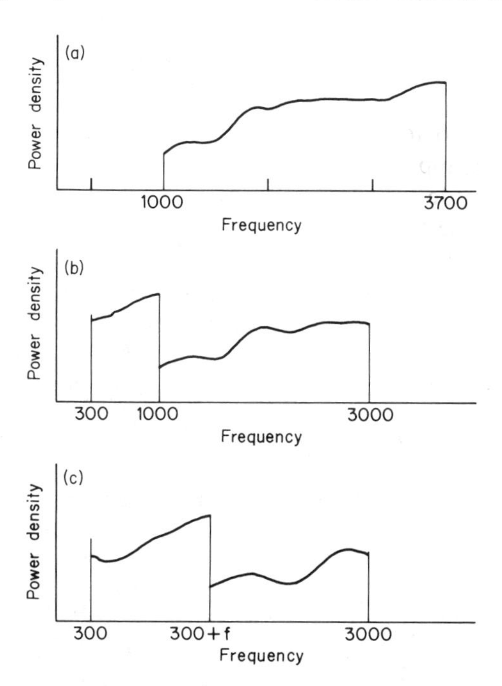

FIG. 4.9. Band-shift inversion. (a) Frequency inversion using a carrier frequency of 4000 Hz. Band-shift inversion using a carrier frequency of (b) 4000 and (c) (3300 + f) Hz.

be, say, 4000 Hz then we obtain an inverted signal whose spectrum is shown in Fig. 4.9(a). This signal is no longer in the same band as our original one, but we can arrange for it to be in this band by taking that part of the signal above 3000 Hz and putting it at the low frequency end. (Note that although the signal of Fig. 4.9(a) occupies a different frequency band it has, of necessity, the same bandwidth as our original signal.) This is the principle of *band-shift inverting* and is illustrated in Fig. 4.9(b). Clearly if, in general, we choose a carrier frequency of $(3300 + f)$ Hz then our band-shifted inverted signal will be as in Fig. 4.9(c). A typical band-shift inverter has been 4 and 16 different carrier frequencies which result in 4–16 different 'shifts'.

There is another technique which is very similar to band-shift inversion and in fact is often confused with it. It is called frequency hopping inversion. As with a band-shift inverter, a *frequency hopping inverter* uses a set of different carrier frequencies but then it simply 'loses' that part of the signal which is outside the original band. In this system there is only a slight variation in the various carrier frequencies, at most about 300 Hz, and it relies on the fact that if the information content at the low frequencies of the signal is lost then the signal will still be highly intelligible.

For either system there must be a precise definition of the rules which decide when and how the set of carrier frequencies is to be used. There are a number of alternatives, which include the following:

(a) Let each key determine a carrier frequency. A frequency will then be used whenever the appropriate key is selected.

(b) Let each key determine an ordering of the possible carrier frequencies. The carrier frequencies will then be used in a given order whenever the appropriate key is chosen. If this method is adopted then a decision has to be taken as to how long the scrambler should use any given carrier frequency before changing to the next one in the chosen ordering.

(c) Let each key initialise a pseudo-random number generator which will then select a different carrier frequency at suitably chosen time intervals.

Any arrangement of frequently changing the carrier frequencies, like for instance (b) and (c) above, is often referred to as a cyclical band-shift inverter. A typical time interval for each carrier frequency in a *cyclical band-shift inverter* is on the order of 10 to 20 msec. Since the carrier frequency is changing so often any cyclical band-shift inverter requires some form of synchronization between transmitter and receiver. If the receiver does not change carrier frequency at the appropriate time, or if it changes to the wrong frequency, the communications system will fail. Thus, some form of timing information must be sent to, or possibly be inherent in, the receiver. We shall not discuss this type of problem now. However, the importance of synchronization, and the problems associated with it, should not be underestimated and will be discussed in Chapter 6.

Systems which rely on band-shift inverters have the obvious failing that, since there are only a limited number of possibilities for the carrier frequency, the original signal can be recovered reasonably easily by using 'trial and error' methods with relatively simple equipment. Thus an interceptor who possesses a band-shift inversion descrambler might be able to try different carrier frequencies until he obtains signals which sound like unscrambled speech.

In earlier discussions we have repeatedly stressed that the human brain can sometimes adapt and essentially descramble parts of scrambled messages. With simple inverters there is a major problem. The residual intelligibility of the output signal is unacceptably high. (The *residual intelligibility* of an output signal is that proportion of the original signal which can be understood directly when listening to the ciphered message.)

Brunner (1980a) gives some results on residual intelligibility tests on cyclic band-shift inverters. For text he claims that the residual intelligibility is in the range 30–50% while for numbers it is in the range 55–85%. These figures are surprisingly poor when compared, for instance, with the results of Jayant *et al.* (1981) who found that a simple frequency inverter produced results in the region of 30% (for untrained listeners). We might have expected the more sophisticated cyclic band-shift inverter to be superior to the simple inverter. Unfortunately we have no details of Brunner's experiments.

The difference between the residual intelligibility for text and numbers is to be expected. Number tests, particularly for numbers in the range 0 to 9, cannot really claim to assess the intelligibility of the scrambled speech. They are only a measure of the effect of the scrambler on the ten signals: zero, one, two, three, four, five, six, seven, eight and nine. The listener is merely trying to differentiate between ten sounds which, with the possible exceptions of five and nine, are totally dissimilar prior to scrambling. Clearly this is an exceptionally severe test of a scrambler. Furthermore it is by no means obvious that the relative performances of two scramblers on a number test in any way reflects their comparative residual intelligibility for scrambled speech. It is, however, very common for users to perform numbers tests, so their results are of interest since they tend to be used as a 'benchmark' for comparing scramblers.

Another interesting, and possibly surprising, observation of Brunner was that, in his experiments, the code variation rate had an optimum value with respect to residual intelligibility, and that any increase in the rate beyond this optimum value actually enhanced the residual intelligibility. (Since the distortion which remains in the speech after descrambling is also intensified, it is clearly undesirable to use rates too far above this value.) In his paper

Brunner compared the trade-off between the change in carrier frequency rate and the residual intelligibility.

One common technique which is often used in an attempt to enhance a band-shift inverter is the addition of a number of tones to *mask* the signal. The particular tones added may be key-dependent or not. If they are not, then an interceptor will be able to filter them out just as easily as the receiver. If they are key-dependent and, as a result, repeatedly changing during the course of a transmission then, as before, the transmitter and receiver must be synchronized. An extra disadvantage of adding masked tones is that, if they are at a high level, severe distortion may occur as the transmitted signal passes through any repeaters. Furthermore, since high level tones are likely to require a high proportion of the carrier energy, the signal energy is reduced and the descrambled signal will have a significantly lower signal to noise ratio. One consequence of this deficiency is that a radio user who switches from clear communications, where there are no such tones, to secure communications will notice a definite decrease in the range over which he can communicate. Of course this energy loss can be countered by using low-level tones. But if this is done then the masking is not so effective. In practice, tone masking does not seem to be popular with users. There is almost universal recognition that any extra security which the masking may provide is not worth the accompanying degradation in the audio quality at the receiver.

IV. Bandsplitters

Each of the techniques discussed so far has offered a very low level of security and is unlikely to be used, except in conjunction with some other technique, by a modern scrambler designer. This is not true of bandsplitters. The *bandsplitter*, also called a *bandscrambler*, is one of the most popular of the current scramblers and is so widely used that it warrants a detailed discussion of some possible implementations and its likely performance.

The basic technique is to divide the spectrum into a number of sub-bands and then to scramble the signal by re-arranging the order of the sub-bands. In some of the more sophisticated systems some of the sub-bands may also be inverted. Figure 4.10 illustrates a simple example with five sub-bands in which the sub-bands 1, 2 and 5 have been inverted as well as displaced. When five sub-bands are used there are $5!$ possible reorderings and 2^5 ways of deciding which, if any, sub-bands to invert. Thus, there are $5! \times 2^5 = 3840$ possible ways of rearranging the sub-bands. If the spectrum were divided into m sub-bands then the number of possible rearrangements would be $(m!) \times 2^m$. However, since the most commonly used number of sub-divisions is five, we will restrict our discussion of possible implementations to the situation where we have five sub-bands.

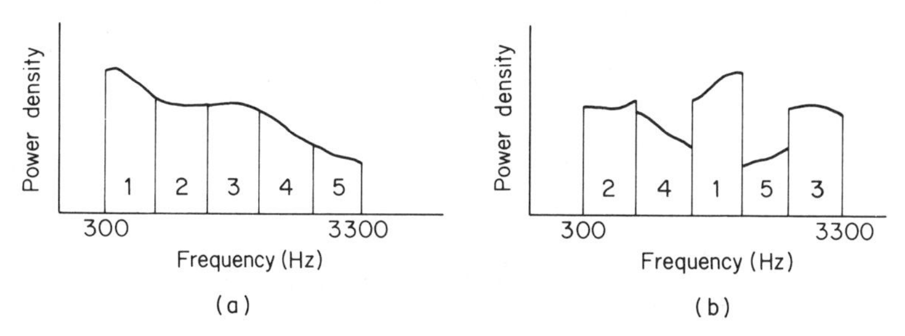

FIG. 4.10. Bandsplitter. (a) Original ordering of sub-bands and (b) scrambled spectrum.

In Fig. 4.11 we exhibit a possible scheme for a five-band bandsplitter. We will assume, for simplicity, that our signal is band-limited to a bandwidth of 3 kHz in the range 300–3300 Hz. We will choose our sub-bands so that they all have equal bandwidths which, for this particular example, must be 600 Hz. Clearly we need to avoid overlaps between adjacent sub-bands and this means that we need good filters, i.e., filters for which the signal outside the band of interest is many decibels lower than the signal within the band. We will also, for simplicity, restrict ourselves to a single filter design. In the system of Fig. 4.11 balanced modulators (or some other means) are used to increase each sub-band frequency so that it falls exactly into the window of

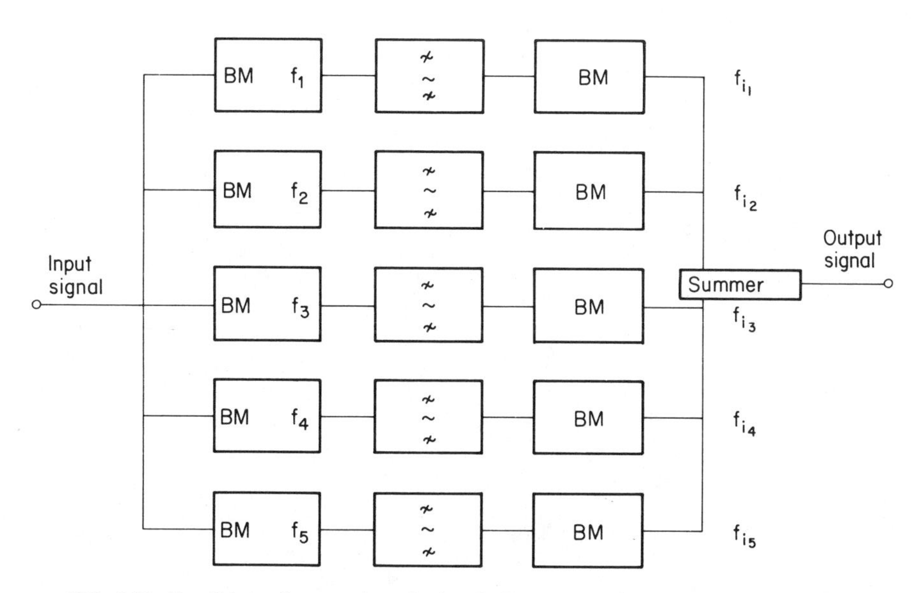

FIG. 4.11. Possible implementation of a bandsplitter. (Each BM is a balanced modulator; the frequencies f_i are the carrier frequencies.)

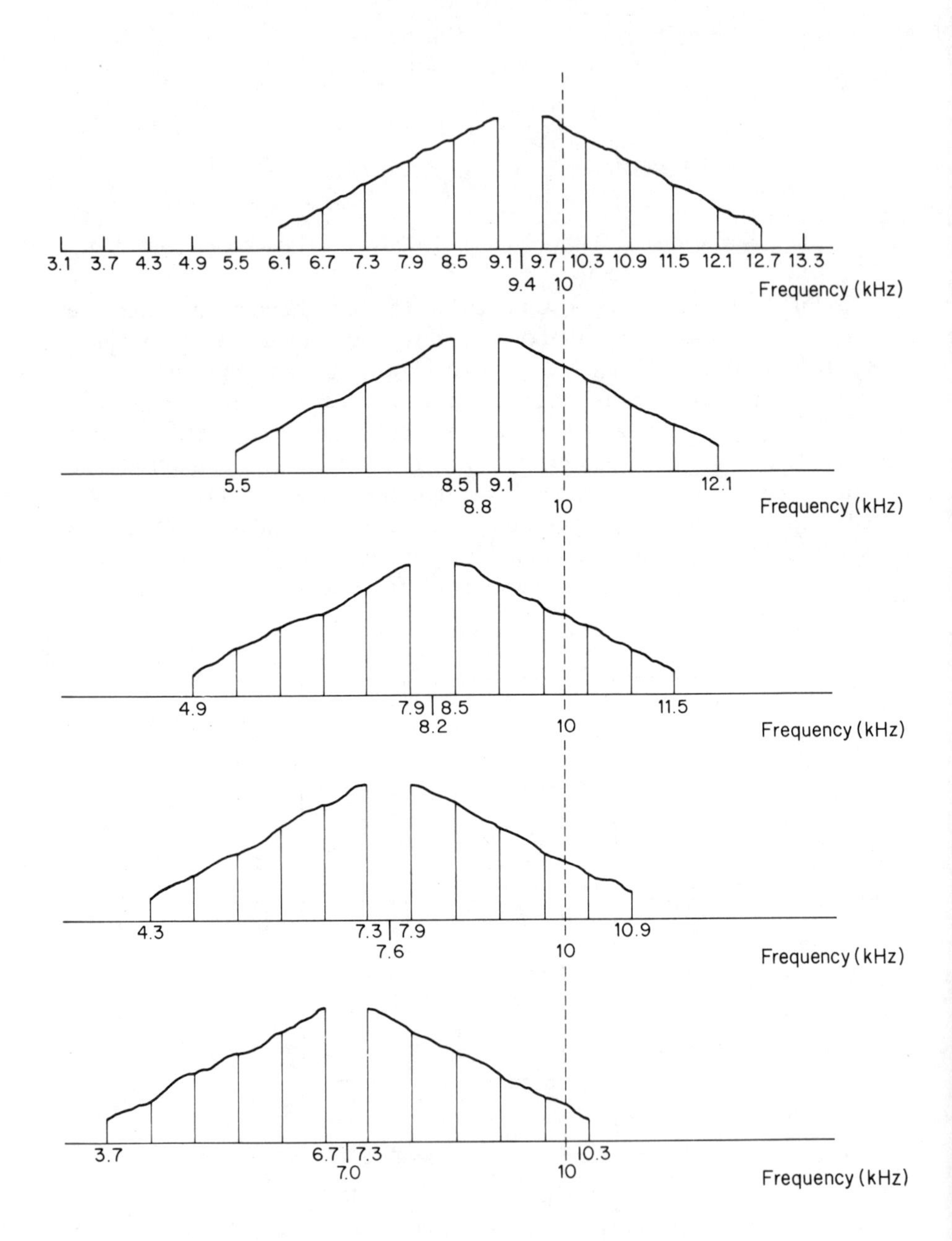

FIG. 4.12. Scheme for obtaining the sub-bands in the range 9.7–10.3 kHz.

our filter. Then, after filtering, each resultant sub-band will be mixed back down to its final position.

In order to work out some specific values for f_1, f_2, f_3, f_4 and f_5 we will assume that our filter is designed as a bandpass filter with a 600-Hz bandwidth centred on 10 kHz. This, of course, means that each sub-band must be moved up to the 9.7–10.3-kHz band. Thus, since band 1 occupies the range from 300 to 900 Hz, we need to use a carrier frequency of 9.4 kHz i.e. we need $f_1 = 9.4$ kHz. Similarly for band 2, which occupies the range 900 to 1500 Hz, we need a carrier frequency of 8.8 kHz. This scheme is shown in Fig. 4.12 from which we can see that $f_1 = 9.4$ kHz, $f_2 = 8.8$ kHz, $f_3 = 8.2$ kHz, $f_4 = 7.6$ kHz and $f_5 = 7.0$ kHz. Clearly the values of f_{i_1} to f_{i_5} will depend upon the permutation chosen and upon which sub-bands are inverted. Thus we need some way of changing the values of f_{i_1} to f_{i_5} each time we change the key. However, for the moment, we will postpone our discussions of how these values might be changed and consider a couple of specific examples.

Suppose that we want to put sub-band 1, uninverted, into the position which was occupied by sub-band 3, i.e., into the range 1.5–2.1 kHz. Immediately after the filter the sub-band we want is, together with all the others, occupying the range 9.7–10.3 kHz. Thus, we must use the value of f_{i_1} which will move the range 9.7–10.3 kHz down to the range occupied by band 3. This is achieved by choosing $f_{i_1} = f_3$; $f_{i_1} = 8.2$ kHz. (To check this, see Section VI of Chapter 2.) Now suppose, on the other hand, we want sub-band 1 to be inverted as well as occupying the position of sub-band 3. In order to achieve the inversion we need a carrier frequency which is above 10 kHz and since we want sub-band 1 to occupy the position of sub-band 3, we want a carrier frequency of $[10 + (10 - f_3)]$ kHz i.e. 11.8 kHz. With this carrier

TABLE 4.1

Carrier Frequency Required for Mixing Down

Position to be occupied by the sub-band under consideration	Carrier frequency required (kHz)
Sub-band 1—not inverted	9.4
Sub-band 2—not inverted	8.8
Sub-band 3—not inverted	8.2
Sub-band 4—not inverted	7.6
Sub-band 5—not inverted	7.0
Sub-band 1—inverted	10.6
Sub-band 2—inverted	11.2
Sub-band 3—inverted	11.8
Sub-band 4—inverted	12.4
Sub-band 5—inverted	13.0

frequency the top part of our band will appear at 1.5 kHz, and the component at 9.7 kHz will appear at 2.1 kHz (see Fig. 2.30).

Although we have been discussing sub-band 1 the same reasoning holds for every sub-band. The reason is that, as we have already observed, prior to mixing down every sub-band is in the range 9.7–10.3 kHz. The situation, i.e., the choice for the value for each of f_{i_1}, f_{i_2}, f_{i_3}, f_{i_4} and f_{i_5}, is given in Table 4.1.

Since filters and balanced modulators can both be realised digitally, the system of Fig. 4.11 can be realised in either analogue or digital form.

Once a permutation has been selected and it has been decided which bands should be inverted, a look-up table, like Table 4.1, is used to choose the carrier frequency. This is essentially the function of the key. However, as with the band-shift inverter, there are a number of ways in which the keys can be used. The choice is the same as before. Namely:

(a) Use the key to select a particular rearrangement.

(b) Use the key to pre-select a set of rearrangements, and then use this set sequentially.

(c) Use the key to initialize a pseudo-random number generator which will then select a different re-arrangement every so often.

When a bandsplitter is used as in (b) or (c) it is often referred to as a *rolling bandsplitter*. The bandsplitter might utilize a particular re-arrangement for any period between a few hundred milliseconds and a number of seconds.

One famous example of a rolling bandsplitter was the *A-3*. This was designed by Bell Telephone Laboratories and used in the late 1930s. In this system the 250–3000 Hz bandwidth was divided into five sub-bands of 550 Hz but, out of the 3840 possible re-arrangements, only six were used. These six rearrangements were employed in a sequential pattern of length 36. [Thus, the A-3 was a system of type (b).] Each rearrangement was used for a period of 20 sec and thus the pattern of rearrangements was repeated every 12 min.

The A-3 was not very secure. Some of the engineers at Bell Telephone Laboratories listened to some speech scrambled by the A-3 and, according to Kahn (1967), were able to recover an average of 47% of the words after just a few trials. In one test the intelligibility is said to have risen to 76%.

In order to discover why the A-3 was so insecure, we must, as always, consider what is happening to the speech. Before we begin to investigate the reason why, we observe that the majority of the 3840 possible rearrangements result in a residual intelligibility that is unacceptably high. It is, for instance, generally accepted that, if one is forced to rely on permutations only and does not invert any sub-bands, then considerably less than 10% of the 120 possibilities provide reasonable security. In his survey paper, Jayant suggests that only 5% of the 3840 rearrangements are 'good' (Jayant, 1982), while

Khan reports that the Bell Telephone Laboratories believed that only 11 of them provided 'adequate security'.

There are a number of technical reasons for the number of 'good' rearrangements being so small. Before we discuss them and show how to identify them, we must mention (yet again!) some of the remarkable properties of the human brain and ear. One particular property is what Kahn calls the 'cocktail party syndrome'. This is the ability of a human to listen to several conversations simultaneously and, although they appear to be at the same level, to isolate one particular conversation on which to 'eavesdrop'. The brain and ear are also able to make such incredible use of the redundancy in speech that we can understand a conversation even if we do not hear most of it very clearly. There are, as we have already seen, many reasons why this is so. McCalmont (1973) claims that it is possible to obtain reasonably good intelligence out of a voice transmission which is bandwidth limited to a 300–500-Hz spectrum. The first formant of a speech signal usually falls within the first two sub-bands and, as a consequence, these contain considerably more than 40% of the energy in the signal. Thus if the speech has been scrambled but a listener is able to 'concentrate' on a single sub-band corresponding to one of the lower frequency sub-bands, he may actually 'hear' the unscrambled speech. Another, more serious, corollary is that if a cryptanalyst is able to find the new positions of the first two sub-bands and translate them back, he will have recovered a sufficient proportion of the content of the signal that he will probably be able to understand the message.

Although we will not concentrate on the time domain until the next chapter, we must mention that delaying the sub-bands is a technique often used to enhance a bandsplitter. The idea is to improve the unintelligibility of the speech by adding a different time delay to each sub-band. Thus, for example, we might decide to delay band 1 by 0 msec, band 2 by 10 msec, band 3 by 20 msec, band 4 by 30 msec and band 5 by 40 msec. The signal would then be recovered at the receiver by reversing the order of the delays. Unfortunately, this has the effect of introducing an overall delay which may be unacceptable to a user and might also prevent the use of the device in certain duplex systems. It also adds to the cost of the system and probably degrades the final audio quality. We will have more to say about this in subsequent chapters.

With or without sub-band delays, a rolling bandsplitter offers more security than one which uses a fixed rearrangement of the bands. The security is increased still further if a pseudo-random number generator is used to change the rearrangement every few milliseconds. There are various alternatives for the way in which this type of scheme can work. The two most widely used schemes are:

(a) For each change of the rearrangement, the pseudo-random number generator generates a number from 1 to 120 to select one of the 5 ! possible permutations on the five sub-bands and then generates five binary digits to decide between inversion or not for each sub-band.

(b) For each change of the arrangement, the pseudo-random number generator generates an address for a look up table which contains a selection of the 'best' rearrangements. Out of the total of 3840 possible rearrangements this look up table is likely to contain as few as 256 entries, but 512 and 1024 are other fairly common values. In practice this look up table is likely to be in *read only memory* (ROM).

Since, in practice, such a large percentage of the possible rearrangements leave too much residual intelligibility, method (b) is usually considered superior to (a). It is important to notice that when (b) is used the period of the device does not depend on the ROM size but on the pseudo-random number generator. As we saw in Chapter 3 we can make this period arbitrarily large. Another important consideration for this type of method is the synchronization scheme, but we shall postpone our discussion of this until Chapter 6.

A. Assessing Rearrangements of the Sub-bands

If we are going to have a ROM to store the most suitable rearrangements then we need some way of deciding the relative merits of the possible rearrangements. As usual, the only way to choose the best is to select them as the result of listening tests. These tests appear to suggest that

(i) bands should be moved as far as possible and if a band is not moved it should be inverted.

(ii) any bands which were adjacent originally should not remain adjacent after scrambling. In fact, they should be separated as far as possible and if they remain near to each other at least one should be inverted.

If we accept this as a basis, then it is possible to invent scoring schemes for arrangements and then use only those which score more than a certain value. Many such schemes have been suggested and we will now give an example of one. However the reader should certainly not assume that this is the best method nor that all rearrangements which score above a certain threshold are 'good'. Our example is merely intended as an example of the type of scheme which might be employed. In practice, any rearrangement which scores more than the accepted baseline would probably be subjected to further rigorous listening tests before being stored in the ROM.

In order to obtain a score for a particular rearrangement we might perform the following calculation.

(1) Calculate the shift factor for the permutation being used. The shift factor, denoted by (SF), is the sum of the absolute differences between the original position of each sub-band and the position which it occupies after the rearrangement. Thus for example, if α is the permutation

$$\begin{bmatrix} 1 & 2 & 3 & 4 & 5 \\ 3 & 5 & 1 & 2 & 4 \end{bmatrix}$$

then $(SF(\alpha)) = |1-3| + |2-5| + |3-1| + |4-2| + |5-4| = 10$. Since bands should be moved as far as possible a high shift factor is obviously desirable.

(2) Count the number of unmoved bands. If we denote this number by (UB) then, since bands should be moved, this number should be small, preferably zero. For our example $(UB(\alpha)) = 0$.

(3) Determine whether the permutation has any bad patterns. Here we might, for instance, decide to count the number of consecutive pairs of sub-bands which are adjacent and in the same order in the final signal. If we denote this score by (BP) then in our example α, since 1 and 2 remain adjacent, we have $(BP(\alpha)) = 1$. For a 'good' arrangement (BP) should be as small as possible.

(4) Calculate the inversion factor (INV) of the rearrangement. This might, for instance, be given by a score of 1 for every pair of adjacent sub-bands in the scrambled signal such that one is inverted and the other is not. A 'good' rearrangement is likely to have a reasonably high value for (INV).

Bearing in mind that a good rearrangement should have high scores for (SF) and (INV) but low scores for (UB) and (BP), and that bad patterns and fixed bands are particularly undesirable, we might then obtain our final score S by the formula

$$S = (SF) - 2(UB) - 3(BP) + (INV)$$

If we look back at the example of Figure 4.10 then the permutation is

$$\begin{bmatrix} 1 & 2 & 3 & 4 & 5 \\ 3 & 1 & 5 & 2 & 4 \end{bmatrix}$$

If we denote the rearrangement by θ then $(SF(\theta)) = |1-3| + |2-1| + |3-5| + |4-2| + |5-4| = 8$, $(UB(\theta)) = 0$, $(BP(\theta)) = 0$ and $(INV(\theta)) = 3$. So far this example our score is given by $S = 8 - 2.0 - 3.0 + 3 = 11$.

Given any scheme like the one we have proposed we need to decide if it does what we want and, provided it does, what we consider to be a good score. For our particular scheme we note that (SF), (UB) and (BP) depend only on the permutation and that (INV) depends solely on the inversion pattern. If we write 1 for inversion and 0 for non-inversion then, clearly, the highest possible value for (INV) is 4 and is given by 10101 or 01010. There are many possible patterns which give (INV) = 3, 2 or 1 and precisely two, i.e., 00000 and 11111, which make (INV) equal to 0.

Clearly the highest possible value for (UB) is 5 which occurs when the permutation is the identity. Similarly the lowest possible value for (SF) is 0 which also occurs when the permutation is the identity. (Note that it might be argued that our formula is essentially counting the unmoved bands twice. Clearly too many unmoved bands cause a low value for (SF) and so (UB) and (SF) are certainly not independent). It is not immediately obvious how large the value of (SF) might be and precisely which permutations obtain this maximum value. Direct calculations show that the maximum value for SF is in fact 12 and that this value is attained by 20 of the 120 permutations.

If we want to know the best arrangements then, clearly, they are obtained by adding an inversion pattern of 10101 or 01010 to one of the best permutations. Again by direct verification we find that the highest possible value for (SF) − 2(UB) − 3(BP) is 12 and that this value is achieved by only 4 of the permutations. Thus, the maximum value for S is 16 and is achieved by 8 different arrangements. For our particular scoring system a reasonable passmark might be 13 or even 14. However, we must stress, yet again, that our formula is not necessarily the best. A ‘good’ rearrangement is determined by the listening tests and the object of any formula is to try to reflect the results of these tests.

Even when he has found a method of generating his good rearrangements and has entered them in a ROM, the designer's problems are not over. He must, as we have already mentioned, not forget that an interceptor is quite likely to obtain a legitimate receiver and, as a consequence, know precisely those rearrangements which are in the ROM. He might then decide to enter an arbitrary key and listen to the resultant deciphered message. Of course, unless he is exceptionally lucky, he will not select the correct key and will not hear clear speech; but how well-scrambled is this new signal likely to be? This is the next problem which the designer must face.

Suppose, for example, that our ROM has 512 rearrangements stored in it and that our pseudo-random number generator is selecting from them. Then we would have to expect that an unauthorised receiver would use the correct rearrangement once in every 512 attempts. This is an inescapable consequence of the type of system we are using and there is nothing we can do about it. What we may be able to do, however, is to prevent him from getting too close to correct descrambling when he uses the wrong rearrangement. There are, as we know, a number of rearrangements which hardly reduce the intelligibility at all. For instance, any permutation which leaves the first two sub-bands unaltered would, if used for scrambling, give a scrambled message which would still be intelligible. Thus, we would like to restrict our set of stored rearrangements so that if we scramble with one and then attempt to descramble with another the resulting signal is still well scrambled. Such a set is called a *mutually secure set*. If A and B are any two rearrangements, then, for instance, scrambling by using A and then descrambling with B is the same as scrambling with $B^{-1}A$. Thus if A and B belong to a mutually secure set, the rearrangements $B^{-1}A$ and $A^{-1}B$ must also yield well scrambled signals. In order to obtain a mutually secure set of rearrangements we must, for all arrangements A and B in the set, subject $A^{-1}B$ and $B^{-1}A$ to a similar scoring test to that which we have just described. In practice the set of tests used for $A^{-1}B$ and $B^{-1}A$ is likely to be less stringent than those applied to A and B. The reason for this is, quite simply, that if the tests are too severe the designer is likely to find himself with an empty ROM!

In order to illustrate mutual security we will ignore possible inversions and restrict ourselves to permutations. Suppose that we let

$$\alpha = \begin{bmatrix} 1 & 2 & 3 & 4 & 5 \\ 5 & 4 & 1 & 3 & 2 \end{bmatrix} \quad \text{and} \quad \beta = \begin{bmatrix} 1 & 2 & 3 & 4 & 5 \\ 4 & 3 & 5 & 2 & 1 \end{bmatrix}$$

Then, referring back to our scoring system, $S(\alpha) = 12$ and $S(\beta) = 12$. Since this is the highest possible score for a permutation, both α and β are candidates to be stored in the ROM. From our discussion of permutations in Chapter 3 we know that

$$\alpha^{-1} = \begin{bmatrix} 1 & 2 & 3 & 4 & 5 \\ 3 & 5 & 4 & 2 & 1 \end{bmatrix} \quad \text{and} \quad \beta^{-1} = \begin{bmatrix} 1 & 2 & 3 & 4 & 5 \\ 5 & 4 & 2 & 1 & 3 \end{bmatrix}$$

If we now encipher using α and decipher with β then, for any i from 1 to 5, the final position of band i is $\beta^{-1}(\alpha(i))$. So, for instance $\beta^{-1}(\alpha(1)) = \beta^{-1}(5) = 3$. Similar considerations give

$$\beta^{-1}\alpha = \begin{bmatrix} 1 & 2 & 3 & 4 & 5 \\ 3 & 1 & 5 & 2 & 4 \end{bmatrix} \quad \text{and} \quad \alpha^{-1}\beta = \begin{bmatrix} 1 & 2 & 3 & 4 & 5 \\ 2 & 4 & 1 & 5 & 3 \end{bmatrix}$$

Since $S(\beta^{-1}\alpha)$ and $S(\alpha^{-1}\beta) = 8$ we would probably feel that α and β are mutually secure. If we put

$$\gamma = \begin{bmatrix} 1 & 2 & 3 & 4 & 5 \\ 5 & 4 & 2 & 1 & 3 \end{bmatrix}$$

then $S(\gamma)$ is also 12. But now

$$\gamma^{-1} = \begin{bmatrix} 1 & 2 & 3 & 4 & 5 \\ 4 & 3 & 5 & 2 & 1 \end{bmatrix} \quad \text{and} \quad \gamma^{-1}\alpha = \begin{bmatrix} 1 & 2 & 3 & 4 & 5 \\ 1 & 2 & 4 & 5 & 3 \end{bmatrix}$$

In this case $S(\gamma^{-1}\alpha) = -6$ and any message scrambled with $\gamma^{-1}\alpha$ is likely to be highly intelligible.

Thus, α and γ are not mutually secure and we do not want to include both α and γ in the ROM. In order to ensure that the set in the ROM is mutually secure we could test each possible entry against each of the permutations which have already been entered. In practice a mutually secure set of permutations would probably be generated on a computer prior to writing it into the ROM. It is perhaps worth noting here, with regard to both testing for mutual security and to descrambling, that for any permutation α, $S(\alpha) = S(\alpha^{-1})$. Thus we can choose our set so that whenever it contains a permutation α it also contains its inverse α^{-1}. This will then enable us to enter them in the ROM, in such a way that we can ensure that the address of any permutation and its inverse differ only in the first bit. The first bit can be used to indicate whether we are enciphering or deciphering while the rest of the address will be identical for α and α^{-1}. In this way deciphering is achieved by merely changing the first bit of each address. There is a slight problem with this suggestion in that any arrangement of order 2 is its own inverse. Thus these must either be included twice, which increases the probability of them being chosen, or arrangements of order 2 must be avoided.

Other possibilities for trying to improve the system include rolling the codes as quickly as possible. However, the signal transmitted may already be saturated with discontinuities which have been created by our tampering. Changing the rearrangement is likely to cause even more discontinuities and make us even more vulnerable not only to the synchronization difficulties but also to any distortion which may occur during transmission.

B. Increasing the Number of Sub-bands

Another option is to increase the number of sub-bands. In our example we used five sub-bands and, clearly, if this number were significantly increased then there would be a corresponding increase in the number of suitable rearrangements available. Unfortunately, any increase in the security which might be anticipated is counteracted by the introduction of many practical difficulties. The filters and other components used introduce extra noise and distortion into the signal. Furthermore their operation is not totally linear. Any modification of the signal always introduces imperfections and a degradation of the quality, and bandscramblers tend to be more susceptible to noise and non-linearities than many other scramblers. The introduction of extra sub-bands may, for many practical transmission links, render the system either unusable or so expensive that it is uneconomical. If, for instance, we look back at Fig. 2.8 we can see the type of differential delay that can occur. If one introduces extra sub-bands and/or rolls them faster, the effects of this delay can be horrendous.

Having pointed out these problems we comment that this is yet another area in which digital signal processing may provide a breakthrough. It may, at some time in the not too distant future, enable us to construct economically some form of channel equaliser within the receiver. However, in the case of bandsplitters, it is not clear that, even if it proves to be possible, any extra security will justify the work involved.

V. An Example Using the DFT

Our next scheme relies on fast digital signal processing and may be considered as a generalisation of a bandsplitter. Thus, in order to consider it, we remind the reader of the basic properties of the DFT. In order to obtain the spectral coefficients X from the sample vector x we use the DFT matrix F (with complex entries). The relation is $X = Fx$. We also saw that, if the spectrally inverted signal is represented by its sample vector y, then $y = F^{-1}PFx$, where P is the appropriate permutation matrix.

If we try to replace the permutation matrix P by another permutation matrix Q then we will get a new vector $z = F^{-1}QFx$. However, if we are going to use Q for some form of scrambling and want z to be the sample vector of the new signal then, obviously, z must be a real-valued vector. This considerably restricts the possible choices for Q. If we are thinking in terms of a bandsplitter then, if our sample has size n, we are actually trying to permute the $\frac{1}{2}n$ spectral coefficients of our signal. This means, for example, that we can choose Q to have a form which ensures that it permutes the first $\frac{1}{2}n$ coefficients amongst themselves, permutes the second $\frac{1}{2}n$ amongst themselves and then interchanges the two halves. Thus Q may be of the form

$$Q = \begin{array}{c} \overbrace{\qquad}^{\frac{1}{2}n} \; \overbrace{\qquad}^{\frac{1}{2}n} \\ \left[\begin{array}{c|c} O & Q_1 \\ \hline Q_2 & O \end{array}\right] \end{array} \begin{array}{l} \}\ \frac{1}{2}n \\ \}\ \frac{1}{2}n \end{array}$$

where each entry of O is 0 and Q_1 and Q_2 are permutation matrices.

Ideally we can think of this technique as splitting the signal's frequency spectrum in $\frac{1}{2}n$ very fine bands and then performing a permutation on them before finally retransforming to an analogue signal. This might suggest that the final signal has exactly the same bandwidth as the original one. If it were possible for n to be infinite, then this would be true; but it cannot be infinite. Not only because of the infinite processing power which would be required but also because of the infinite delay which would occur between transmitter and receiver. (Recall that we need all the n samples before we can perform our DFT!) Thus, since n is finite, the process creates discontinuities in our signal in the same way that a conventional rolling bandsplitter does. Consequently we cannot assume that our output signal will have the same bandwidth as the input. Indeed all the comments which we made about rolling faster or increasing the number of sub-bands in the bandsplitter apply here. Furthermore, as we have already observed, the process also creates an extra delay between transmitter and receiver. It may also cause synchronization problems. Despite all these snags this technique may give a higher security level than the conventional bandsplitter, and the security may be increased still further by changing the permutation matrix every so often, i.e., by using it in a rolling fashion.

The example discussed above is just one of many transformations which may be used in this type of technique. Another possibility, which uses discrete prolate spheroidal sequences for the transform, is described by Aaron Wyner (1979a,b).

In the past, scrambling in the frequency domain has been considered to be solely a privacy technique. Most publications on the subject have suggested that it is not practicable to obtain a high level of security. On the other hand scrambling of the type which we have just described, i.e., systems which use transforms like the DFT, have only recently become viable. There is plenty of scope for research in this area. The major problem is, probably, to decide whether or not such systems can remain secure while simultaneously offering an adequate recovery of the audio signal at the receiver.

VI. Spread Spectrum

We end this chapter by discussing a technique which, although not really a scrambling system, offers a certain level of security. It involves spreading the spectrum which the signal occupies. This, of course, is in direct contrast to the other systems in this chapter where the aim has been to preserve the signal bandwidth. In order to introduce the technique we will look at a privacy system which was devised by James Roberts as long ago as 1881. This system uses the simple idea of switching a message between two or more channels.

The motivation was the observation that if someone intercepts one of the channels he will not obtain enough of the signal to enable him to understand, or reconstruct, it. Roberts, who was thinking in terms of the telephone, decided that if he employed two or more lines, using different routes, then he would thwart any effort to 'tap' his entire message. Clearly the security of such a system depends on the number of channels used and how long is spent on each channel.

The basic philosophy behind modern *frequency hopping radio* is fairly similar to Roberts' idea. Here, rather than transmit continuously on a single frequency, the radio will repeatedly change frequency. It is likely to change its frequency at regular intervals according to some pattern determined by a pseudo-random number generator which is seeded by a key. Thus, for example, a VHF frequency hopping radio might use a large part of the VHF band for its hopping. The time spent on each frequency will vary but will usually be short and, for a good system, may be just a few milliseconds.

Once frequency hopping is introduced, the bandwidth used by a radio is likely to be enormous. However, since the time spent in each frequency is so short it can share a frequency band with a number of other radios. Even if a number of the frequency slots which it would like to use are occupied by other radios, perhaps with more power than the frequency hopping radio, its dwell time in each slot is so short that the intelligibility may not be seriously impaired. In practice it can be shown that even with as much as 40% of the band blocked a good frequency hopping radio will still provide communication. This, of course, is an important advantage of such radios. It means that, if an enemy is trying to jam communications, he has to jam almost the entire band before he seriously inconveniences the user.

For true speech security a user might consider scrambling his speech as well as hopping it. The interceptor would then be faced with a daunting task. To listen to the communication he must not only find some method for descrambling, but first he has to find the constituent elements and piece them together.

The popularity of frequency hopping radios has increased significantly during the past few years. However, it should be pointed out that one of the most difficult design aspects of a frequency hopping radio is to devise a method of maintaining synchronization between transmitter and receiver. This is, of course, essential to ensure that they both hop simultaneously. These problems are similar to the synchronization requirements for scramblers and will be considered, in some detail, in Chapter 6.

5. Time Domain Scrambling

I. Introduction

One important characteristic of time domain scramblers is that they may imply a significant delay between the speaker's utterance at the transmitting terminal and the reconstructed message being output from the receiving terminal. This effect can be similar, or in some cases much worse, than that which we experience when making a transatlantic telephone call via satellite. Most users regard any appreciable delay as being detrimental to the system. It is certainly possible for someone who is consistently using a system with delays to become accustomed to them and, as a result, not be seriously inconvenienced. However, anyone who is repeatedly changing from a system with a negligible delay to one with a substantial delay is likely to have problems.

The problems caused by delays are likely to be particularly acute in the context of a duplex system. Users of half-duplex systems are usually very disciplined in their use of the system and this helps nullify the effect of the delays. For instance, users of half-duplex systems are likely to use the word 'over' to clearly define when one of them has finished talking. In such systems it is common to differentiate between the overall system delay and the 'over–over' delay. The former refers to the time difference between one communicant speaking at the start of a message and the other hearing. The latter refers to the time difference between one speaker finishing his message and beginning to receive the reply. These may or may not be identical. However the mere existence of the over–over protocol means that the users are much less likely to object to a slight extra delay.

Typical delays can vary from a few milliseconds to several hundred milliseconds. (Note that we saw some of the former in Chapter 4.) The precise time depends on the type of system used and then, once the type is determined, on the parameters of the particular system.

Time domain scramblers fall into three broad categories:

(a) reversed time segmentation
(b) time element scramblers
  (i) hopping window
  (ii) sliding window
(c) time sample scramblers.

Hopping and sliding window scramblers are currently the most widely used speech scramblers. This is a consequence of both their robustness and their relatively low cost for a medium-to-high security level. Although most of the chapter is devoted to them, we begin with a discussion of reversed time segmentation. In the final section we look at time sample scramblers which, as a result of recent advances in digital signal processing, are likely to become more popular.

II. Reversed Time Segmentation

Reversed time segmentation offers very little security and, as a consequence, is generally regarded as merely a voice privacy technique. However, it adapts well to an 'implementation' with a microprocessor and the simplicity and low

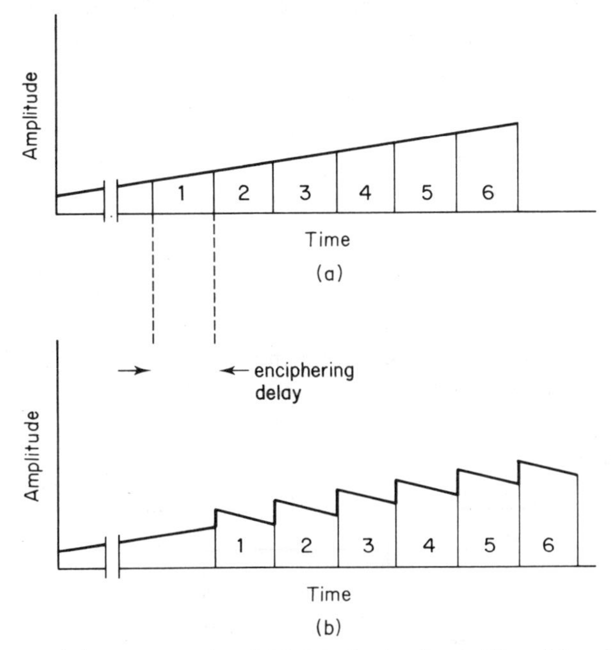

FIG. 5.1. Reversed time segmentation. (a) Original voice signal; (b) enciphered voice signal.

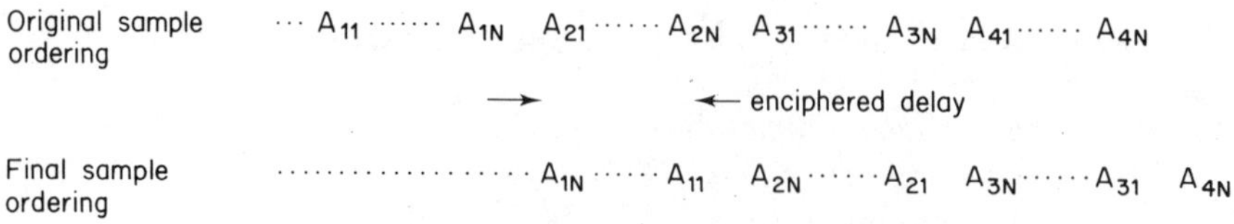

Original sample ordering $\cdots A_{11} \cdots\cdots A_{1N} \quad A_{21} \cdots\cdots A_{2N} \quad A_{31} \cdots\cdots A_{3N} \quad A_{41} \cdots\cdots A_{4N}$

$\longrightarrow$ $\longleftarrow$ enciphered delay

Final sample ordering $\cdots\cdots\cdots\cdots A_{1N} \cdots\cdots A_{11} \quad A_{2N} \cdots\cdots A_{21} \quad A_{3N} \cdots\cdots A_{31} \quad A_{4N}$

FIG. 5.2. Reordering of samples for reversed time segmentation.

cost of this implementation often lead to its use in situations where the security is not of paramount importance.

As a first step in *reversed time segmentation*, the analogue signal is sampled using, for example, PCM. The samples are divided into time segments which are stored in memory, and then the samples in each segment are delivered to the D/A converter in reverse temporal order. A typical system with the time segments labelled 1 to 6 is illustrated in Figs. 5.1 and 5.2 then shows the final order of the samples for this scheme when each segment contains N samples. The duration of the time segments is likely to vary according to the system requirements but might, typically, lie between 50 and 400 msec. From the figure it is clear that longer time segments cause longer delay times but, to balance this, they appear to provide lower residual intelligibility.

In this system the aim is to handle the incoming and outgoing speech simultaneously and this means that to generate the signal represented in Fig. 5.2 it is sufficient to have storage for just one segment of speech. As each sample is output from the store it is then replaced by the incoming sample. The system might be implemented by using *random access memory* (RAM) as shown in Fig. 5.3. If this is the case then the size of the RAM clearly restricts the length possible for the time segment. In order to illustrate how the memory size might affect the length of the segments we will look at a specific example. Suppose that an 8-bit PCM is used and that the sampling rate is 8 kHz. If we had an 8-kbit RAM, then we could use time segments which correspond to 1000 samples. Thus, for our particular sampling rate, the maximum possible segment length is $\frac{1}{8}$ sec or 125 msec.

Clearly if we perform reverse time segmentation on a signal for which the segments have already been reversed then, provided we do not change the

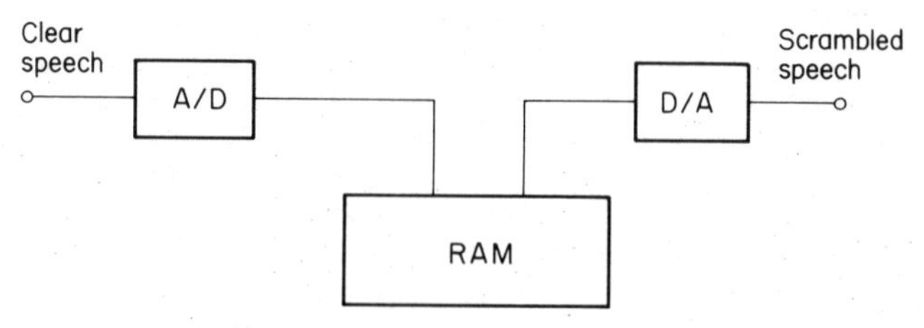

FIG. 5.3. Possible implementation of reversed time segmentation.

length of the segments, we will obtain the original signal. Thus, in this system the descrambler is identical to the scrambler. However, since they must use the same time boundaries, it is obviously crucial that the transmitter and receiver are synchronized. This is a problem we have already encountered and, as before, we will do no more than mention the problem, stress its importance and postpone our discussion until Chapter 6.

Now that we have described the system we must ask the same questions that we posed for the systems of Chapter 4. How well does the signal become scrambled? What is the quality of the reconstructed speech? To answer them we rely on the published results of Belland and Bryg (1978) who implemented reversed time segmentation for segment lengths varying from 50 to 400 msec. Their conclusions were

(a) the delivery rate of the speaker was a significant factor in deciding the residual intelligibility of the ciphered speech;
(b) with very slow speech rates a segment length of at least 250 msec was required to obscure the message content;
(c) 150-ms segments were too short to render even conventional speech unintelligible;
(d) there was no observable degradation in the quality of the recovered speech.

Their comments about the correlation between the delivery rate of the speaker and the residual intelligibility are not really surprising. In Section IV of Chapter 2 we saw how slowly speech can change with time (see, for instance, Fig. 2.19). In fact we noted there that a typical vowel sound is likely to last 100 msec. Given this, we should certainly not expect reversed time segmentation with segments of less than 100 msec to seriously affect the vowels. Of course speakers vary considerably and it is clear that the residual intelligibility for this type of system is likely to differ according to the characteristics of the various speakers.

Their conclusion about the voice quality may be rather more unexpected. However they are supported by Udalov (1980) who describes the small spectral distortion of the signal as one of the major advantages of the system. Using a segment size of 260 msec, Udalov says "Although a definite syllabic content was present in the encoded message, the sounds themselves were totally devoid of meaning. The recovered voice, however, was of excellent quality".

In our description of the system we talked about reversing the order of samples and assumed PCM to be the A/D converter. Clearly this is not a necessary requirement for the system and the basic concept should be possible with any type of A/D converter. However these different systems are likely to produce slightly varying performances. In particular, if we use a lower bit rate we are more likely to create spectral distortions.

The system that we have described so far has no key and is, therefore, a code rather than a cipher system. The situation is similar to the one we met when discussing frequency inversion. Now, as then, we can introduce a key and this is achieved by allowing the segment size to vary. However, the RAM size in the transmitter and receiver will, as we have seen, restrict the possibilities for the segment size. Thus the lengths of the segments are likely to be limited to a very small range. The extra security obtained in this way is also likely to be limited. One reason for this is that if an interceptor were to have a receiver adjusted to a fixed segment length, which was about the average size of all the possibilities, then he would obtain a signal which, although not sounding perfect, would exhibit a very high residual intelligibility.

Since it has the advantage of being relatively cheap and simple to implement, reversed time segmentation has been suggested for use in hand-held radios. It also appears to be insensitive to many potential channel deficiencies including, in particular, group delay variations which, as we have seen, cause the downfall of many other scrambling schemes. This insensitivity is a consequence of using reasonably long segment lengths. (We will say more about group delay when we discuss segment lengths for time element scramblers in Section III.) But, as we have already observed, these long segments have the disadvantage that they introduce system delay which, end-to-end, is twice the segment length i.e., typically about $\frac{1}{2}$ sec. We must point out however that, compared to some of the other systems we shall discuss, a system delay of $\frac{1}{2}$ sec might not appear to be too disastrous.

We will say more about reversed time segmentation in Chapter 6.

III. Time Element Scrambling

The basic idea behind the *time element scramblers* which we shall discuss in this chapter is quite similar to the bandsplitting which we discussed in Chapter 4. The technique is often referred to as *time division multiplexing* (TDM) or *time segment permutation* (TSP). The aim is to permute a number of time segments of the speech signal. There are essentially two different techniques, called the *hopping* (or *fixed*) *window* and the *sliding window*. We shall discuss them both.

A. The Hopping Window Technique

In this technique the analogue signal is divided into (equal) time periods called *frames*. Each frame is then sub-divided into smaller equal time periods called *segments*. Once this has been done the input is scrambled by permuting the segments within each of the frames. This process is illustrated in Fig. 5.4 where we have divided the frame into eight segments.

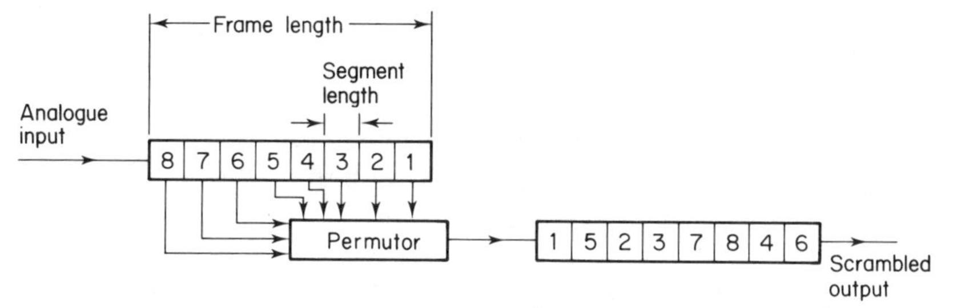

FIG. 5.4. Hopping window technique.

When setting up a hopping window system it is necessary to decide upon values for the lengths of the frames and segments. Clearly this decision is important. In this type of scrambling the signal within any given segment is not distorted and, furthermore, the segment length determines how much information is contained within that segment. This suggests that it is desirable to keep the segments as short as possible and, obviously, they must be short enough that complete words cannot be contained within a segment. Unfortunately the segment length also has a significant bearing on the audio quality of the recovered signal and this quality decreases as the segment lengths get smaller. Thus, as we saw so often in the earlier chapters, there is a balance to be made between the level of security and the audio quality. This balance is rather delicate and it is, perhaps, helpful to see why the degradation of the audio quality increases as the segment length decreases. The first reason is that permuting the segments causes discontinuities in the signal which, in turn, lead to an expansion in the bandwidth. Whenever we take a speech signal, 'cut it' up and then put it back differently we will, as can be seen clearly from Fig. 5.5, get discontinuities at the boundaries of the time segments. These sudden changes imply a high frequency component in our transmitted signal and, as a consequence, an increase in the bandwidth. Since these discontinuities only occur at the segment boundaries, the number of discontinuities is directly proportional to the number of segments. Thus if the segment length is decreased the number of discontinuities per unit time will increase and the distortion of the transmitted signal will get worse.

A second, but not unrelated, disadvantage of having short time segments can be seen by considering the system's sensitivity to the delay characteristics of the transmission channel. In Fig. 2.8 we saw a typical group delay characteristic for a voice channel. If the channel input is continuous speech then the effect of this is perceptually negligible. However the periodic discontinuities in permuted speech mean that, after the received signal segments have been reassembled in the correct order, the quality of the signal will be degraded. Furthermore an increase in the number of discontinuities

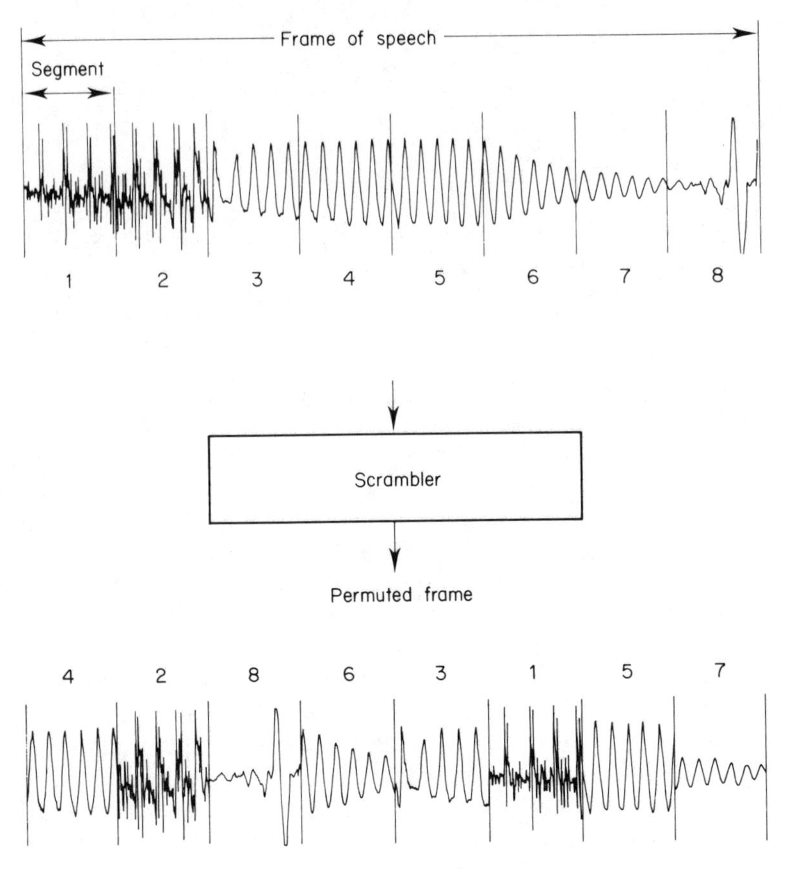

FIG. 5.5. Permutation of a frame of speech.

per unit time causes a corresponding increase in the degradation. The explanation of this is straightforward. The effect of the channel group delay variation is to smear the segment boundaries. This effect is illustrated in Fig. 5.6 from which it is clear that the segment length should certainly exceed the difference between the maximum and minimum delay with respect to frequency. This should then ensure that transient effects in the descrambled speech are not too objectionable.

In order to obtain some acceptable compromise between the security and audio quality requirements, most of the types of equipment which are currently available use a segment duration somewhere in the range of 16 to 60 msec.

The choice of the frame length is equally important. This choice affects the delay between the analogue signal being fed into the equipment and the

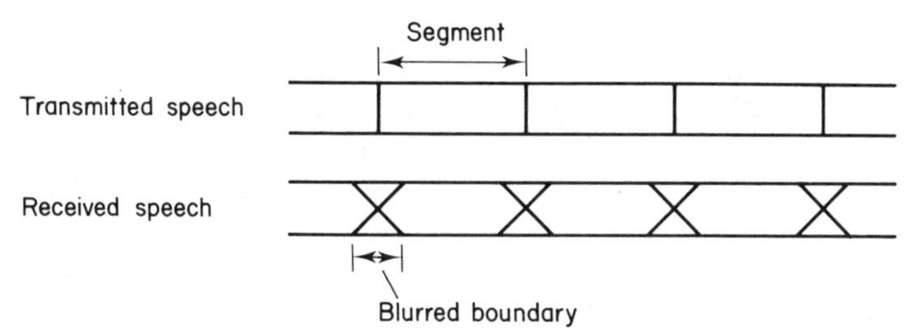

FIG. 5.6. Effect of group delay on boundaries.

signal being reconstructed as 'clear speech'. To see why this delay occurs we will look back at the example in Fig. 5.4. If, in this example, the segment length is T seconds then it takes $8T$ sec for all eight speech segments to enter the device. Although it is not so in our specific example, we may wish to permute the segments in such a way that segment 8 will be transmitted first. Consequently we will not start to transmit until all 8 segments are in the device. Thus since, for instance, segment 1 must be delayed by at least $8T$ sec, delays have already occurred. If we wish to allow all possible permutations of the 8 segments then we must be prepared for the possibility, as in fact actually happens in our example, that the last segment received may be the first one to be output. This means that the receiver cannot begin to decipher until he has received all 8 segments and implies a delay of another $8T$ sec. Thus, even if we assume that the actual transmission time is negligible, there is a time delay of $16T$ sec for each speech segment. (This is illustrated in Fig. 5.7 which shows what happens during the first $24T$ sec of transmission for the example of Fig. 5.4.) It is important to note here that, for our particular example, we only deduced that the delay had to be $16T$ sec because we wanted to be able to use all permutations of the 8 segments. In particular we were prepared to transmit segment 8 first and segment 1 last. In general if we wish to use all possible permutations of the segments then for a system with m segments per frame the time delay is $2mT$ sec.

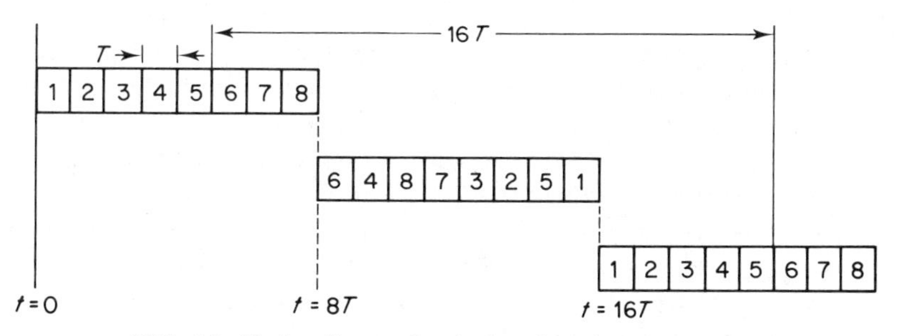

FIG. 5.7. Timing diagram for the hopping window process.

As we have already said, this delay is similar to that experienced on international telephone calls which are transmitted via satellite. From the user's point of view they are undesirable and present a case for making the number of segments per frame as small as possible. Unfortunately, (yes, you've guessed it!) from the security point of view we need long frames. One reason is, quite simply, that if we have m segments per frame than we have $m!$ possible permutations to use. Clearly if we have too few permutations then an interceptor will be able to try them all. The larger the number of possible permutations the less likely an interceptor is to be able to guess the correct one. Another reason is that, as we saw when discussing phonemes, a speech sound can last for quite a long time. To see this we merely have to look back at Fig. 2.19 which shows how slowly the speech spectrum changes. This was also a problem for reversed time segmentation. To illustrate how disastrous short frames can be, we have only to consider an example in which there is a frame which consists of a single tone. No matter which permutation is used the resultant signal will still be a single continuous note, (but almost certainly degraded in quality as a result of our tampering). Although this example is extreme it nevertheless shows that, if we make our frames too short, we may not be able to achieve sufficient dispersement of the segments. This may result in significant parts of words being unaltered and allow a listener to guess part, or even all, of the message.

There is no obvious mathematical way for choosing optimal values for the lengths of the segments or frames. In practice it is necessary to test any given choice experimentally. One good, and very demanding, test for a time element scrambler is to read out, in an arbitrary order, some numbers between one and ten and for a group of listeners to write down what they 'hear' when listening to the scrambled message. We have already met this test and know that, since the listener is only trying to distinguish between ten possible sounds, it is a considerably more demanding test of the scrambler than asking listeners to understand scrambled messages for which they do not know the context. Experiments show that, unless there are a large number of segments per frame, most time element scramblers perform badly against this test.

As a general rule the frame length should be as long as the user will accept. Within most of these types of equipment which are currently available a frame comprises between eight and sixteen segments.

When the lengths of the segments and frames have been chosen the final 'ingredient' for a hopping window time element scrambler is the permutation. As we saw when discussing bandsplitters, some permutations are better than others and we must now try to decide which ones are most suitable for our system. We must also decide how to use these permutations. As in the case of band-shift inverters or bandscramblers there are a number of ways in which we can use our basic system. We can, for instance, have a key which selects one fixed permutation and then use this given permutation for every frame. Another possibility is to let our key select several permutations and then repeatedly use them in some fixed order. We discussed these possibilities in section III of Chapter 4 and, as we said in that discussion, a better idea is to employ some form of pseudo-random number generator to select a different permutation for each frame. If we have 8 segments per frame then the total number of available permutations is $8! = 40{,}320$. So, if each segment has a duration of 40 msec, after about 3.6 h of continuous usage we must be using some of the permutations for at least the second time. However, as we saw in Chapter 4, the pattern of permutations used will not begin to repeat until the sequence repeats i.e., the period of the pseudo-random number sequence determines the period of the sequence of permutations used. Although with 8 segments there are 40,320 possible permutations, some will offer more security than others and we may not wish to use them all. This, of course, is precisely the situation which we encountered in Chapter 4. We must, just as we did then, decide what constitutes a 'good' permutation and then use only those which pass some form of 'scoring test'. If α is a permutation on the 8 segments such that the ith segment is moved to the $\alpha(i)$ position then, as usual, we will write

$$\alpha = \begin{bmatrix} 1 & 2 & 3 & 4 & 5 & 6 & 7 & 8 \\ \alpha(1) & \alpha(2) & \alpha(3) & \alpha(4) & \alpha(5) & \alpha(6) & \alpha(7) & \alpha(8) \end{bmatrix}$$

So the permutation which represents the example of Fig. 5.4 is

$$\begin{bmatrix} 1 & 2 & 3 & 4 & 5 & 6 & 7 & 8 \\ 8 & 6 & 5 & 2 & 7 & 1 & 4 & 3 \end{bmatrix}$$

The criteria for good permutations in this context are slightly different to those which were appropriate for bandsplitters. However one common necessity is that a suitable permutation for a hopping window time domain scrambler must have a high shift factor. Before discussing the general principles for determining good permutations we will give two examples.

Example 1 $\begin{bmatrix} 1 & 2 & 3 & 4 & 5 & 6 & 7 & 8 \\ 1 & 3 & 2 & 4 & 5 & 7 & 6 & 8 \end{bmatrix}$

Example 2 $\begin{bmatrix} 1 & 2 & 3 & 4 & 5 & 6 & 7 & 8 \\ 8 & 3 & 1 & 6 & 4 & 2 & 7 & 5 \end{bmatrix}$

If we were able to listen to the effects of each of these two we would find that the first has a very high residual intelligibility. In fact, after only a few repetitions we would probably begin to understand the message. The second permutation would give a far lower residual intelligibility and it is doubtful whether our understanding would increase after the first few hearings. One reason for this disparity is, clearly, that the shift factor of the first permutation is only 4 while the second has a shift factor of 20. But this is not the only reason and we must try to determine some others. The situation is obviously very similar to the one we considered for bandsplitters. Once again we need to be able either to apply listening tests to decide which permutations are good or else to devise some type of scoring system based on a sample of listening tests. It is the latter alternative which is usually adopted, particularly as the number of possible permutations starts to increase. We have already seen an example of a scoring scheme in Chapter 4. Rather than simply give another one here we will list some steps which need to be taken before a sensible scheme can be devised. They are:

(a) Perform some listening tests to determine a set of general rules concerning the correlation between the various properties of the permutations and the residual intelligibility of the resultant signal.
(b) Devise a scoring scheme based on these general rules.
(c) Rank a random set of permutations according to this scoring scheme and perform a further set of listening tests to examine the correlation between the scores of the permutations and the residual intelligibility.
(d) Use the results of the tests in (c) to determine a threshold score above which a permutation may be considered 'good'.

As we have already observed, the tests in step (a) show that, without doubt, a high shift factor is necessary for low residual intelligibility. However, a high shift factor, alone, does not offer any guarantees. As an illustration we will give a third permutation which has a very high shift factor of 32 but which leaves a high residual intelligibility. (The reasons will soon become apparent!)

$$\text{Example 3} \qquad \begin{bmatrix} 1 & 2 & 3 & 4 & 5 & 6 & 7 & 8 \\ 8 & 6 & 5 & 7 & 1 & 3 & 2 & 4 \end{bmatrix}$$

Apart from its low shift factor, Example 1 has a number of other undesirable properties. Consider, for instance, the consecutive segments 4 and 5. In the scrambled frame they appear in the same consecutive order. Thus if segments are approximately 40 msec long, this gives about 80 msec of the original speech signal. As we have already observed, most phonemes can be clearly recognized within this sort of time interval. Now look at the segments 6 and 8. In both Examples 1 and 3 they appear as consecutive elements and, although it is not immediately apparent, this is also undesirable. Perception trials have established that if the scrambled signal has two consecutive segments of the type i and $i + 2$, for some i, then the listener will usually be able to deduce the corresponding part of the message; the human brain is able to improvise and 'fill in' the missing segment. (The reader should not find this too surprising. As we have already observed, if we hold a telephone conversation on a 'noisy' line then we are usually able to understand the entire conversation although we do not actually hear every syllable.) As well as being able to 'fill in' missing segments the brain also naturally rejects superfluous segments. Thus patterns like $i?(i + 1)$ in the scrambled signal also lead to a high residual intelligibility. To a lesser extent the patterns $i?(i + 2)$, $i?(i + 3)$, $i??(i + 2)$ and $i??(i + 3)$ also yield some residual intelligibility. [In case it is not clear, when we say that the scrambled signal has a pattern like $i??(i + 3)$ for some i, we mean that it contains two segments which, in both the original and scrambled message, are only separated by two other segments. For instance in Example 3 the scrambled frame contains 5768 in positions 1 to 4. This is of the form $i??(i + 3)$ with $i = 5$. Similarly Example 3 has 324 in positions 5 to 7 and this is of the form $i?(i + 1)$ with $i = 3$.]

It is perhaps worth mentioning here that there is another way of writing permutations which, in this particular context, has the definite advantage that it exhibits the patterns more clearly. If we look back at Fig. 5.4 we actually see the segments in the order in which they appear. In other words, since segment 1 is moved to the 8th position and segment 2 goes to position 6 etc., we actually see the pattern 6 4 8 7 3 2 5 1. If we chose to write our permutations in this way, then Example 1 would be written as (1 3 2 4 5 7 6 8), Example 2 would be (3 6 2 5 8 4 7 1) and Example 3 would be (5 7 6 8 3 2 4 1). With this representation statements like, for instance, "segments 6 and 8 appear as consecutive elements in Examples 1 and 3" become easier to verify. This notation is not, however, quite so convenient for a number of other purposes including, for instance, computing the shift factor.

Once we have decided what determines a good permutation we must try to find some. Suppose we decided that we wanted permutations on eight segments which have no patterns of the following types:

$$i(i + 1),\ i?(i + 1),\ i(i + 2),\ i?(i + 2),\ i??(i + 2),\ i?(i + 3),\ i??(i + 3).$$

Suppose, furthermore, that we asked for a shift factor of at least 20 and that the first segment was moved. (This last demand is to ensure that two consecutive segments which occur at the end and beginning of consecutive frames are not adjacent in the scrambled message.) Anyone who tries to achieve this by merely writing down permutations and then checking to see if they have the desired properties will probably find himself writing down a large number of permutations. This is because a very small proportion of the 40,320 permutations satisfy them. Even if a permutation satisfies them all, it must still be subjected to listening tests before we can be confident it will have a low residual intelligibility.

The precise conditions which must be demanded of a permutation are highly subjective and various people suggest different criteria. As a consequence there are considerable discrepancies in values for the number of good permutations. For instance it is claimed (Telsy Systems, 1979) that about 20,000 of the permutations on 8 letters are useful. MacKinnon (1980), on the other hand, says that only about 3000 are good and Jayant (1982) reports that, in certain circumstances the number may be as low as about 40. Clearly these three authors are applying somewhat different criteria and/or standards.

In order to see how we might try to reach a conclusion for ourselves, we will assume that we have devised a scoring scheme to rank the permutations and see how we might try to assess it. One obvious means by which the closeness of our scoring system to actual residual intelligibility might be estimated is to order the permutations using each of the two criteria and then compare the rankings. As an example suppose that we have a set of 20 permutations on which we have performed listening tests and have obtained

TABLE 5.1

Rank Correlation Using Spearman's Coefficient

Listening test	Scoring system	D	D^2	$\sum_{i=0}^{n} D^2$
1	1	0	0	0
2	2	0	0	0
3	3	0	0	0
4	5	−1	1	1
5	11	−6	36	37
6	8	−2	4	41
7	4	3	9	50
8	12	−4	16	66
9	7	2	4	70
10	20	−10	100	170
11	6	5	25	195
12	17	−5	25	220
13	9	4	16	236
14	16	−2	4	240
15	10	5	25	265
16	18	−2	4	269
17	14	3	9	278
18	19	−1	1	279
19	15	4	16	295
20	13	7	49	344

the ordering shown in column 1 of Table 5.1. (In practice we would probably obtain such an order by averaging the orders proposed by a number of listeners.)

Thus we are essentially using the listener's ordering to label the permutations so that permutation 1 gave the highest residual intelligibility and permutation 20 gave the least. Suppose that our scoring system is designed so that a high score corresponds to a high residual intelligibility and that column 2 of Table 5.1 has ranked the permutations according to this system. So, for instance, permutation 1 has the highest score, permutation 7 has the fourth highest score and permutation 10 has the lowest score. There are a number of methods for measuring the correlation between two different rankings like those in this table. One such method is to calculate *Spearman's rank order correlations*, r, which is given by

$$r = 1 - [6 \sum D^2/n(n^2 - 1)]$$

where D is the difference in the rank orders for any given permutation. In Table 5.1, column 3 shows the values for D, column 4 shows D^2 and column 5 then shows the sum of the values of D^2. For our example $n = 20$, so we have $r = 1 - (6 \times 344)/20(400 - 1) = 0.74$.

It is fairly easy to show that, for any two orderings, the value of r always lies between -1 and 1. A value of 1 corresponds to perfect correlation, 0 implies no correlation and -1 indicates an 'inverse' correlation. In order to decide whether a particular value of r is good enough we can refer to published tables of critical values for Spearman's coefficient. As an example we show, in Table 5.2, a list of the values of r for 5% and 1% significance levels for some possible values of n. For our particular example we had $n = 20$ so from the table we can see that a 5% significance level corresponds to $r = 0.450$ and a 1% significance level corresponds to $r = 0.591$. Thus, with our value of 0.74 we can certainly claim 99% confidence in the correlation between listening tests and this particular scoring system. We might now try various other scoring systems to see which give the best value for r.

There are, of course, many other tests for comparing different rankings. One particular example is to calculate *Kendall's coefficient* $\varkappa$ which is given by

$$\varkappa = 1 - (4\tau)/n(n - 1)$$

where τ is the minimum number of transpositions of adjacent characters to go from one ranking to another. Kendall's coefficient is much more difficult to calculate than Spearman's coefficient and, consequently, this test is used less frequently. For a comparison of various tests of this type we refer the reader to Kak (1983).

TABLE 5.2

Critical Values for Spearman's Coefficient

n	5%	1%
5	1.000	—
6	0.886	1.000
7	0.786	0.929
8	0.738	0.881
9	0.683	0.833
10	0.648	0.794
12	0.591	0.777
14	0.544	0.715
16	0.506	0.665
18	0.478	0.628
20	0.450	0.591
22	0.428	0.562
24	0.409	0.537
26	0.392	0.515
28	0.377	0.496
30	0.364	0.478

Once we have chosen our particular scoring system and are happy with its performance, we can then set a threshold and, since we are assuming that a high score corresponds to a high residual intelligibility, decree that any permutation whose score exceeds this threshold is unacceptable. Thus we will use only those permutations which score less than the threshold. (Note that with some schemes, like the one used in Chapter 4, a low score corresponds to a high residual intelligibility. For these schemes we reject permutations which score less than the threshold.) Once this is agreed then we have to decide how our key is going to select the good permutations. Since there is obviously an advantage to be gained from changing the permutation after every frame, we have basically two choices. We can allow the sequence generator to produce arbitrary permutations and then screen them in some way, probably using our scoring system, to ensure that we only use those which meet our requirements. The other possibility is to generate some (or all) of the good permutations, store them in a ROM within the equipment and then let the sequence generator select pseudo-randomly from the ROM. Not surprisingly these are two of the options which we met in the last chapter. However, our situation is now slightly different and we will consider the relative merits of each alternative in our current context.

The main disadvantage of the first alternative is the time factor. By the end of each frame we must have selected a 'good' permutation for the next frame. But if we merely let our sequence generator choose permutations pseudo-randomly then, although statistically the probability may be very high, we cannot guarantee that it will produce a 'good' one in time. So, in this case, we need to incorporate some contingency plan to protect ourselves from this possibility. This could, for example, allow the use of a previous permutation for a second time. Other possibilities include relaxing the screening conditions as time runs out or simply allowing extra time to wait for a 'good' permutation. But all are undesirable. On the other hand the system has one big advantage. This is that, once we have a reasonable sequence generator and algorithm for generating permutations from that sequence, all the good permutations can be used. In contrast the ROM method only allows the use of those permutations which are stored. If our store is not big enough then this will not be all the good permutations. Furthermore we must assume that a determined interceptor will know the contents of our ROM. (This corresponds to our worst case condition WC1.) When there are only 8 segments/frame then, if we take the 'strictest' definition of 'good', the number of such permutations is small enough that we can probably store them all. When this happens the ROM method is usually considered preferable. But, as soon as we start using more than eight segments per frame, the limitation on the number of permutations, which can actually be used, is certainly a disadvantage of our second method.

One definite advantage of the ROM method is that, just as we did for bandsplitters in Chapter 4, we can introduce the concept of mutual security. If we are adopting the first alternative and using our sequence generator to generate permutations directly, then there is nothing we can do to eliminate the possibility of someone with a similar device using the wrong key but, nevertheless, generating inverse permutations which will partially descramble our permutation. All we can do is rely on the fact that the number of permutations is so large that the probability of the interceptor succeeding in this way is small. However, with only eight segments to a frame, the total number of good permutations is, in our opinion, not large enough for us to trust to 'luck' and the system is liable to be broken by straightforward trial and error. If, however, we are only using permutations which we have selected and stored in a ROM then, at the cost of further reducing the number of usable 'good' permutations, we can protect ourselves by ensuring that the sorted permutations are mutually secure. Testing mutual security can be achieved either in the direct way described in Chapter 4 or by using a rank correlation test. This latter scheme involves testing permutations for 'closeness' by means of a rank correlation test similar to Spearman's coefficient. It also seems to be possible to choose a method of permutation generation which will ensure a low correlation between the permutations produced, see for example Kak (1983). However, certainly when the number of segments per frame is small, a direct testing scheme seems preferable.

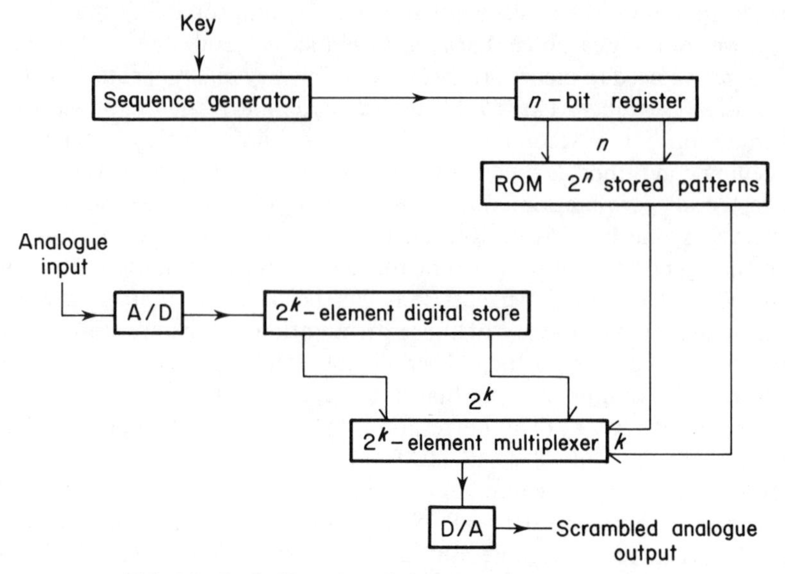

FIG. 5.8. Typical hopping window time element scrambler.

Clearly the selection and generation of the good permutations is a fundamental aspect of the hopping window technique. However, we have probably said all that we can on the topic and will now return to discussing the overall system. Figure 5.8 is a block diagram for a typical hopping window time domain scrambler. The A/D conversion at the input facilitates the storing and processing of the speech. Once it is converted to digital form, the signal is fed into a store of 2^k elements, where 2^k is the number of segments per frame. (So in our example, where we have been using 8 segments/frame, $k = 3$.) Each element of this store contains the number of digital samples appropriate to a particular segment. The segments are then removed from the store according to addresses from the ROM containing the permutation. Finally the signal is reconverted to analogue form for transmission. In practice, the 2^k-element digital store will be a RAM and the multiplexing, i.e., selecting the correct elements from the store at any given time, will be microprocessor based with the store addresses held within the ROM. If the sequence generator is used to generate patterns in real time then the n-bit register and ROM must be replaced by a processor (or complex piece of hardware) to determine permutations and screen them for low residual intelligibility.

As an example of the above process we will consider a system with $k = 3$ and assume that our 8-element store is as in Fig. 5.9(a). Each time a segment is withdrawn all those to the left of it are shifted one position to the right

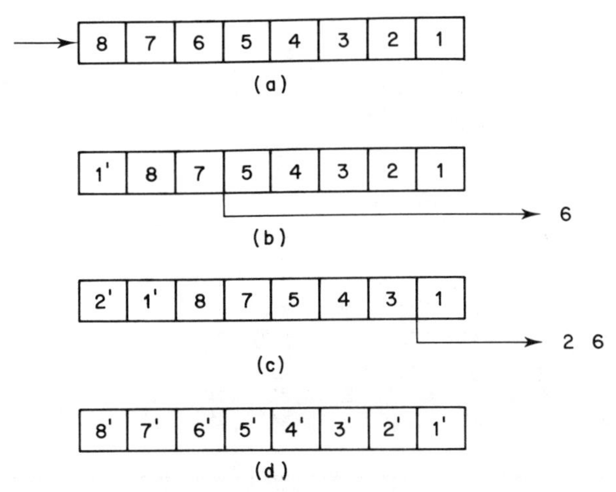

FIG. 5.9. Example of storage organisation. (a) 8-element store, (b) segment 6 removed, (c) segment 2 removed and (d) new window ready for permuting.

and a new segment is introduced on the left. Thus if, for instance, we were to withdraw segment 6 first then the store would be as in Fig. 5.9(b), where $1'$ represents segment 1 of the next frame. If we then withdrew segment 2 our store would be as in Fig. 5.9(c) and eventually we would reach the situation of Fig. 5.9(d), where we have a new window of 8 segments ready for permuting. If we let α be the permutation for this example then, so far, we know $\alpha(6) = 1$ and $\alpha(2) = 2$. Suppose that α was the permutation

$$\begin{bmatrix} 1 & 2 & 3 & 4 & 5 & 6 & 7 & 8 \\ 4 & 2 & 6 & 5 & 8 & 1 & 3 & 7 \end{bmatrix}$$

Then the order in which the segments leave the store would be 6, 2, 7, 1, 4, 3, 8, 5, i.e., 7 would be withdrawn third, 1 would be fourth, etc. The succession of states is shown in Table 5.3. It is important, here, to note that the ROM would not actually contain the permutation itself but the address from which each segment should be withdrawn. Thus from Table 5.3 we see that, for this particular example, the ROM would contain 6, 2, 5, 1, 2, 1, 2, 1. Of course the system we have just described is just one of many possibilities for organising the store.

Before leaving hopping window systems to discuss the sliding window technique we must investigate the security of a hopping window system. This, as we have already stressed, is dependent on the length of the time delay which the operator is prepared to accept. One of the designer's major problems is to find the appropriate balance between time delay and residual intelligibility.

TABLE 5.3

The Succession of States of the Store

Cells								
8	7	6	5	4	3	2	1	Output
1′	8	7	5	4	3	2	1	6
2′	1′	8	7	5	4	3	1	2
3′	2′	1′	8	5	4	3	1	7
4′	3′	2′	1′	8	5	4	3	1
5′	4′	3′	2′	1′	8	5	3	4
6′	5′	4′	3′	2′	1′	8	5	3
7′	6′	5′	4′	3′	2′	1′	5	8
8′	7′	6′	5′	4′	3′	2′	1′	5

One important fact in this context is the variation between different languages. When considering the English language most authors recommend that the segment length should not be longer than 50–60 msec. However Beth *et al.* (1983) considered the German language and concluded that, since most Germans tend to talk slowly, the segment length should be 75 msec. For an 8-segment frame this implies a frame length of 600 msec and, consequently, a system delay of 1.2 sec. In order to reach this conclusion, Beth *et al.* performed a number of listening tests using their experimental hopping window time element scrambler. Their results are interesting and we will discuss them so that we can then compare them with other results in Chapter 6.

One of the tests which they performed was to record seven 'texts' of 20 four-digit numbers. Each digit in each of these four-digit numbers was spoken individually, e.g., 3-8-6-4, and after each four-digit number there was a pause of about two seconds. The texts were designed so that each digit

TABLE 5.4

The Sets of Three Texts Used

Scheme	First text heard	Second text heard	Third text heard
1	1	2	4
2	2	3	5
3	3	4	6
4	4	5	7
5	5	6	1
6	6	7	2
7	7	1	3

occurred eight times, twice in each of the four possible positions. Each listener was asked to listen to three texts and the schemes for doing this were as shown in Table 5.4. (This arrangement ensured that each text occurred once in each position within the three texts. The permutations used for each of the seven texts are shown in Table 5.5. Here, as when discussing our scoring system earlier in this chapter, we represent the permutation by listing the segments in the order in which they actually appear. Thus, for example, (7 1 3 4 5 2 6 8) is the permutation

$$\begin{bmatrix} 1 & 2 & 3 & 4 & 5 & 6 & 7 & 8 \\ 2 & 6 & 3 & 4 & 5 & 7 & 1 & 8 \end{bmatrix}$$

TABLE 5.5

The Permutations Used for Each Text

Text	Permutation used
1	random permutation changing every frame
2	fixed permutation: (1 2 3 4 8 6 5 7)
3	fixed permutation: (7 1 3 4 5 2 6 8)
4	fixed permutation: (7 2 6 3 4 5 8 1)
5	fixed permutation: (6 4 8 1 2 7 3 5)
6	fixed permutation: (5 6 7 8 1 2 3 4)
7	fixed permutation: (6 5 8 7 2 1 4 3)

The listeners were asked to write down their best guess for each number and to avoid leaving blanks. The results are given in Table 5.6. The most dramatic result is the significantly better performance of text 1 for which the changing permutations were used. (Do not forget that someone who did not even hear the texts would get about 10% of the digits correct by random guesswork.)

TABLE 5.6

The Results of the Listening Tests

Text	Number of identified digits	Percentage of digits identified
1	708	29.5
2	2173	90.5
3	2144	89.3
4	1486	61.9
5	1609	67.0
6	1949	81.2
7	1415	59.0

Another question mark against the security of the hopping window concerns the resistance to 'parallel listening'. We have already discussed the cocktail party syndrome and noted the brain's remarkable ability to concentrate on one particular conversation even when the level of that particular conversation is no higher than several others within close proximity. This suggests one possible method of attack for an interceptor. He could playback all the segments simultaneously during each segment period of the frame and attempt to hear what was being said. Not surprisingly the success rate for this type of attack is dependent on the number of segments per frame. If there are only four segments per frame then it appears that this line of attack is likely to be, at least partially, successful. However, we have seen no evidence to suggest that it is successful for eight or more segments per frame.

Another possible approach for the cryptanalyst is to attempt, via various techniques like listening or unscrambling spectrograms, to unscramble enough frames that, with his assumed knowledge of the ROM or screening process, he can deduce sufficient output from the sequence generator that he may be able to deduce the entire key used. But this is precisely the situation we discussed in Chapter 3. To counteract this we need a sequence generator that is difficult to break; i.e., one for which knowledge of a section of the sequence does not enable the cryptanalyst to determine the key within any reasonable time.

Let us assume that our system is secure against this approach. This means that the only way in which the cryptanalyst can deduce our message is by unscrambling each individual frame. Clearly, then, the time required to obtain the message is directly proportional to the number of frames. Having said that we must stress that it is often possible to determine the information within a frame without a perfect unscrambling. Furthermore if the cryptanalyst knows the ROM contents or screening process, then he knows precisely which permutations he needs to try for the unscrambling. He might even be able to build an automatic system to try each possibility and analyse which possibilities give a signal most like speech.

This may, for example, involve writing a program to analyse a spectrogram and then use a jigsaw approach to fit the pieces together in the correct order. Another interesting possibility is to use the computer to match the beginnings and endings of the shifted segments. This might then lead to the correct rearrangement necessary to unscramble the speech. One such strategy, which has been suggested, is to consider each pair of segments in a frame and assign to them a value which reflects the probability, based on the beginnings and endings of those segments, that they should follow each other in the unscrambled speech. Once these values have been assigned an algorithm can be produced to rearrange the segments in such a way as to be most consistent with them.

TABLE 5.7

The Assigned Values

Segment A	Segment B	Likelihood that B followed A
1	2	6
1	3	1
1	4	3
2	1	4
2	3	4
2	4	2
3	1	1
3	2	7
3	4	2
4	1	2
4	2	3
4	3	5

As an example we will consider a four-segment scrambled frame whose segments are labelled 1, 2, 3, 4. We shall suppose that, based on some kind of scoring scheme, we have been able to assign the values shown in Table 5.7 to indicate the likelihood that segment B follows segment A in the unscrambled speech. Using this table we can consider each of the 24 possible rearrangements of these four segments to see which provides the 'best fit'. So, for instance, we may decide to assign to each rearrangement a number which is the product of the numbers assigned to its three component pairs. Thus, for example, in the frame 2413 we have 2 followed by 4, 4 followed by 1 and 1 followed by 3. So, since from Table 5.7, the numbers assigned to 24, 41 and 13 are 2, 2 and 1 respectively we assign 4 ($= 2 \times 2 \times 1$) to the arrangement 2413. The complete set of values assigned to each possibility for the unscrambled frame is given in Table 5.8. From this table we would deduce that 4321, with a score of 140, was the most likely rearrangement of the unscrambled speech.

It is important to realise that assigning numbers to the possible rearrangements by multiplying the numbers for the three 'components' of pairs may not be the optimum way of determining the best fit. We may have to try other possibilities and then test them practically.

It is also possible to devise methods of obtaining a spectrogram in real time by using a Fourier transform; a coding device could convert the spectrum to a digital form and a fast computer could then do the matching. This, however, represents an extremely sophisticated and rather expensive strategy for the cryptanalyst. It is likely to be beyond the ability of most interceptors and its efficiency would decrease rapidly as the number of

TABLE 5.8

The Assigned Numbers

Segment ordering	Assigned number
1234	48
1243	60
1324	14
1342	6
1423	36
1432	105
2134	8
2143	60
2314	12
2341	16
2413	4
2431	10
3124	12
3142	9
3214	84
3241	28
3412	24
3421	24
4123	48
4132	14
4213	12
4231	12
4312	30
4321	140

available permutations grew larger. Thus to guard against this possibility we need as large a number of 'good' permutations as possible which, in turn, requires a larger frame. But, as we have already seen, this type of time division system can cause a time delay which is twice the frame length. Thus, when we increase the frame we also have the undesirable effect of increasing the delay. But, if we now look back to Fig. 5.7 and the accompanying discussion, we see that a time delay of twice the frame length was only necessary because every permutation was allowed and, as a consequence, a segment could be delayed for the entire duration of the frame. Thus, if we limit our permutations so that no segment is delayed for 'too long' we can reduce the delay time. This is called a *sliding window system*. Before we discuss sliding window systems we must make one important observation. In our discussions, so far, we have regarded the segments as indivisible. Consequently we assumed that a segment could not be transmitted until it had all been received. In practice, of course, this is not necessarily true.

However, our aim is merely to illustrate the type of considerations involved and so, since it simplifies the discussion considerably, we will continue to make this assumption. Referring back to Fig. 5.7 again, we see that there were two causes for the delay. First the transmitter had to wait for all segments to arrive before he could start his transmission (this was to allow for the possibility that the permutation might 'shift' the last segment to the first position). Then the recipient had to wait for all of them to be received before he could start to decipher (this was in case the permutation had shifted the first segment to the last position). The principle behind a sliding window system is to choose only those permutations which do not shift any segment too far and, in this way, the time is reduced.

B. The Sliding Window Technique

There are a number of variations of the sliding window principle. We shall begin this section with a fairly detailed discussion of a simple example and then extend our arguments to consider some alternative strategies.

If we look back at Fig. 5.9 and Table 5.3 it is interesting to note that, in our example of a possible method for organising the storage of segments in the scrambler, there were nearly always segments in memory that could not be accessed. These were the segments which belonged to the next frame. This must, in some sense, be considered an uneconomical use of the store and a sliding window scrambler attempts to make use of all the segments in the store at any given moment. Suppose, for example, that we have a four-segment store at the transmitter then, at any given time, we would like to be able to select any element from that store. We shall soon see that this is achieveable provided that we are prepared to impose constraints in order to ensure that the time delay does not become too excessive. In Table 5.9 we show one possibility for the process at the scrambler store. In this table the first column shows the new segment of speech being input to the scrambler, the next four columns show the contents of the store, the sixth column shows the store being selected at any given time and the final column shows the segment being output. Note that in this case, unlike the example of Table 5.3, we are simply replacing each segment which is output by inputting the next segment in the vacant storage element. This is certainly feasible with a RAM and, although not the only possible strategy, we will adopt it to simplify our explanation of the overall system.

At the start of the process depicted in Table 5.9 we simply fill the four storage elements. The next store to be selected is 4 and segment 4, which is the content of that storage element, is passed to the output while segment 5 enters the fourth store. If we look, for instance, at the seventh time slot we see that store 1 is selected, its content, which is element 6, is passed to the

TABLE 5.9

The Scrambling Process

Input segment	Storage elements 4	3	2	1	Store selected	Output segment
1	—	—	—	1	1	—
2	—	—	2	1	2	—
3	—	3	2	1	3	—
4	4	3	2	1	4	—
5	5	3	2	1	4	4
6	5	3	2	6	1	1
7	5	3	2	7	1	6
8	5	3	8	7	2	2
9	5	9	8	7	3	3
10	5	9	8	10	1	7
11	11	9	8	10	4	5
12	11	9	12	10	2	8
13	11	9	13	10	2	12
14	11	9	14	10	2	13
15	11	9	15	10	2	14
16	11	16	15	10	3	9
17	11	16	15	17	1	10
18	18	16	15	17	4	11
19	18	19	15	17	3	16
20	18	19	20	17	2	15
—	18	19	—	17	2	20
—	—	19	—	17	4	18
—	—	—	—	17	3	19
—	—	—	—	—	1	17

output and the new segment, which at this time is segment 7, is inserted into store 1. Since each element is erased from the store as soon as it has been transmitted, it is impossible for the same element to be transmitted twice. However, with the scheme as it is at present, it is certainly possible for us never to access a particular store. Were this to happen one of the elements would never be transmitted which, of course, would cause horrific problems at the receiver. Not only would there be an infinite delay but the receiver would also need an infinite store to accommodate the remainder of the message. This potential hazard can be avoided by setting a maximum delay on any segment which, in turn, can be achieved by ensuring that each store is reselected within a predetermined number of segment periods. This number will probably be related to the number of stores at the receiver.

In this system the task of the descrambler is to replace each element in its correct position relative to the remainder of the message. If this is done then the elements enter the scrambler and leave the descrambler in the same order which means they must all suffer the same delay. Thus if we let d represent the total delay, in terms of segment periods, and if a given element is delayed for d_s segment periods at the scrambler then it must be delayed for d_d segment periods at the receiver, where $d = d_s + d_d$.

In Table 5.10 we give one possible descrambling process for the scheme of Table 5.9. Although we have chosen to put four storage elements in the descrambler there is no reason why the scrambler and descrambler should contain the same number of elements. Having the same number does, however, often simplify the operation and also makes practical sense since, if two way communications are required, a scrambler may also be required to act as a descrambler. By comparing Tables 5.9 and 5.10 we can see that the total time delay is 8 segment periods, (corresponding to the total storage in receiver and transmitter), and that, as predicted, each time segment is

TABLE 5.10

The Descrambling Process

	Storage elements					
Input segment	4	3	2	1	Store selected	Output segment
4	—	—	—	4	1	—
1	—	—	1	4	2	—
6	—	6	1	4	3	—
2	2	6	1	4	4	—
3	2	6	3	4	2	1
7	7	6	3	4	4	2
5	7	6	5	4	2	3
8	7	6	5	8	1	4
12	7	6	12	8	2	5
13	7	13	12	8	3	6
14	14	13	12	8	4	7
9	14	13	12	9	1	8
10	14	13	12	10	1	9
11	14	13	12	11	1	10
16	14	13	12	16	1	11
15	14	13	15	16	2	12
20	14	20	15	16	3	13
18	18	20	15	16	4	14
19	18	20	19	16	2	15
17	18	20	19	17	1	16
—	18	20	19	—	1	17
—	—	20	19	—	4	18
—	—	20	—	—	2	19
—	—	—	—	—	3	20

delayed in the descrambler by $8 - d_s$ segment periods. So, for example, segment 7 spends three segment periods in the scrambler and five in the descrambler. Since we are assuming that each segment must be fully received before it can be output, we are assuming that each segment must spend at least one period in the descrambler which, for our example, implies a maximum delay of seven segment periods in the scrambler. Thus, we must ensure that each store is selected at least once within every seven segment periods, and this must override all our other requirements. So if a pseudo-random number generator is being used for store selection then it must be interrupted if any of the stores has not been accessed for 'too long'. We now look at some scrambling and descrambling algorithms which will ensure that the system works.

1. *A Scrambling Algorithm*

In Fig. 5.10 we show the flow diagram of a possible scrambling algorithm. Although, for this diagram, we have restricted ourselves to our small example it should be clear how to generalise this approach to larger, more complicated systems. If we label the counters corresponding to the storage elements

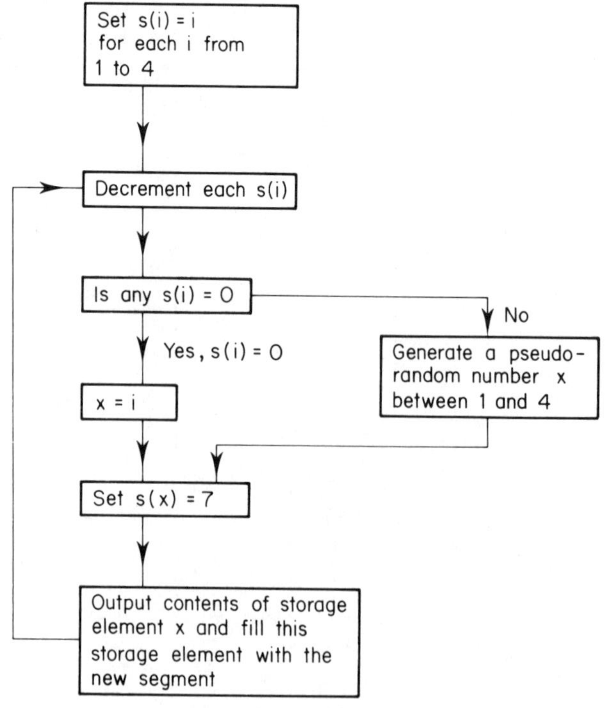

FIG. 5.10. Flow diagram for the scrambler.

$s(1)$, $s(2)$, $s(3)$ and $s(4)$, then to initialise our program we set $s(i) = i$. At the start of each round we decrement each $s(i)$ and check to see if any $s(i) = 0$. If there is a store j with $s(j) = 0$ then we must use store j. If not, we generate a pseudo-random number to indicate which store we should use. Whichever store, x say, is used, we set the counter $s(x)$ equal to 7 and then start the next round. Note that by starting with $s(i) = i$, for $i = 1, 2, 3, 4$, we guarantee that the first four stores selected are 1, 2, 3, 4 and also that, at any given time, at most one of the $s(i)$ can be 0.

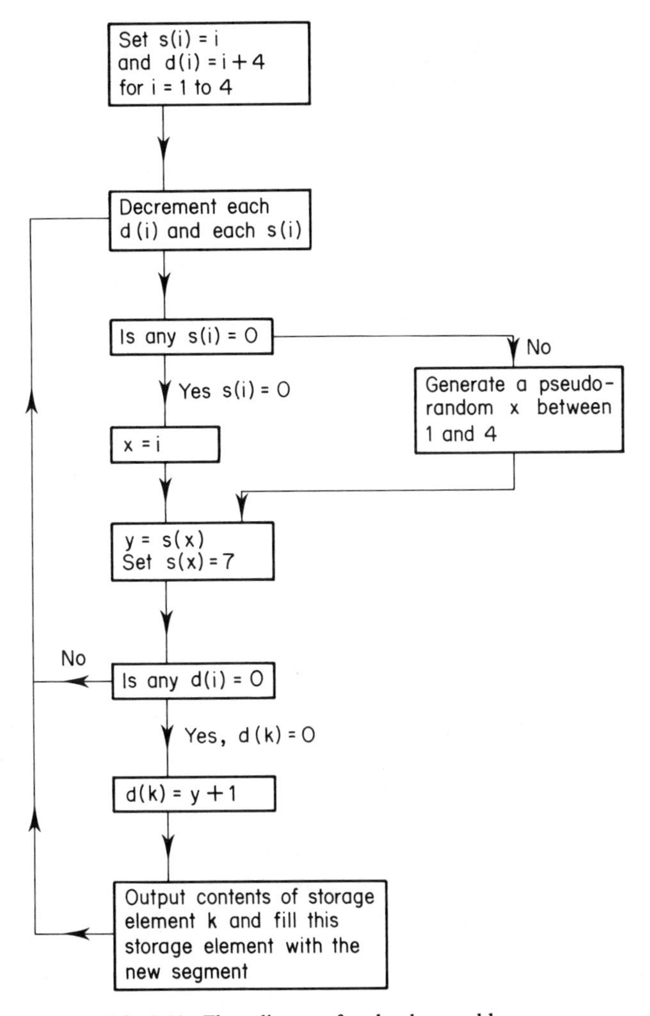

FIG. 5.11. Flow diagram for the descrambler.

TABLE 5.11

A Worked Example Utilizing the Scrambling and Descrambling Algorithms

	Scrambler						Descrambler								
Segment period	$s(1)$	$s(2)$	$s(3)$	$s(4)$	Random number	Output store	$s(1)$	$s(2)$	$s(3)$	$s(4)$	$d(1)$	$d(2)$	$d(3)$	$d(4)$	Output store
	1	2	3	4			1	2	3	4	5	6	7	8	
1	0	1	2	3	—	1	0	1	2	3	4	5	6	7	—
	7						7								
2	6	0	1	2	—	2	6	0	1	2	3	4	5	6	—
		7						7							
3	5	6	0	1	—	3	5	6	0	1	2	3	4	5	—
			7						7						
4	4	5	6	0	—	4	4	5	6	0	1	2	3	4	—
				7						7					
5	3	4	5	6	4	4	3	4	5	6	0	1	2	3	1
				7						7	7				
6	2	3	4	6	1	1	2	3	4	6	6	0	1	2	2
	7						7					3			
7	6	2	3	5	1	1	6	2	3	5	5	2	0	1	3
	7						7						7		
8	6	1	2	4	2	2	6	1	2	4	4	1	6	0	4
		7						7						2	
9	5	6	1	3	3	3	5	6	1	3	3	0	5	1	2
			7						7			2			
10	4	5	6	2	1	1	4	5	6	2	2	1	4	0	4
	7						7							5	
11	6	4	5	1	4	4	6	4	5	1	1	0	3	4	2
				7						7		2			
12	5	3	4	6	2	2	5	3	4	6	0	1	2	3	1
		7						7			4				
13	4	6	3	5	2	2	4	6	3	5	3	0	1	2	2
		7						7				7			
14	3	6	2	4	2	2	3	6	2	4	2	6	0	1	3
		7						7					7		
15	2	6	1	3	2	2	2	6	1	3	1	5	6	0	4
		7						7						7	
16	1	6	0	2	—	3	1	6	0	2	0	4	5	6	1
			7						7		1				
17	0	5	6	1	—	1	0	5	6	1	0	3	4	5	1
	7						7				1				
18	6	4	5	0	—	4	6	4	5	0	0	2	3	4	1
				7						7	1				
19	5	3	4	6	3	3	5	3	4	6	0	1	2	3	1
			7						7		5				
20	4	2	6	5	2	2	4	2	6	5	4	0	1	2	2
		7						7				3			
21	3	6	5	4	2	2	3	6	5	4	3	2	0	1	3
		7						7					7		
22	2	6	4	3	4	4	2	6	4	3	2	1	6	0	4
				7						7				4	
23	1	5	3	6	3	3	1	5	3	6	1	0	5	3	2
			7						7			4			
24	0	4	6	5	—	1	0	4	6	5	0	3	4	2	1
	7						7				1				
25							6	3	5	4	0	2	3	1	1
26												1	2	0	4
27												0	1		2
28													0		3

2. *A Descrambling Algorithm*

Since the descrambler has to be able to deduce the delay incurred by each element in the scrambler, the descrambler and scrambler must use identical pseudo-random number generators. As well as having a set of counters to tell it which storage element to use, the descrambler also keeps a record of the counters at the scrambler. However, instead of simply re-setting $s(x)$ to 7 whenever the scrambler utilizes storage element x, the descrambler also makes use of the contents of $s(x)$ prior to it being reset. This information essentially tells the descrambler how long the segment has remained in the scrambler which, of course, determines how long it must remain in the descrambler. In Fig. 5.11 we give a flow diagram for the descrambler. In this diagram $s(i)$ is as in Fig. 5.10 and $d(i)$ represents the counter for the ith storage element of the descrambler.

In order to see that our algorithms are successful we have worked through the scrambler and descrambler for our example of Tables 5.9 and 5.10. The results are shown in Table 5.11, which should be compared with the two earlier tables.

3. *The Security Level*

In our discussion we have concentrated on the maximum delay of any segment through the transmitter–receiver and have shown that descrambling is possible. We will now turn our attention to the security level. If we refer back to Table 5.9 we can see that, in the sequence of transmitted segments, segments 2 and 3 are transmitted consecutively. The same applies to segments 12, 13 and 14; 9, 10 and 11; 18 and 19. From earlier remarks we know that this is undesirable and is likely to lead to a greater residual intelligibility in the scrambled signal.

There are a number of ways for trying to avoid adjacent segments of the clear speech remaining together in the scrambled speech. We will look at two of them. The first, due to Jayant *et al.* (1983), is based on the concept called temporal distance. If the transmitted sequence of segments is $a_0, a_1, a_2, \ldots$, then, for any i, the *temporal distance* $t(i)$ between a_i and a_{i+1} is defined as $|a_i - a_{i+1}|$. Thus, in our example of Table 5.9, the transmitted sequence is 4, 1, 6, 2, 3, 7, 5, 8, 12, 13, 14, ... and the temporal distances are 3, 5, 4, 1, 4, 2, 3, 4, 1, 1, ... Clearly for unscrambled speech $t(i) = 1$ for all i, while for scrambled speech $t(i) \geqslant 1$ for all i. If we are to avoid consecutive segments of the clear speech being consecutive in the scrambled speech than we must avoid transmission sequences which have any temporal distances equal to 1. Jayant *et al.* suggested the specification of a minimum value for $t(i)$ in the output of the sequential scrambler. If we call this value t, then the pseudo-random number generator is successively sampled until it achieves an output which has t for its minimum temporal distance. (Note that if a segment has spent its maximum permitted time in the scrambler store then it will have to be released no matter what the value of its temporal distance. Thus, in certain circumstances the condition of imposing a minimum value for $t(i)$ may have to be violated.)

If we refer back to Fig. 5.10 then we can see that the implementation of this scheme requires the insertion of a subroutine after the generation of x via the pseudo-random number generator. This subroutine should compare the segment in the specified store with the one which has just been transmitted and if the condition $t(i) \geqslant t$ is violated should produce a new number from the generator. Clearly, since the descrambler can perform the same process, this extra subroutine will not inhibit the descrambling.

The choice of t is important. Great care must be taken to ensure that a suitable value is chosen. In order to illustrate the type of complication which can arise from a bad choice of t, we will look at a small example. Suppose that we choose $t = 3$ for a four-segment store system in which the process started by selecting segment 3. Since $t = 3$ the next segment selected would have to be at least 6 but, as is clear from Table 5.12, segment 6 would still be unspoken. According to Jayant *et al.*, this particular problem can be avoided by choosing $t \leqslant [(s + 1)/2]$, where s is the number of storage elements in the scrambler. (Jayant assumes that the descrambler also has the same number of storage elements.) So, in our example, since $s = 4$, t should be at most $[(4 + 1)/2] = 2$.

By introducing a minimum temporal distance we are limiting the number of possibilities for the segment which can be selected at any given time. This, unfortunately, means that we are not the only people to gain from its introduction. Any decrease in the number of possibilities automatically makes the cryptanalyst's task easier. The designer has to decide whether he will confront the cryptanalyst with a very low residual intelligibility but a comparatively small number of potential output sequences or whether he will

TABLE 5.12

A Bad Choice for t

Input segment	Storage elements				Store selected	Output segment
	4	3	2	1		
1	—	—	—	1	1	—
2	—	—	2	1	2	—
3	—	3	2	1	3	—
4	4	3	2	1	4	—
5	4	5	2	1	3	3
6					?	

concede a little residual intelligibility in order to keep a high number of possibilities for the output sequence. The two options must be carefully balanced.

In their paper, Jayant *et al.* produce histograms of the temporal distance using $s = 8$ with $t = 1$ and $t = 4$. (Note that taking $t = 1$ is, essentially, having no minimum temporal distance.) These histograms are based on a simulation involving 132 segments. When $t = 4$ the histogram peaks at $t(i) = 4$ but there are still a significant number of $t(i) < 4$ caused, as we noted earlier, by the scrambler being forced to release segments which have "overstayed their welcome". From listening tests performed, as in Beth's experiments, using balanced sets of four-digit numbers, Jayant *et al.* obtained intelligibility scores which indicated that there was no obvious advantage in using values of t which are greater than 1. They attributed this surprising result to some kind of threshold effect in the perception of temporally scrambled speech. Furthermore they also found that, using 16 msec segments with a total delay time of up to 384 msec, their sliding window system showed no appreciable advantage, in terms of residual intelligibility, over a hopping system with the same overall delay. However, when the delay time was increased to 512 msec then, in comparison with a hopping system having the same delay, the sliding approach produced a significant reduction, about 10%, in the residual intelligibility.

C. Another System

None of the sliding window systems which we have met so far have involved dividing the signal into frames. The signal has been treated continuously and they have used techniques which, essentially, involve infinite permutations. In this section we describe a system, due to Beker and Mitchell (to be submitted), in which frames are introduced. This then enables the designer to use the properties of finite permutations to control the residual intelligibility etc.

We will begin our discussion of their system by looking at it purely in terms of permutations. If α is a permutation on $\{1, 2, \ldots, n\}$ then we can regard α as moving each integer i a certain number of positions to the "right". (Here the convention is that if $\alpha(n) = 1$ then α has moved n one position to the right.) For any given positive integers k and n, with $k \leqslant n$, we define $A(n, k)$ to be the set of all permutations on $\{1, 2, \ldots, n\}$ with the property that every element is moved between 1 and k positions to the right. So, for example, if

$$\alpha = \begin{bmatrix} 1 & 2 & 3 & 4 & 5 & 6 & 7 & 8 \\ 2 & 5 & 4 & 7 & 6 & 1 & 8 & 3 \end{bmatrix}$$

or, using our alternative notation $\alpha = (6\ 1\ 8\ 3\ 2\ 5\ 4\ 7)$, then α is in $A(8, 3)$. (This is established by straightforward verification. For instance $\alpha(1) = 2$ so

1 is moved one position to the right, while $\alpha(6) = 1$ so 6 is moved three positions to the right.) A more precise mathematical definition of $A(n, k)$ is given by $A(n, k) = \{\alpha \in S_n \mid \alpha(i) \in \{\overline{i+1}, \overline{i+2}, \ldots, \overline{i+k}\}\}$ where S_n is the set of all permutations on $\{1, 2, \ldots, n\}$ and $\overline{i+j} \equiv i + j (\text{mod } n)$. In other words $\overline{i+j} = i + j$ if $i + j \leqslant n$ and $\overline{i+j} = i + j - n$ if $i + j > n$.

In order to see how our permutation α might be used in a sliding window system and to see what delay is incurred we can consider the timing diagram of Fig. 5.12. In this diagram we have used different letters to distinguish between the segments of the different frames. So the segments of the first frame are each preceded by A, those of the second frame by B, etc. Because of the condition imposed on our permutation we know that each segment will be transmitted within at most three segment time slots which, of course, means that the receiver can begin to unscramble the speech signal after four time slots. Thus, if each time slot is T sec, our permutation α incurs a total time delay of $4T$ sec. In general if we use a permutation from $A(n, k)$ then each segment will be transmitted within kT sec and the total time delay will be $(k + 1)T$ sec. Note that if we wish to change the permutation then the new permutation must be chosen so that it 'matches' the existing one. They must agree at the beginning and end of the frames to make the 'change over' possible.

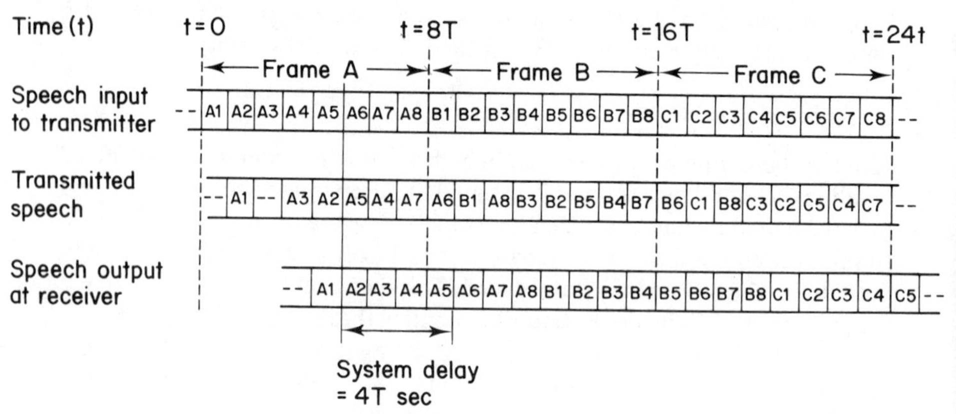

FIG. 5.12. Timing diagram for the sliding window.

This technique has the advantage that we can, in advance, generate 'good' permutations while still enjoying many benefits of the sliding window system as opposed to hopping. For instance, in this system the delay time depends on k, which is related to the store size, and not on the frame size n. Since we are now working with finite permutations it should be possible to calculate the total number available to us, i.e., the number of permutations in $A(n, k)$, and also to preselect (or screen) them to ensure that we only use permutations which result in a low residual intelligibility. Unfortunately it is not at all easy to determine the size of $A(n, k)$. However Beker and Mitchell have recently devised an algorithm which computes $A(n, k)$ for reasonably large values of n and k. The values for $A(n, k)$ soon become surprisingly large. Here are a few examples,

$$|A(8, 4)| = 264$$

$$|A(16, 8)| = 5.67 \times 10^8$$

$$|A(24, 8)| = 8.75 \times 10^{12}$$

$$|A(24, 8)| = 3.68 \times 10^{25}$$

$$|A(48, 12)| = 1.67 \times 10^{33}$$

The fact that $|A(n, k)|$ is large does not, of course, give any guarantee about the number of permutations which result in a sufficiently low level of residual intelligibility. As an example of a particularly bad permutation in $A(8, 3)$ consider

$$\begin{bmatrix} 1 & 2 & 3 & 4 & 5 & 6 & 7 & 8 \\ 4 & 3 & 5 & 6 & 7 & 8 & 1 & 2 \end{bmatrix}$$

or, in our other notation, (78213456). The effect of this permutation is shown in Fig. 5.13 from which it is quite clear, without any need to perform any listening tests, that a high level of residual intelligibility will result. Experimentation has indicated that, as in the case of our earlier hopping systems,

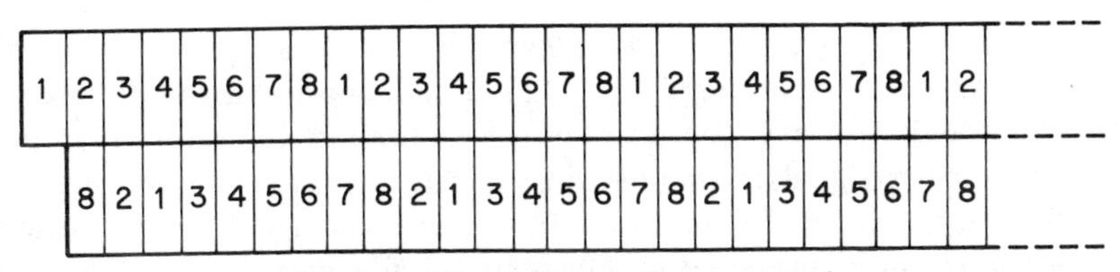

FIG. 5.13. Timing diagram for our example.

the most important property to avoid is that two segments which were originally consecutive should remain so. Thus we should restrict our permutations still further by considering only those permutations α with the property that, for every i, $\alpha(i + 1)$ does not immediately follow $\alpha(i)$. Various computations concerning the number of permutations which satisfy this extra criterion have been performed and we refer to Bromfield and Mitchell (to be submitted).

IV. Time Sample Scramblers

The sampling theorem asserts that a band limited signal of bandwidth B Hz between frequencies f_1 and f_2 Hz ($f_2 > f_1$) can be characterised by samples taken at a frequency of $2f_2/m$ samples/sec, where m is the largest integer not exceeding f_2/B. One possible method for scrambling is simply to sample the signal, operate on the samples and retransform to an analogue signal. This approach can be very successful. In fact, to quote Jayant (1982) "The technique is so effective that even simple systematic permutations rather than pseudo-random ones, are sufficient to realise extremely low levels of intelligibility". We will, in due course, describe some of the techniques which have been suggested for using the method and will look at their level of performance. Before that, however, we must focus attention on the limitation of such a strategy and explain why such systems have not been universally adopted.

There are essentially two major drawbacks to adopting this method. One is the accompanying bandwidth extension and the other is the need for preservation of individual sample integrity. We shall discuss each in turn.

Suppose that we have a signal which is band limited from 300 Hz to 3.3 kHz and that we sample it at 8 kHz. Then the maximum frequency in the scrambled speech, obtained by passing the scrambled samples through a bandpass filter, could be as high as 4 kHz. If this happened then the bandwidth would have expanded. To avoid this, in practice, we would have to prefilter the analogue signal, using a filter with a cut-off frequency of less than 3 kHz, sample at 6 kHz and hence obtain a scrambled signal with a highest frequency of about 3 kHz. If we do this, then, although some degradation will have occurred, the bandwidth extension problem can be overcome.

The problem of preserving sample integrity is considerably more difficult. Over any real communications channel, it is almost inevitable that the signal will be distorted. However, because of the continuous and slowly varying nature of speech signals, for unscrambled signals these distortions are normally not perceptually objectionable. The same levels of distortion become significantly more noticeable when made discontinuous by the inverse operation of the descrambler. (This was precisely the reason that segment length was such a critical factor in the time element scramblers of Section III. Their robustness in the face of bad channel distortions is what has made them so popular). Despite this obvious handicap there is no need to completely abandon the idea of time sample scrambling. Recent advances in digital signal processing mean that channel equalisation at a low cost may soon be a practical reality.

Some of the most interesting work in the area of time sample scrambling has been done by Phillips *et al.* (1971) and we shall consider some of their results.

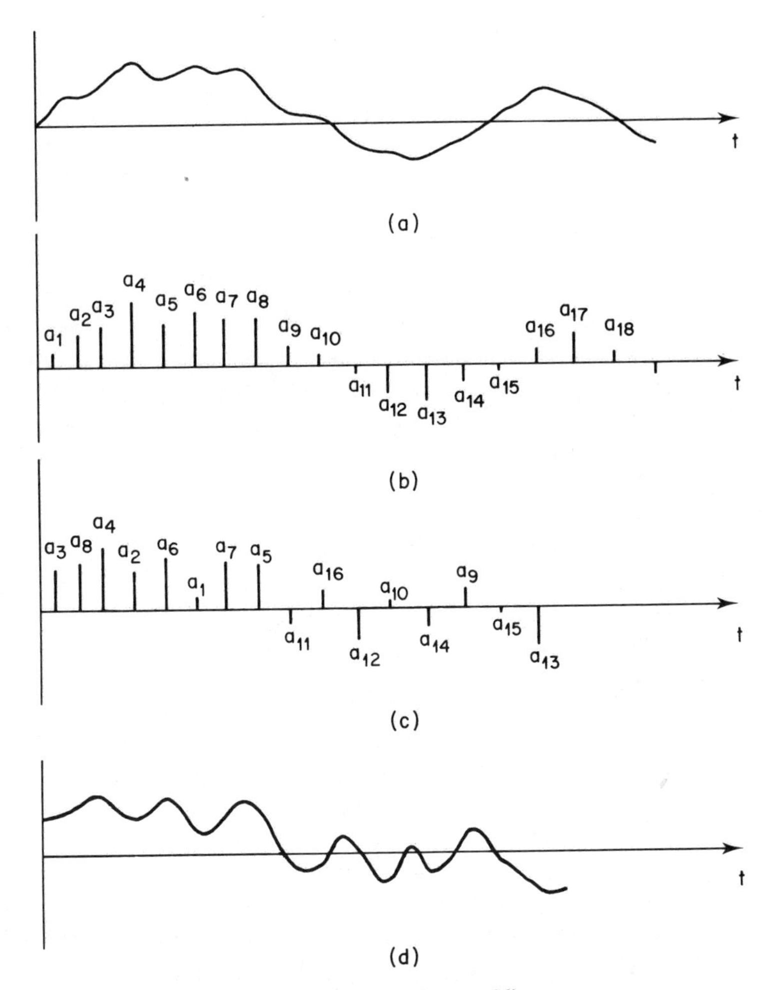

FIG. 5.14. Time sample scrambling.

In Fig. 5.14 we illustrate the basic idea of *time sample scrambling*. Figure 5.14(a) shows the original speech and Fig. 5.14(b) shows the scrambled speech. For the example illustrated in these diagrams we used 8-sample blocks and repeatedly use the permutation

$$\begin{bmatrix} 1 & 2 & 3 & 4 & 5 & 6 & 7 & 8 \\ 6 & 4 & 1 & 3 & 8 & 5 & 7 & 2 \end{bmatrix}$$

Thus Fig. 5.14(c) shows the permutation applied to the first two blocks of samples and the resulting waveform is then shown in Fig. 5.14(d).

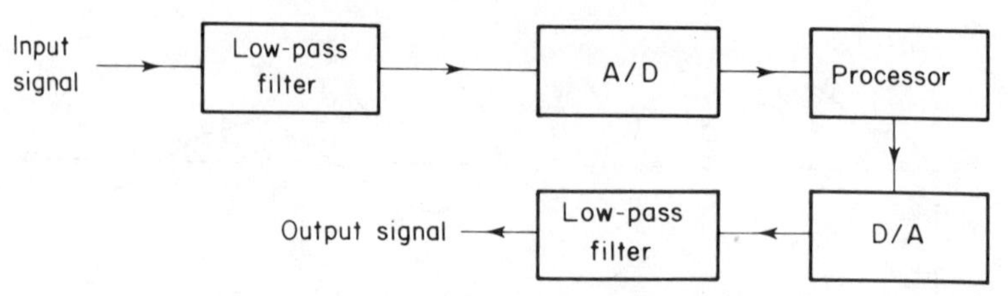

FIG. 5.15. Experimental time sample scrambler.

Phillips *et al.* performed a number of experiments to determine the effect of various permutations and block sizes on the residual intelligibility of the signal. They were particularly interested in the effects of the block size and the shift factor of the permutation. Not surprisingly the problem concerning the choice of permutation is similar to that of the frequency band scrambler or the time element scrambler. In Fig. 5.15 we give a block diagram for their experiment. The input signal was prefiltered, sampled using a 12-bit/sample A/D converter at a sampling rate of 7 kHz, processed, reconverted to an analogue signal and then post filtered. They used filters with cut-off frequencies of 3.1 kHz. Some spectrograms showing a portion of unscrambled speech and the effect of scrambling using a permutation on 10-sample blocks and increasing the shift factor Γ are shown in Fig. 5.16.

In intelligibility tests using monosyllabic words as test material, Phillips *et al.* subjected their listeners to short passages of continuous scrambled speech before presenting them with a word list. As a 'benchmark' zero scrambling produced only 92% intelligibility. Although we cannot be sure, we must assume that this was a direct result of the bandlimiting introduced by the experimental set-up. They found that a 10-sample block with a shift factor of about 40 produced about 2% intelligibility, while the intelligibility of even a simple 2-sample block was only 22%. They concluded that the permutations should be chosen subject to the following considerations.

(1) The block size should be as large as possible, not forgetting that this will increase the delay time.

(2) Permutations with either very small or very large shift factors should be avoided.

(3) Permutations in which certain consecutive samples remain consecutive should be avoided.

(4) Permutations which essentially consist of a number of permutations of smaller block size should be avoided. One such example is

$$\begin{bmatrix} 1 & 2 & 3 & 4 & 5 & 6 & 7 & 8 \\ 3 & 2 & 1 & 4 & 7 & 6 & 5 & 8 \end{bmatrix}$$

which is, essentially, $\left[\begin{smallmatrix} 1 & 2 & 3 & 4 \\ 3 & 2 & 1 & 4 \end{smallmatrix}\right]$ and $\left[\begin{smallmatrix} 5 & 6 & 7 & 8 \\ 7 & 6 & 5 & 8 \end{smallmatrix}\right]$.

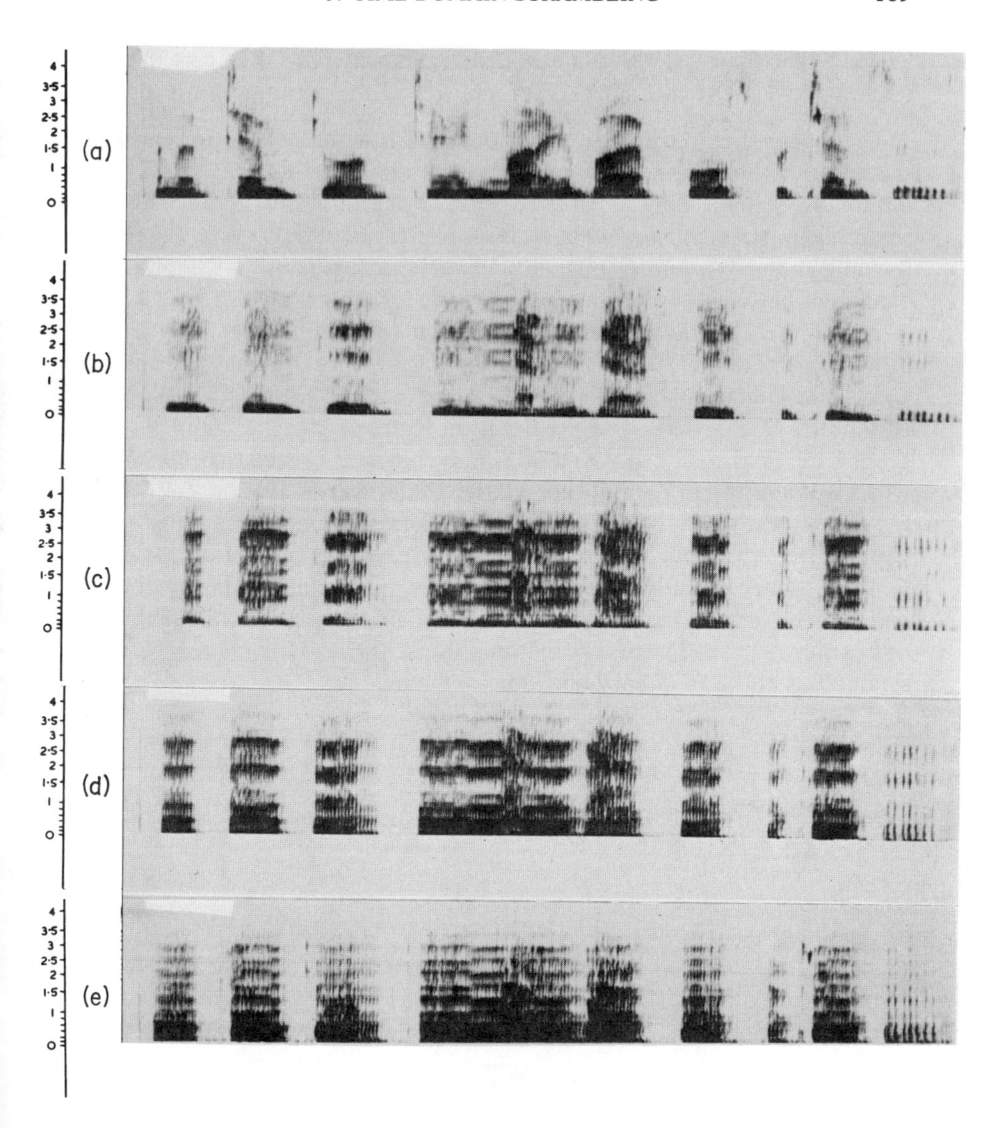

FIG. 5.16. Frequency spectra of scrambled speech signals. Vertical scales are in kilohertz. (a) Speech unscrambled, (b) after block 10 scramble $\Gamma = 14$, (c) after block 10 scramble $\Gamma = 26$, (d) after block 10 scramble $\Gamma = 44$ and (e) after block 10 scramble $\Gamma = 50$. [From Phillips *et al.* (1971).]

(5) If the permutation is changed at regular intervals then care must be taken to ensure that the shift factor changes as the permutation is altered.

The reader should compare these conclusions with the rules for choosing permutations in frequency bandscramblers and time element scramblers. Although we have only considered sample permutations it is possible to scramble by performing other operations on the samples. We refer the reader to Phillips and Watkins (1973), and also to the discussion in Chapter 4 on changing the signs of alternate samples.

To end this chapter we mention briefly the relation between time sample scrambling and the frequency technique using the DFT as described in Chapter 4. That technique was described by $z = F^{-1}QFx$ where x is the block of samples, F the DFT, Q a permutation matrix and z the samples representing the final signal. If we could find a choice of Q such that $QF = FP$, where P is a different permutation matrix, we would obtain $z = F^{-1}QFx = F^{-1}FPx = Px$ which, of course, is simply the time sample scrambler which we have just discussed. Since there are, in fact, appropriate choices for P and Q, these two apparently different techniques, one in the frequency domain and the other in the time domain, can be identical on occasions. This explains our earlier remarks that it is sometimes nonsensical to distinguish between scrambling in the frequency and time domains.

6. Two-Dimensional Scrambling and General Implementation Techniques

I. Introduction

In Chapters 4 and 5 we considered scrambling in the frequency and time domains separately and, as we saw, each had relative advantages and disadvantages. In practice a designer will probably try to capitalize on the strong points of each technique and is likely to try to combine them in some way. We are now in a position to start comparing the various analogue techniques and to consider how they might be combined. This is one of the main aims of this chapter. In Section IV we introduce some of the possible ways of combining different techniques and in Section V we will give a detailed comparison of various aspects of a number of the techniques which we have introduced.

In this chapter we also consider some of the implementation problems of analogue scramblers and, when doing this, we pay particular attention to synchronization. This topic has been mentioned many times; for instance, whenever we considered systems for which the scrambling permutations could change during transmission, such as with rolling bandsplitters or time element scramblers for which the permutation changed every frame, etc. In Section VI we (at long last!) discuss some of the techniques which are used for synchronizing the sequence generators at the transmitter and receiver. Then, in Section VII, we consider the implications of these synchronization techniques on the range of a radio to which the scrambler might be fitted.

We begin the chapter with two short sections, one on amplitude scrambling and the other on time delays.

II. Amplitude Scrambling

Although there are three relevant parameters associated with a speech signal, (namely time, frequency and amplitude), we have only discussed techniques which rely on operations in the time or frequency domain. This is not just an indication of bias on our part. There is, as far as we know, only one commonly used scrambling technique which works on the signal amplitudes. It is known as *masking* and the basic idea is to mask the signal by the linear addition of pseudo-random amplitudes.

One of the major advantages of this method is that it is possible to make the resultant signal sound like white noise. Another advantage of this technique is that, since we can produce a virtually unlimited number of pseudo-random noise amplitudes, it does not impose any restriction on the key size. In fact it is possible to obtain a security level comparable to that of the digital techniques to be described in Chapter 7. Unfortunately there are also a number of disadvantages associated with this type of system.

The first disadvantage is that there is a significant loss in the signal-to-noise ratio at the receiver which, for radio applications, causes a decrease in the effective range. This loss in the signal-to-noise ratio arises because, for any given level of total input, part of the energy has to be given to the masking code and this energy will then (hopefully!) be subtracted from the received signal. A further disadvantage is that, since further noise will have been added during transmission, the mask will be altered before reaching the receiver and consequently the subtraction at the receiver will be imperfect. This can be particularly serious if the signal which results from the scrambling procedure has some large amplitudes. The reason is that these may then be 'limited' by the dynamic range of the transmission path and of the transmitting and receiving terminals. This, in turn, means that non-linearities will occur which might result in the final unscrambled signal being significantly different from the original one. Yet another problem is that, as with many other techniques, including, for example, time scrambling, the receiver requires perfect synchronization if the mask is to be removed from the correct part of the signal. Here even a small loss in sample integrity may result in the receiver failing to descramble the signal sufficiently well to make it intelligible.

Some of these problems can be overcome by using a method similar to that suggested by Weinstein (1980). This method uses the addition of amplitudes with a modulo operation and, if we assume that the operation is performed digitally, can be described mathematically. To obtain this description we assume that the digital samples of the speech waveform are constrained to a $(-A, A)$ amplitude range and that the pseudo-random noise amplitudes are uniformly distributed over the same interval. Before performing any arithmetic we add A to each speech and noise amplitude and thus represent them by numbers in the range 0 to $2A$. The scrambled speech is then produced by modulo-$2A$ adding the numbers, determining these amplitudes, and subtracting A from the result. If we let x_n and k_n represent corresponding speech waveform and pseudo-random noise samples, with $0 \leqslant x_n < 2A$ and $0 \leqslant k_n < 2A$ for each x_n and k_n, then the scrambled signal is represented by y_n where y_n is given by

$$y_n = x_n + k_n (\text{mod } 2A)$$

The scrambled amplitude is, of course, $y_n - A$ and lies in the range $(-A, A)$ and, despite the statistics of the x_n, it will be uniformly distributed in this range. The descrambling operation is given by

$$x_n = y_n - k_n (\text{mod } 2A)$$

and the descrambled speech amplitude is, of course, given by $x_n - A$.

Since, in this type of scheme, the signal amplitude is limited by the scrambling process, no limiting should occur. Thus, one of the problems which concerned us is no longer troublesome. Similarly we are no longer necessarily reducing our range by spending power on the pseudo-random noise. The reason for this is that, when using this technique, roughly half of the transmitted amplitudes become smaller rather than increasing. The presence of a limited amount of ambient noise should present no major difficulties. However, channel distortions and losses in sample integrity may have significant effects on the receiver and descrambler. It is certainly possible to overcome these problems by using sophisticated and expensive equalization and synchronization techniques. However, given that a very high level of security is required, it is necessary to compare the expense of designing and building such a piece of equipment with that of utilizing a greater bandwidth and hence allowing a fully digital system to be adopted.

III. Time Delays and Full-Duplex Operation

In this section we re-emphasize some of the problems, which we first noted in Chapter 2, involved in using a scrambler that exhibits time delays. If time delay is a problem with a user's network then that user should ignore all time domain techniques. This is likely to be the case if, for instance, full-duplex operation is required. Although we touched upon this problem in Section II of Chapter 2 we will now consider the problem a little more fully and, for this discussion, we will assume we are using a telephone system.

A standard telephone contains a transformer system called a *hybrid*, which is used to isolate the microphone from the earpiece and to connect both to a two-wire line. In practice most users do not like the hollow effect which results if the earpiece is totally decoupled from the microphone, so the connections are made to allow a certain amount of feedthrough from the microphone to the earpiece. This is called *sidetone* and has the extra advantage that it also helps the speaker to keep the level of his voice within the dynamic range of the system. This two-wire line then goes to the local exchange where another hybrid converts the two-wire line to a four-wire line permitting amplifications in each direction. The system is illustrated in Fig. 6.1. One aim in the design of a hybrid is to attenuate interactions between the transmit and receive paths. However, it is almost certainly not perfect and reflections, or *echoes*, occur. As we explained in Chapter 2, if these delayed versions of the message signals reach the speaker's earphones they can be very distracting. Furthermore the longer the time delay, the greater the distraction will be. In fact Fig. 2.10 shows how dramatically the user's difficulties increase as the delay gets longer. In general most users will grudgingly accept delays of up to 60–80 msec, but delays of more than 100 msec are usually unacceptable.

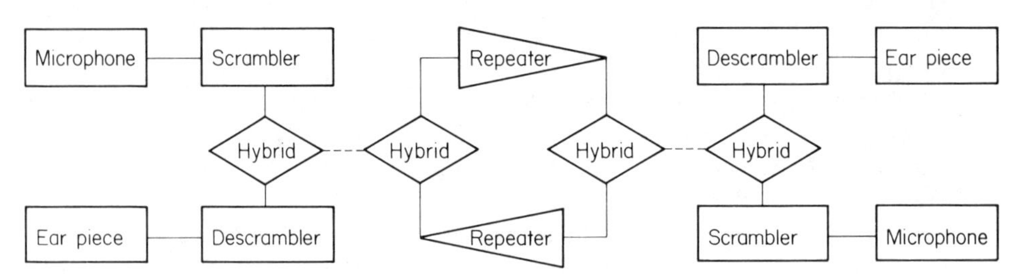

FIG. 6.1. Duplex scrambler in a telephone network.

As we have already stressed, if a scrambler is employed in a system with echoes, then the echoes themselves will also be scrambled. If we use a fixed code bandscrambler then, provided both the scrambler and descrambler employ the same key, this does not cause any additional problems. But if we use a rolling bandscrambler then an echo might arrive after the permutation has been changed and if this occurs then the received echo will be incorrectly descrambled, causing additional disturbance and distraction to the recipient. However, if we ensure that the rate of changing permutations is relatively slow compared with the echo delay then the chances of this happening are probably low enough for it to be acceptable.

If, on the other hand, we consider using a time element scrambler with a delay of half a second, then we have a problem. The echoes will not be heard until at least half a second later and will almost certainly be descrambled incorrectly because they will be out of synchronization with the descrambler.

One way of trying to overcome this problem is by providing a local sidetone directly from the microphone to the earpiece, i.e., before scrambling, and trying to configure the hybrid circuit in the transmitter to 'fully' suppress echoes. This does not, however, solve the problem of echoes coming down the line. It might be possible to overcome that problem by using, in the terminal, signal processing circuitry which uses some kind of training sequence at the start of the transmission to provide echo cancellation. Since telephone transmissions are reasonably static, they do not usually need the echo cancellers to be adaptive. However, they certainly can be made adaptive and for some channels, radio transmissions for instance, they have to be. At the present time, echo cancellation is still an expensive technique and full-duplex communications tend to be available only for scramblers with very short delay.

IV. Combination Techniques

Most of the common ways of designing systems to utilize two or more scrambling techniques tend to combine a frequency technique with a time technique. There is, however, one important exception to this which involves the coupling of reversed time segmentation with time element scramblers.

A. Combining Time Domain Techniques

Almost all time element scramblers are implemented digitally and, as a consequence, the speech segments are stored digitally in RAMs. This means that it is easy to perform a reversed time operation on each segment as it is withdrawn from the store for transmission. Many systems even use a key to determine, via a pseudo-random number generator, which of the segments should be reversed and which should be left alone. Most designers tend to regard this type of system as a time element scrambler with the extra bonus of some reversed time segmentation. If we adopt this attitude then, unfortunately, the decrease in the residual intelligibility is not as great as we might hope. The reason for this is that for reversed time segmentation to be effective we need time segments of the order of 250 msec, whereas time element scramblers require much shorter segments; of the order of 30 msec. Since we start with a time element scrambler, the segments are usually kept short and, as a result, the effectiveness of the reversed time segmentation is minimised. In practice, tests we have conducted suggest that a listener's success rate is reduced by about 5–10% when reversed time segmentation is added to a time element scrambler. Despite this small improvement we stress that, since there is almost no cost penalty, it is common practice to combine reversed time segmentation with time element scrambling.

B. Two-Dimensional Techniques

If a technique combines some forms of frequency and time domain scrambling then it is often referred to as a *two-dimensional scrambler*. There are many possibilities for obtaining a two-dimensional scrambler and, in principle, any of the frequency techniques of Chapter 4 can be coupled with a time element scrambler. However the robustness and effectiveness of the resulting system is likely to vary dramatically according to the particular techniques used. We will discuss a few of the possibilities.

1. *Time Element Scrambling/Varying Clock Rates*

Our first example uses a frequency scrambling method which, since on its own it provides virtually no security, we did not discuss in Chapter 4. This method relies on the fact that, within a small interval, it is possible to vary the clock rate of an A/D or D/A converter without significantly affecting the resulting signal's bandwidth. Varying this clock is essentially merely adding a form of frequency modulation to the signal. Since, in order to process it, the time element scrambler will have to convert the analogue signal to digital form, the implementation is very simple. By slightly altering the clock rates of the A/D and D/A converters, the segments will be represented by varying numbers of samples and the overall effect is to marginally blur the boundaries between the segments. This, of course, increases the difficulty of cryptanalysis by the jigsaw method. Use of the numbers test indicates that this method reduces the listener's success rate by between 10 and 15%. If the channel conditions are bad then the recovered signal may also suffer distortion and, as a result, devices operating in this way are often provided with a switch which allows the user to select whether or not to employ the frequency domain scrambling.

2. *Time Element Scrambling/Frequency Inversion*

Another simple addition to a time element scrambler is frequency inversion. Here, once again, we can capitalize on the fact that the time element scrambler produces the signal in digital form. Since, as we saw in Chapter 4, frequency inversion can then be achieved by simply inverting alternate samples, the implementation is straightforward. As in our last example the residual intelligibility is reduced by about 10–15%, but this can be increased slightly by employing a pseudo-random number generator to provide a key which selects the segments to be inverted.

3. *Time Element Scrambling/Bandsplitting*

Possibly the most natural, and attractive, idea for a two-dimensional system is to couple a bandscrambler with a time element scrambler. We will now investigate this possibility and, for simplicity, begin by assuming that our time element scrambler is a hopping window system. The first observation to make is that the bandscrambler should be rolling since otherwise the only true advantage is in terms of residual intelligibility. If it is not rolling then the scrambling which we can perform and the security obtained is very limited. For a non-rolling bandscrambler, a cryptanalyst would be able to attack the overall system by first breaking the bandscrambler and then attacking the time element scrambler. As we saw in Chapter 4, he is likely to be able to break the bandscrambler in a relatively short time by, possibly, a jigsaw approach on the spectrograph or filtering and listening to only a smaller part of the spectrum.

For our discussion we shall assume that both the bandscrambler and the hopping window time element scrambler are changing codes every frame and that the bandscrambler frame length is synchronized to the segment length of the time element scrambler. In any system of this type we get discontinuities at every segment boundary for the time element scrambler and at every permutation change for the bandscrambler. However, by making the bandscrambler change permutations at segment boundaries, we can keep the number of discontinuities to a minimum. If, in order to consider a particular example, we assume that we have a five-band bandscrambler and that the time element scrambler has 8 segments/frame, the situation is as shown in Fig. 6.2. In this figure we have labelled the sub-bands of segment j by A_{1j}–A_{5j}

	A_{51}	A_{52}	A_{53}	A_{54}	A_{54}	A_{55}	A_{57}	A_{58}	
	A_{41}	A_{42}	A_{43}	A_{44}	A_{45}	A_{46}	A_{47}	A_{48}	
...	A_{31}	A_{32}	A_{33}	A_{34}	A_{35}	A_{36}	A_{37}	A_{38}	...
	A_{21}	A_{22}	A_{23}	A_{24}	A_{25}	A_{26}	A_{27}	A_{28}	
	A_{11}	A_{12}	A_{13}	A_{14}	A_{15}	A_{16}	A_{17}	A_{18}	

FIG. 6.2. Matrix for two-dimensional scrambling.

and the segments of frame i by A_{i1}–A_{i8}. In order to illustrate the technique we will assume that our time scrambling permutation is

$$\begin{bmatrix} 1 & 2 & 3 & 4 & 5 & 6 & 7 & 8 \\ 3 & 7 & 6 & 2 & 8 & 5 & 1 & 4 \end{bmatrix}$$

A_{27}	A_{44}	A_{41}	A_{48}	A_{26}	A_{43}	A_{52}	A_{15}
A_{47}	A_{34}	A_{51}	A_{18}	A_{36}	A_{13}	A_{12}	A_{25}
A_{57}	A_{14}	A_{31}	A_{58}	A_{46}	A_{23}	A_{32}	A_{55}
A_{17}	A_{54}	A_{11}	A_{28}	A_{56}	A_{33}	A_{42}	A_{45}
A_{37}	A_{24}	A_{21}	A_{38}	A_{16}	A_{53}	A_{22}	A_{35}

FIG. 6.3. Example of T–F scrambling.

and that our eight successive band scrambling permutations are $\begin{bmatrix}1&2&3&4&5\\2&5&1&4&3\end{bmatrix}$, $\begin{bmatrix}1&2&3&4&5\\3&1&4&5&2\end{bmatrix}$, $\begin{bmatrix}1&2&3&4&5\\2&1&3&5&4\end{bmatrix}$, $\begin{bmatrix}1&2&3&4&5\\4&2&1&5&3\end{bmatrix}$, $\begin{bmatrix}1&2&3&4&5\\1&5&4&3&2\end{bmatrix}$, $\begin{bmatrix}1&2&3&4&5\\4&3&2&5&1\end{bmatrix}$, $\begin{bmatrix}1&2&3&4&5\\4&1&3&2&5\end{bmatrix}$, $\begin{bmatrix}1&2&3&4&5\\5&4&1&2&3\end{bmatrix}$.

If we assume that the bandscrambling takes place after a segment has been selected then the final situation is shown in Fig. 6.3. To see how this figure is obtained we will consider two of the time segments. The first segment to be transmitted is segment 7 so the first column of Fig. 6.3 must correspond to segment 7 and this is reflected in the fact that its elements are A_{17}, A_{27}, A_{37}, A_{47} and A_{57} in some order. The order in which they appear is determined by our first permutation. Using this permutation the sub-bands are re-arranged in the order A_{37}, A_{17}, A_{57}, A_{47}, A_{27} which, since from Fig. 6.2 we see that we are putting the first subband at the bottom of the column, gives the first column of Fig. 6.3. Similarly the fourth segment to be transmitted is segment 8 and for this segment the subbands are permuted using the fourth of our eight permutations. Thus the order of the subbands is A_{38}, A_{28}, A_{58}, A_{18} and A_{48} which gives the fourth column of Fig. 6.3.

If, on the other hand, we apply the bandscrambling to the segments before they are permuted then the result will be slightly different. If, for instance, our first permutation is applied to segment 1 then we would obtain A_{31}, A_{11}, A_{51}, A_{41}, A_{21} and this, under time element permutation would be the third sample transmitted. The total effect is shown in Fig. 6.4. (To avoid confusion we have labelled Fig. 6.3 as T–F scrambling, to indicate that the time scrambling was performed first, and labelled Fig. 6.4 as F–T scrambling.) Clearly the only real effect is to change the order in which the bandscrambling permutations are used. In each case we have merely used the same permutation on the columns and then used different permutations on the elements of each individual column. The result is that in each time slot we are still sending the permuted sub-bands of a single time element. Clearly this information is likely to prove useful to a cryptanalyst. He would find his task much more difficult if we were able to 'break-up' the columns and find a

A_{57}	A_{44}	A_{21}	A_{18}	A_{46}	A_{43}	A_{42}	A_{25}
A_{17}	A_{14}	A_{41}	A_{28}	A_{16}	A_{53}	A_{32}	A_{35}
A_{37}	A_{54}	A_{51}	A_{58}	A_{26}	A_{33}	A_{12}	A_{45}
A_{47}	A_{24}	A_{11}	A_{48}	A_{36}	A_{13}	A_{52}	A_{55}
A_{27}	A_{34}	A_{31}	A_{38}	A_{56}	A_{23}	A_{22}	A_{15}

FIG. 6.4. Example of F–T scrambling.

technique which treated all 40 cells of our matrix as elements to be permuted amongst themselves, i.e., if we could use one permutation on 40 elements rather than a number of separate permutations on either 5 or 8 elements. This would also mean that there were a larger number of possibilities for the final matrix; i.e., more possibilities for the scrambled message. An example of such a matrix is shown in Fig. 6.5. In order to obtain a scrambled signal of the form represented by Fig. 6.5 we merely take our 40 components and divide them into batches of five for transmission but, unlike the system earlier, we no longer require that the individual components of an given batch belong to the same time element. Furthermore this type of system can be implemented by using any one of the sliding window techniques described in Chapter 5. There is clearly no theoretical difficulty since the only difference between this and the normal sliding window system is that segments arrive in batches of five, which obviously causes no real problems, and we need to release five from the store before we can transmit anything. Just as in Chapter 5, the size of the store will affect the precise number of

A_{23}	A_{37}	A_{22}	A_{38}	A_{32}	A_{54}	A_{15}	A_{46}
A_{36}	A_{56}	A_{13}	A_{48}	A_{24}	A_{42}	A_{53}	A_{17}
A_{57}	A_{16}	A_{12}	A_{21}	A_{45}	A_{58}	A_{25}	A_{55}
A_{11}	A_{47}	A_{35}	A_{51}	A_{14}	A_{26}	A_{43}	A_{33}
A_{41}	A_{27}	A_{28}	A_{44}	A_{31}	A_{52}	A_{18}	A_{34}

FIG. 6.5. Example of two-dimensional scrambling using a 40-element permutation.

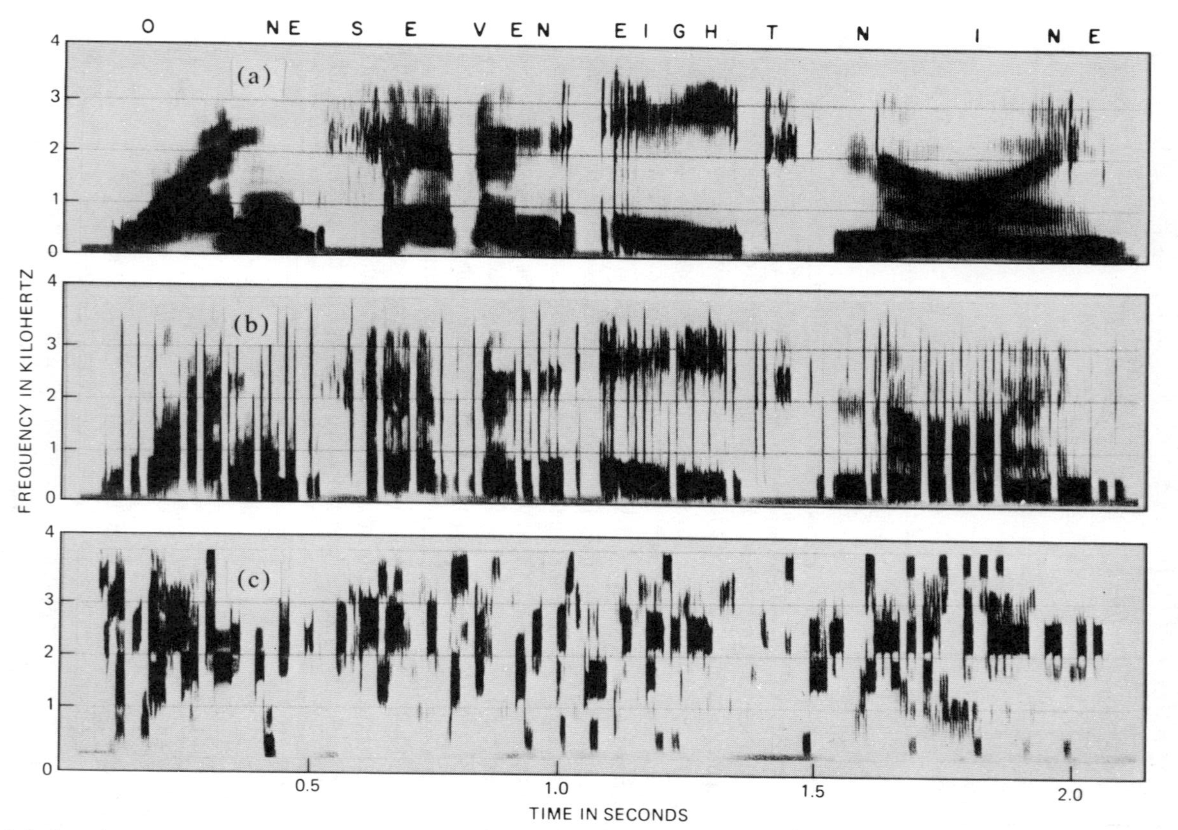

FIG. 6.6. Speech spectrograms: (a) unscrambled speech (female speaker, digit sequence '1978'), (b) output of sliding window element scrambler with communication delay of 128 msec and (c) output of sliding window combined time and frequency scrambler with the same communication delay of 128 msec. [From Jayant *et al.* (1983). Reprinted from The Bell System Technical Journal. Copyright 1983, AT&T.]

permutations which we can use and we must decide upon rules to decide how long a segment may remain in the store. We can also, at least in theory, improve the system still further by using techniques like frequency inversion or reversed time segmentation to include some extra scrambling. However we should not get too carried away. We now have sufficient knowledge of transmission paths and the effects of various techniques to realise that as we add extra 'goodies' to our scrambler the chances of our message actually getting to the receiver with good fidelity are likely to decrease rapidly. Furthermore the cost is also likely to increase dramatically and become prohibitive. At the present time two-dimensional scramblers of the type we have just described tend to be rather expensive and are not particularly robust in their performance over poor channels. However they do offer a fairly high level of security and so, when a high-security-level analogue system is required, they have to be considered. But, as always, if a high security level is absolutely crucial then a digital system might be better and the user will be faced with a difficult decision.

Figure 6.6. shows spectrograms of unscrambled speech, a sliding window time element scrambler with 16-msec segments and a total delay time of 128 msec and a sliding window and frequency scrambler utilizing 16-msec segments, four sub-bands and a total delay time of 128 msec. The effect of scrambling in both domains simultaneously is clearly visible.

Jayant *et al.* call the system we have just described a *sequential TFSP scrambler* and subjected it to a number of intelligibility tests. As in the earlier tests they used four digit numbers spoken by both a male and female speaker.

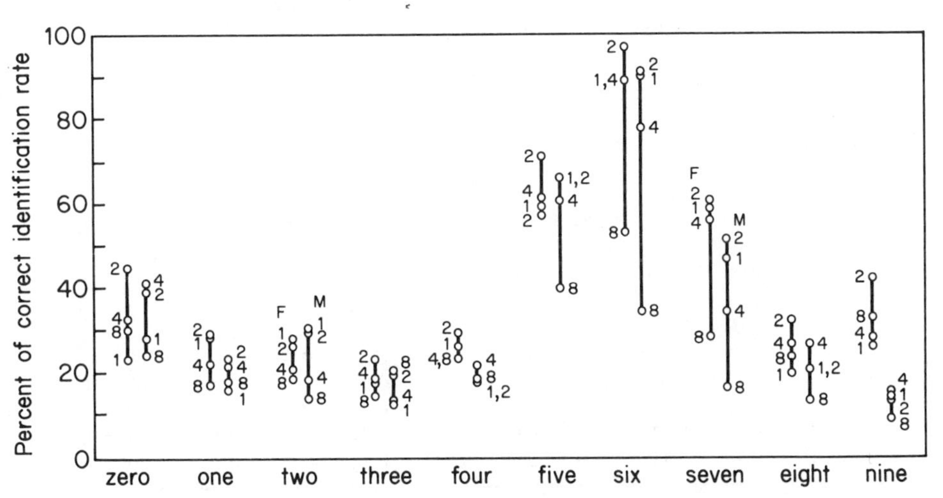

FIG. 6.7. Correct identification rates. [From Jayant *et al.* (1983). Reprinted from The Bell System Technical Journal. Copyright 1983, AT&T.]

For these tests they used four sub-bands in the frequency domain and varied the time storage elements over the range 1, 2, 4 and 8. This meant that their matrices contained 4, 8, 16 and 32 entries and their time delays were 32, 64, 128 and 256 msec. In all these tests they employed a total of eighteen listeners. Their results are published in Jayant *et al.* (1983) and we show them in Fig. 6.7. With the 256-ms delay they found that the residual intelligibility when averaged over all ten digits was about 25%. However there was a significant variation in the performance of the individual digits. This is clear from Table 6.1 where, for instance, we can see that, for a time delay of 256 msec, the

TABLE 6.1

Matrices Showing Digit Confusion in a TFSP Scrambler with a Time Delay of 256 msec.[a]

Female speaker

Scrambler input	Listeners' response									
	0	1	2	3	4	5	6	7	8	9
0	*0.30*	0.08	0.05	0.05	0.10	0.09	0.05	0.11	0.05	0.11
1	0.09	*0.17*	0.05	0.05	0.06	0.10	0.03	0.10	0.07	0.27
2	0.14	0.05	*0.18*	0.19	0.02	0.07	0.18	0.07	0.05	0.05
3	0.14	0.08	0.15	*0.14*	0.11	0.07	0.15	0.07	0.05	0.03
4	0.08	0.12	0.04	0.05	*0.23*	0.18	0.10	0.06	0.08	0.05
5	0.03	0.06	0.02	0.04	0.07	*0.57*	0.03	0.06	0.07	0.07
6	0.03	0.05	0.03	0.04	0.08	0.09	*0.53*	0.09	0.04	0.03
7	0.06	0.11	0.03	0.07	0.07	0.15	0.10	*0.28*	0.07	0.07
8	0.06	0.13	0.07	0.06	0.06	0.14	0.15	0.07	*0.23*	0.03
9	0.08	0.10	0.04	0.06	0.04	0.22	0.02	0.06	0.06	*0.32*

Male speaker

Scrambler input	Listeners' response									
	0	1	2	3	4	5	6	7	8	9
0	*0.24*	0.12	0.08	0.05	0.08	0.11	0.09	0.08	0.09	0.06
1	0.08	*0.17*	0.06	0.08	0.09	0.19	0.06	0.09	0.09	0.09
2	0.22	0.10	*0.13*	0.08	0.10	0.05	0.18	0.08	0.04	0.03
3	0.14	0.11	0.09	*0.20*	0.10	0.06	0.10	0.10	0.04	0.06
4	0.08	0.13	0.07	0.07	*0.18*	0.15	0.11	0.10	0.03	0.07
5	0.09	0.11	0.02	0.03	0.06	*0.40*	0.04	0.11	0.08	0.08
6	0.11	0.07	0.09	0.09	0.07	0.05	*0.35*	0.08	0.06	0.04
7	0.15	0.12	0.06	0.06	0.08	0.07	0.16	*0.16*	0.09	0.05
8	0.09	0.13	0.09	0.07	0.09	0.09	0.12	0.12	*0.13*	0.08
9	0.18	0.11	0.04	0.09	0.09	0.12	0.08	0.10	0.10	*0.08*

[a] From Jayant *et al.* (1983). Reprinted from The Bell System Technical Journal. Copyright 1983, AT&T.

spoken digits five and six seemed exceptionally difficult to scramble and their residual intelligibility ranged from 35 to 57%. Interestingly they found their female voice harder to scramble but they attributed this to the fact that she spoke more slowly than their male speaker. On the whole their results confirmed that, as expected, increasing the delay resulted in an improvement in the scrambling. Figure 6.7 summarizes the results of their experiments by plotting the percentage of correct identifications for each spoken digit. In each case there are two vertical bars; the one on the left refers to the female voice and the other refers to the male. Each bar has the four values 1, 2, 4, 8 which correspond to delays of 32, 64, 128 and 256 msec, respectively.

We must stress yet again that the numbers test, although it certainly provides us with useful guidelines, does not reflect the scrambler's performance with normal speech. Further experimentation suggests that a scrambler of the above type will yield virtually 0% intelligibility for normal speech.

4. *Other Possibilities*

Brunner (1980a) describes two different two-dimensional scramblers which both use frequency inversion and cyclic bandshifting with 16 possible values for the shift. Since the first of these uses a time technique which we have not yet discussed we will begin our discussion of Brunner's work by looking at his time domain technique. It is called *dynamic time reverberation* and is a bandpreserving operation in the time domain. One simple form of reverberation consists of multiple time-discrete echoes with an envelope which, typically, decays exponentially. The interecho interval is controlled and varied at periodic intervals; possibly several times per second. Thus, at any given moment, the scrambler output is a function of the present speech amplitude together with its past amplitudes. But, and this is important, the contribution of each amplitude is decreased by a factor which depends upon the time which has elapsed since the amplitude first appered, i.e., the greater the time which has passed since the amplitude was used the lower its contribution to the scrambler output. This simple form is often called *forward reverberation*. *Reverse reverberation* is the case when, rather than decaying, the speech sounds gradually build up to their full values. Since the human ear tends to be less accustomed to hearing evolving sounds than it is to hearing decaying sounds, reverse reverberation tends to yield a lower residual intelligibility. However, with reverse reverberation, the scrambler output clearly depends on future amplitudes and thus, as a consequence, there is an inevitable time delay. Forward reverberation, while yielding a higher residual intelligibility, involves no time delay.

In the first of the two systems described by Brunner, forward reverberation is employed in addition to the cyclical frequency bandshift operation. Brunner says that this technique, which involves performing the frequency domain scrambling prior to the scrambling in the time domain, produces digit intelligibilities in the range of 18–28% and a word intelligibility of zero. He recommends this technique for telephone and vhf/uhf half-duplex radio channels. The second system combines cyclical bandshift scrambling with time shifting of speech between two sub-bands. We have already discussed the differential delaying of sub-bands, (see Chapter 4). In this technique the frequency spectrum is split into two halves and the lower half is delayed by t sec. The upper sub-band is then delayed by t sec at the descrambler. Thus there is an overall delay of t sec. This time Brunner found that the system provided digit intelligibilities in the range of 25–38% and word intelligibilities of 2–3%. He recommends it for use over lower-quality radio and telephone channels which introduce heavy signal distortion and interference, such as SSB, fading and large frequency offsets. In this system the time scrambling takes place prior to the frequency scrambling.

V. Comparisons of Techniques

For the last two and a half chapters we have discussed a number of different scrambling techniques. As far as analogue systems are concerned, the list is now more or less complete. In this section we will now look back at the various examples, compare them and see what conclusions we can reach. The reader must accept that we cannot possibly reach any firm conclusion about which is the 'best' system.

A. A Statistical Comparison

As we have repeatedly emphasized, in any given situation there is a balance to be made between audio quality and residual intelligibility together with the overall cryptographic strength. This is the user's decision and, as we saw in Chapter 1, will vary dramatically. So, of course, as the user's priorities change then so will our assessment of the 'best' system. However, no matter what his priorities may be, every user will require a reasonably low residual intelligibility from his system and this is why we have placed such emphasis on this asect. For each of the systems that have been introduced the reader should have some idea of the approximate level of residual intelligibility.

We have, on a number of occasions, discussed the statistical information which a number of authors have published in reports on various listening tests. Although these tests are very important they are, unfortunately, not particularly helpful for comparing systems. Most of the tests which we discussed were conducted by different people in different places at different times. They used different equipment, different speakers and different subjects. In some instances they even used different languages. Thus, although each is interesting in its own right, it is not easy to use their results to make any direct comparisons. Clearly if we wish to compare a number of systems then we need some tests specifically designed for the purpose. Such a set of tests were performed by Jayant *et al.* of Bell Laboratories and we will now report on their work (Jayant *et al.*, 1981).

In their tests Jayant *et al.* compared time sample scramblers, hopping window time element scramblers, frequency inversion and a two-dimensional system which combined frequency inversion with a hopping window time element scrambler. We will first explain the format of their tests and then, after discussing the various parameters which they measured, we will present their results.

Their tests for measuring the residual intelligibility were very similar to those which we have already discussed. They began by recording the scrambled speech of two speakers, one female and one male. As in the earlier tests, each sample consisted of four digit numbers with each digit spoken separately. We must stress yet again that this type of test is very harsh on the scrambler and, furthermore, that it is not clear that the relative performances of scramblers in this test will give an accurate indication of their relative performances when scrambling normal speech. We must also point out that the authors were aware of the limitations of their analysis. Nevertheless the results are still of immense interest. Each speaker recorded a list of 200 four-digit numbers and the lists were balanced so that each of the ten digits occurred four times within each set of ten numbers. It was also arranged that each digit was in a different position within each group of four. In order to compare the various techniques directly, five sets of ten numbers recorded by each speaker were processed by each type of scrambler.

In these tests a total of twenty five different scramblers were used. Eighty listeners were divided into five groups of sixteen and each group heard the speech processed by five of the twenty five scramblers. They judged two scramblers per day for five days and, on each day, heard one tape from the male speaker and one from the female. In order to reduce the ambient noise and various other distractions the subjects listened to the recordings through headphones. They were told to listen to each number and then to write down their best guess for that number. Finally they were instructed to avoid giving no answer and to guess if necessary.

The parameters recorded for each scheme were

(1) digit intelligibility,
(2) subject variability,
(3) learning,
(4) fatigue
(5) learning and fatigue.

Also recorded were delay time and bandwidth required for each scheme.

TABLE 6.2

The Experimental Results[a]

Scrambling scheme	1% energy bandlimits W_L	W_H	Encoding delay in 8 kHz samples	Digit intelligibility (%)	Subject variability (%)	Learning (%)	Fatigue (%)	Learning fatigue (%)
Clear speech	120	1920	0					
1	120	1920	0	30	8	37	7	0
2(a)	120	3640	2	92	4	0	0	0
2(b)	120	3480	8	69, 89	10, 4	35	4	0
2(c)	120	3640	32	20, 31	6, 6	33	0	11
2(d)	280	3680	128	16, 32	8, 7	21	14	14
3(a)	80	2240	256	100	<1	0	0	0
3(b)	40	2600	256	100	<1	0	0	0
3(c)	40	3040	256	96	2	0	0	0
3(d)	40	3440	256	63, 74	9, 5	35	3	0
3(e)	120	2040	1024	98	2	0	0	0
3(f)	120	2080	1024	100	<1	0	0	0
3(g)	80	2320	1024	96	2	0	0	0
3(h)	80	2640	1024	90	5	14	0	0
3(i)	80	2920	1024	45	11	41	24	21
3(j)	40	3360	1024	21, 13	12, 6	3	3	10
4(a)	80	2240	256	23	4	4	8	4
4(b)	40	2600	256	25	6	23	4	8
4(c)	40	3040	256	20	3	0	21	0
4(d)	40	3440	256	21	4	13	13	3
4(e)	120	2040	1024	20	4	20	7	3
4(f)	120	2080	1024	20	5	4	0	8
4(g)	80	2320	1024	17	4	4	4	0
4(h)	80	2640	1024	12	2	0	11	0
4(i)	80	2920	1024	13	2	0	6	0
4(j)	40	3360	1024	11	3	6	3	0

[a] From N. S. Jayant, B. J. McDermott, and S. W. Christensen, A comparison of four methods for analog speech privacy. IEEE Trans. Commun. **COM-29**, 18 (1981). Copyright © 1981 IEEE.

Before we consider the results we will briefly consider each of the parameters which were measured and which are recorded in Table 6.2.

1. *Digit Intelligibility*

The *digit intelligibility score*, *I*, for each scheme is the percentage of the 200 digits that were correctly identified, averaged across all subjects. As always with such tests it should be appreciated that with pure guessing we would expect a result of 10%. Occasionally the difference in intelligibility between the male and female sources was statistically greater than chance variability. When this occurred two scores were recorded, the first score corresponding to the male.

2. *Subject Variability*
Subject variability is measured by means of the standard deviation, σ. Roughly speaking one can assume that 68% of individual scores would be within $I \pm \sigma$; 95% of scores would be within $I \pm 2\sigma$ and 99% of scores within $I \pm 3\sigma$.

3. *Learning*
With all scramblers, as we have seen, something of interest is whether or not a subject can 'learn' to understand. To provide some measure of this a record was kept of each individual's scores for the five sets of 10 numbers to which they listened. If the intelligibility between sets of ten numbers showed a statistically significant increase and thereafter remained constant (statistically speaking) then the behaviour was classified as learning. The figure shown is the percentage of the listeners who appeared to 'learn'.

4. *Fatigue*
Another point of interest with scramblers is how tired listeners became as a result of trying to understand the scrambled speech. Obviously, from the designer's point of view, the concentration needed to try to understand the signal can be regarded as an indication of the effectiveness of his technique. In a similar way to that used for learning, it was decided whether intelligibility showed a significant decrease over the five sets of ten numbers. The figure shown is the percentage who appeared to become 'fatigued'.

5. *Learning and Fatigue*
Many subjects showed significant increases in their scores followed by decreases. This was classified under this category.

If the figures for learning, fatigue, and learning and fatigue are summed and subtracted from 100 we will get the percentage of subjects whose scores showed no appreciable change.

6. *Delay*
This refers to the enciphering delay; the time between the speech entering the scrambler and emerging as scrambled speech.

7. *Bandwidth*
The bandwidth expansion was measured using two parameters W_L and W_H. They are shown in Fig. 6.8. They are the low and high frequency tails of 1% energy. The energy in the output signal was measured and averaged over several seconds to obtain values for W_L and W_H. We shall see that for

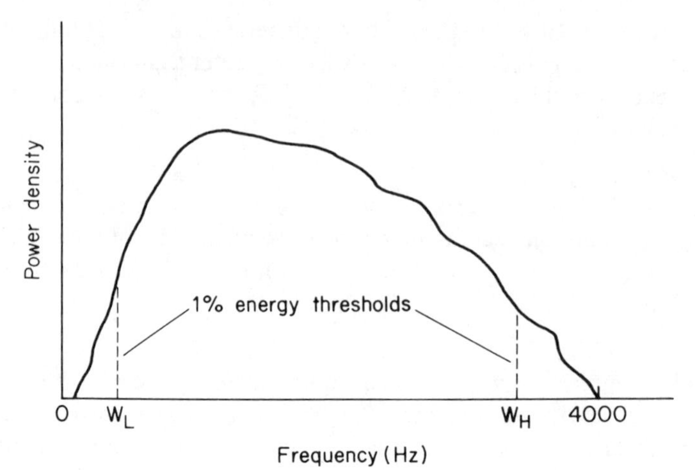

FIG. 6.8. 1% energy thresholds.

clear speech, W_H in particular is much lower than might be expected, resulting from the fact that voiced segments of speech tend to be of lower frequencies than unvoiced segments and, also, tend to dominate most speech. Throughout these tests an 8-kHz sampling rate was used for the 200–3200 Hz bandwidth of the signal. The scramblers compared were

(1) frequency inversion
(2) time sample scramblers using the following block sizes:
    (a) 2 samples/block
    (b) 8 samples/block
    (c) 32 samples/block
    (d) 128 samples/block
(3) hopping window time element scramblers with
    (a) 64 samples/segment; 4 segments/frame
    (b) 32 samples/segment; 8 segments/frame
    (c) 16 samples/segment; 16 segments/frame
    (d) 8 samples/segment; 32 segments/frame
    (e) 256 samples/segment; 4 segments/frame
    (f) 128 samples/segment; 8 segments/frame
    (g) 64 samples/segment; 16 segments/frame
    (h) 32 samples/segment; 32 segments/frame
    (i) 16 samples/segment; 64 segments/frame
    (j) 8 samples/segment; 128 segments/frame
(4) 2-dimensional scrambling using frequency inversion and hopping window time element scrambling with
    (a) 64 samples/segment; 4 segments/frame

(b) 32 samples/segment; 8 segments/frame
(c) 16 samples/segment; 16 segments/frame
(d) 8 samples/segment; 32 segments/frame
(e) 256 samples/segment; 4 segments/frame
(f) 128 samples/segment; 8 segments/frame
(g) 64 samples/segment; 16 segments/frame
(h) 32 samples/segment; 32 segments/frame
(i) 16 samples/segment; 64 segments/frame
(j) 8 samples/segment; 128 segments/frame.

The results from their tests are shown in Table 6.2.

There are a number of interesting points that arise from Table 6.2.

(i) The variation between the listeners' performances tended to be negligible if the intelligibility was either very high or very low.

(ii) Frequency inversion did not produce any bandwidth expansion, had reasonably low residual intelligibility but enabled the listeners to show a 'learning' tendency. This is very much as we predicted in our discussions of frequency inversion of Chapter 4.

(iii) Time sample scrambling increased the bandwidth of the signal. There appeared, not surprisingly, to be a significant correlation between the amount of residual intelligibility and the number of samples per block; i.e., as one increased the other decreased. This technique also appears to be subject to learning characteristics.

(iv) The hopping window time element scramblers exhibited a high residual intelligibility for digits. It was also clear that the bandwidth expanded as the segments became smaller. The residual intelligibility also decreased as the number of segments per frame increased.

(v) Combining frequency domain scrambling with time domain scrambling showed a definite increase in performance with respect to residual intelligibility. Again, it appeared that on the whole an increasing bandwidth was associated with a decreasing segment length and an increasing number of segments per frame reduced the residual intelligibility.

It is encouraging to note that these results are basically in agreement with the theory of the various scramblers we have considered. As we have repeatedly remarked in this book, a great deal of the skill in scrambler design is concerned with making trade-offs between the various parameters and their effects on the performance of the system with respect to security and recovered audio quality.

Unfortunately, Jayant *et al.* did not publish a confusion matrix such as Table 6.1. However, it is worth noting one interesting fact which they reported. This was that "six" had a very high residual intelligibility within all schemes. Apparently, with few exceptions, correct identification of ''six'' was 10–30% higher than any other digit. In one scheme, where the mean intelligibility for all digits was only 25%, the intelligibility of ''six'' was 92%, (the values for the other nine digits ranged from 15–40%). They claim no evidence that ''six'' was the most frequent response for all the digits. It is interesting to note that this was also true to some extent with the results of the tests on the sliding window two-dimensional system which we described in this chapter.

B. A Quantitative Comparison

We shall now consider an atempt by McCalmont (1980) to produce a theoretic quantification of the security offered by an analogue scrambler. His basic aim was to produce a means for quantatively measuring the effectiveness of various schemes and the degree of communications security they provide. He made no attempt to quantify their robustness in the face of a bad communications channel but concentrated only on the security they might provide. It is interesting to consider the parameters that McCalmont felt were important. Hopefully, it will also show the reader just how difficult a theoretical quantification really is! It is hard enough to develop a consistent measure, i.e., one for which someone cannot find a system which is obviously insecure but does well on the measure. To try to prove that your measure is right is virtually impossible. McCalmont restricted his discussion to analogue scramblers that utilize a key which, via a sequence generator, change codes at regular intervals. Thus, only rolling code bandscramblers, as opposed to fixed code ones, were considered. Similarly he considered only those time element scramblers that change permutations, i.e., do not use the same one for each frame. He also did not consider the type of masking techniques which we considered at the start of this chapter. Instead he restricted himself to time and frequency domain scrambling. Following the pattern which we adopted for the Jayant *et al.* experiments we shall begin by describing each of the parameters that McCalmont used.

(1) *TWF*—This is a dimensionless value for the 'time/bandwidth product of a frame'. Essentially, if we let F be the frequency band within which elements of speech might be moved, and let T be the time over which elements of speech might be moved then TWF is defined by $TWF = F \times T$. As an example, if we look back to Fig. 6.2 and assume a frequency band of 3000 Hz and a time duration of 256 msec, i.e., sub-bands of 600 Hz and segments of 32 msec, then $TWF = 3000 \times 0.256 = 768$.

(2) *TWE*—This is the average time/bandwidth product of an element and is calculated by dividing *TWF* by the number of elements in a frame. For values given in Fig. 6.2. we have $TWE = 768/40 = 19.2$.

<table>
<tr><td rowspan="4">A_{21}</td><td>A_{32}</td><td>A_{53}</td><td>A_{44}</td><td rowspan="4">A_{25}</td><td>A_{36}</td><td>A_{57}</td><td>A_{48}</td></tr>
<tr><td rowspan="2">A_{22}</td><td>A_{43}</td><td>A_{34}</td><td rowspan="2">A_{26}</td><td>A_{47}</td><td>A_{38}</td></tr>
<tr><td>A_{33}</td><td>A_{24}</td><td>A_{37}</td><td>A_{28}</td></tr>
<tr><td rowspan="2">A_{12}</td><td>A_{23}</td><td rowspan="2">A_{14}</td><td rowspan="2">A_{16}</td><td>A_{27}</td><td rowspan="2">A_{18}</td></tr>
<tr><td>A_{11}</td><td>A_{13}</td><td>A_{15}</td><td>A_{17}</td></tr>
</table>

FIG. 6.9. Example of an irregular two-dimensional scrambler.

(3) *D—D* represents what McCalmont calls the *TWE* displacement and is given by *TWE/TWF*. Its aim is to define the range or area over which an element may be moved or relocated. Essentially the smaller the value for *D*, the larger the displacement that can be given to an element of speech. Again for our simple example, $D = 1/40 = 0.025$.

(4) *E—E* represents a measure of the irregularity or variation in shape of the elements. An example of variation in shape might, for instance, occur by allowing frequency inversion or reversed time segmentation to be used on the elements. Irregularity of shapes of elements is not something we have considered in detail, but might occur, for instance, by using a matrix like Fig. 6.2. but with less regularity. An example of such a matrix is shown in Fig. 6.9. This might be achieved for instance by varying the number of sub-bands utilized from segment to segment. *E* is then calculated according to the formula $E = E_{\text{min}} \times 0.5 \times (1 + V)/E_{\text{max}}$, where E_{min} is the smallest 'size' of an element and E_{max} is the largest 'size' of an element. *V* is equal to 1 if there is no variation in shape of elements and 0 if elements may change shape during scrambling. For the example of Fig. 6.2 we have $E_{\text{min}} = E_{\text{max}}$ and $V = 1$, so $E = 1$. In the case of Fig. 6.9 the segment A_{21} has largest 'size' 4 and so we have $E_{\text{min}}/E_{\text{max}} = 1/4$ and if $V = 1$ then $E = 0.25$. If we were to further assume that reverse time segmentation took place then $V = 0$ and *E* would equal $1/4 \times 0.5 \times (1 + 0) = 0.125$.

The remaining parameters which McCalmont considered are all concerned with the permutation and sequence generators.

(5) *R—R* is a measure of how often the coding permutations change. He introduced this parameter because increasing the rate of change produces a corresponding increase in the security of the system. *R* is defined simply as the amount of time between permutation changes. Thus, for instance, in Fig. 6.2, if we were to assume a 32-msec segment and to change the permutations

every frame then we would have $R = 0.256$. (It is not clear what value should be given to R in a sliding window system—presumably, since a new permutation is generated for each segment, the segment length would be an appropriate choice).

(6) C—This is a measure of the time which lapses before the scrambling patterns begin to repeat themselves. This will generally depend on the sequence generator, if one is used, but may also depend on the permutation store (if there is one). McCalmont suggests the following method for assigning C:

If the time before repetition is 0 h put $C = 10$
If the time before repetition is 0–1 h put $C = 5$
If the time before repetitions is 1–12 h put $C = 1$
If the time before repetitions is 13–24 h put $C = 0.9$
If the time before repetitions is 25–1000 h put $C = 0.8$
If the time before repetitions is 1000–5000 h put $C = 0.7$
If the time before repetitions is > 5000 h put $C = 0.6$.

(7) A—The parameter A refers to 'automatic code change'. This measures the system's ability to change the coding pattern without the user changing the key, i.e., it refers to the presence of some kind of message key/time of day technique being employed. We have not as yet discussed message keys but they will arise in the next chapter. For the moment we merely make the obvious observation that a scrambler either has or does not have this ability. If no such feature is incorporated in the system then we put $A = 1$; if it is included we put $A = 0.5$.

McCalmont suggests quantifying the degree of security of the system by calculating $S = TWE \times D \times E \times R \times C \times A$. The idea is that the smaller the value of S the higher the security level. In theory his formula seems appropriate. We will now use it to calculate the security of the following three systems:

(a) A rolling bandscrambler with 5 sub-bands, each of 600 Hz; a memory store of 32 permutations (no frequency inversion used) selected via blocks of 5 bits at 32-msec intervals. The five bits are taken from a 16-bit word generated by a non-linear sequence generator. The non-linear sequence generator produces a binary sequence of period 2^{64} and always starts from the same position when switched on.

(b) A hopping window time element scrambler with 8 segments/frames each segment of length 32 msec and a memory store of 1024 permutations selected via blocks of 10 bits from a 16-bit word. This word is generated by a non-linear sequence generator which provides a new word for each frame. The non-linear sequence generator produces a binary sequence of period 2^{64} and always starts from the same position when switched on.

(c) A two-dimensional scrambler made up of a five-band (600-Hz/band) rolling bandscrambler and a hopping window time element scrambler with 8 segments/frame and 32-msec segments. A memory store contains 1024 permutations on the 40 elements selected, via blocks of 10 bits, from a 16-bit word generated by the same sequence generator as described in (a) and (b). Again the sequence generator always starts from the same position when switched on.

In order to assess the security of each system we now compute the appropriate value for each of McCalmont's parameters.

(a) $TWF = F \times T = 3000 \times 0.032 = 96$
$TWE = TWF/5 = 19.2$
$D = TWE/TWF = 19.2/96 = 0.2$
$E = E_{\min} \times 0.5 \times (1 + V)/E_{\max} = 1$
$R = 0.032$

C—We must first calculate the repetition time. The sequence produced by the sequence generator is of length 2^{64} bits and 2^4 bits are used to select each permutation. Thus 2^{60} permutations will be produced before repetition begins. One of these is used every 0.032 sec. Thus, repetition begins after $2^{60} \times 0.032$ sec, i.e., after $2^{60} \times 0.032/3600$ h which is more than 10^{13} h. Thus, from the table of values, $C = 0.6$

$A = 1$

Therefore $S = 19.2 \times 0.2 \times 1 \times 0.032 \times 0.6 \times 1$, i.e., $S = 0.073728$.

(b) $TWF = F \times T = 3000 \times 0.256 = 768$
$TWE = TWF/8 = 96$
$D = TWE/TWF = 0.125$
$E = 1$
$R = 0.256$

C—This calculation is precisely as it was for system (a) and thus $C = 0.6$

$A = 1$

Therefore $S = 96 \times 0.125 \times 1 \times 1 \times 0.256 \times 0.6 \times 1$, i.e., $S = 1.8432$.

(c) $TWF = F \times T = 3000 \times 0.256 = 768$
$TWE = TWF/40 = 19.2$
$D = TWE/TWF = 0.025$
$E = 1$
$R = 0.256$
$C = 0.6$
$A = 1$

Therefore $S = 19.2 \times 0.025 \times 1 \times 0.256 \times 0.6 \times 1$, i.e., $S = 0.073728$.

If we now compare our three values for S we find that both systems (a) and (c) give $S \cong 0.07$ whilst (b) gives $S \cong 1.84$. But now we note that, since for all of these three systems the keystream generator was identical, we can only be comparing residual intelligibilities. In this case, these results clearly do not compare favourably with the statistical results which were presented earlier. Furthermore, nothing has been said regarding the permutations employed in the three examples. We may have deliberately filled some or all of our stores with just a handful of bad permutations, thus rendering the system very insecure!

McCalmont was, of course, aware of the limitations of such a procedure for measuring security levels and pointed out how arbitrary his formula for S was. There is no real doubt that all the parameters considered by McCalmont are relevant when trying to assess a security level. However our three worked examples force us to conclude that the set of parameters which need to be considered is, in practice, far larger than those which he employed. We have, for instance, already seen how difficult it is to measure the likely performance of a permutation or a sequence generator. Somehow these extra parameters need to be incorporated into the final formula. The user of a speech scrambler must be aware of all comparisons of the above type and perform his own tests to estimate the security level offered by any particular system. We know of no scheme which will guarantee a consistent answer.

VI. Synchronization

Any scrambler which offers a reasonable security level relies on some form of pseudo-random number generator to provide sequence addresses for stores etc. Clearly the scramblers in a network can only operate if they have the appropriate keys to initialise these pseudo-random number generators. Equally it is clear that, if it is to descramble correctly, the descrambler must know the precise moment at which to start its own pseudo-random number generator. Without this knowledge it will not be in step with the scrambling device which sent the message and, as a consequence, will be unable to completely decipher the cryptogram. In fact it may not even be able to start deciphering. (Some of the less robust systems may require even more synchronization to allow the receiver to adjust its frequency and, perhaps, to provide some channel equalization, i.e., to compensate for some of the transmission characteristics like, for instance, group delay. These comments apply to a large variety of receivers and are not restricted to those incorporating scramblers. However, they are really beyond the scope of this book.)

In this chapter we will concentrate on the form of synchronization signal required by the receiver so that it can recognise when a message is beginning and can start its own sequence generator. It must then also ensure that its sequence remains in step with that of the transmitter. There are two standard techniques for doing this. In the first, known as *initial synchronization only*, the receiver relies on initial synchronization, at the start of the message, and then relies on a clock to keep them in step. The alternative, known as *continuous synchronization*, is to send frequent updatings of synchronization information for which the receiver then searches. This system has two obvious advantages over initial synchronization only. First it permits *late entry*, i.e., it allows someone to start receiving the message even if he has missed the beginning. If we look back at the system of Fig. 5.8, or indeed if we consider any initial synchronization only system, we can see that it is impossible for anyone to join a secure conversation once it has begun. He has absolutely no way of knowing how far the receiver's sequence generator has moved from its initial position and, therefore, does not know how to initialise his own. With continuous synchronization late entry is possible since at each update, we can tell how far the sequence generator has progressed. Unfortunately continuous synchronization also has a great disadvantage. The same information which allows late entry to a genuine receiver may also enable an interceptor who misses the beginning of the message to deduce how much he has missed. One possibility for avoiding this risk is, at each update, to reload the sequence generator with a combination of a key and a '*time of day*' (TOD) signal which is included as part of the synchronization. (The signal is called 'time of day' because it changes each time that synchronization information is transmitted.) This reloading of the sequence generator also gives the system the added advantage that the sequence generator repeatedly starts in different places. This means that if, for instance, the sequence is selecting a permutation for the scrambling process, then at each update the system will start to use a different pseudo-random sequence of permutations. Thus any cryptanalyst who has managed to deduce the permutations used for a few of the frames prior to the update will not be able to use the knowledge to attack the message after it. Yet another advantage of this method is that fewer bits of the sequence which has been produced by the pseudo-random number generator are used for each key loaded.

The use of a TOD is illustrated in Fig. 6.10. In this situation any person joining the network will, provided he has the correct key, be able to descramble

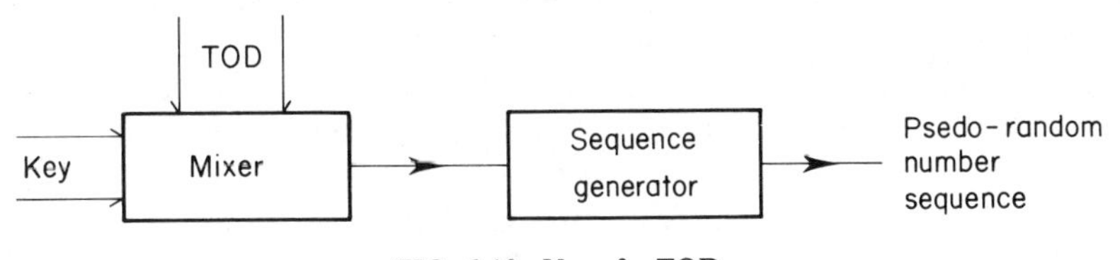

FIG. 6.10. Use of a TOD.

the cryptogram simply by extracting the TOD from the synchronization information and then mixing it with his own key to obtain the appropriate key for loading into the sequence generator. In practice, of course, this entire operation is carried out automatically as part of the descrambling technique. In fact if we look back at McCalmont's 'measure' we can see that the value of his parameter A was determined by whether or not this technique was employed.

If we use the system exactly as shown in Figure 6.10 then we will have introduced another disadvantage. If, for instance, there is a poor-quality link, then one of the synchronization updates may be lost; but if an update is lost, then the new TOD may be also missed and the receiver will be unable to load the correct key into his sequence generator. Once again, however, we have a problem which we can overcome. All that we need to do this time is to ensure that the TODs themselves form a predictable sequence; one possibility might be the outputs from a linear feedback shift register. Once this is done then the transmitter begins by choosing a random TOD but from then onwards the choices follow a predictable sequence. At the receiver, as soon as one TOD is correctly received, he can generate for himself all the other TODs which the transmitter is expected to send. This means that if, at any update time, the receiver misses the new TOD he can deduce what it should have been. Of course he can only do this under the assumption that the previous one used was correct. If this assumption is valid then he will stay in synchronization, but if it is wrong then he will lose it. In the latter case, he was 'in trouble' anyway and his false deduction of the next TOD will not make his situation any worse. This process if called *flywheeling*. The length of time for which a receiver can flywheel depends on the accuracy of his clock but, typically, it can be several hours.

In the situation described above, there is always the possibility that the receiver will obtain a synchronization update signal which contains the wrong TOD, i.e., one that was not expected. This might, (and we will discuss the possibility in more detail later), be a false synchronization in the sense that the receiver might be interpreting some extra signal, e.g., noise, as synchronization. If the receiver is in the process of flywheeling then it can safeguard against this. To do so it notes any update which it receives with the supposedly 'wrong' TOD and then, if the next update received ties up with the latter TOD, it will admit he was wrong and go over to the new one. If it does not tie up, it will remain as it was.

We will now summarise the method of continuous synchronization using a TOD which we have described in the last few paragraphs. At the start of a transmission, the transmitter will generate a random TOD and include it in the synchronization signal. All future synchronization updates will then contain predictable TODs (based on the first one), perhaps generated as the successive states of a linear feedback shift register. As soon as the receiver obtains a TOD it will then, in the event of not receiving a synchronization update when expected, flywheel and load the TOD which had been expected. If it receives an unexpected TOD it will not update its sequence generator immediately but will wait to see if there is another TOD which corresponds to it.

The second advantage of continuous synchronization is that, if a machine allows both scrambled and clear messages, the receiver can deduce for himself whether or not a message is scrambled simply by locating the synchronization updates. (These synchronization updates will not appear in clear messages.) Once he has recognised an update, he switches in the sequence generator and deciphers the message. This facility is often referred to as *clear voice override*. If the receiver is in clear voice override and, due to corruption of the data, the synchronization data is not received, then, of course, it will receive the scrambled message as if it were clear. To avoid this situation most sophisticated devices incorporate a 'hang' of a second or two which keeps the receive unit in secure mode for the time appropriate to a few synchronization signals. Thus, it will only receive scrambled messages as if they were clear if a considerable number of consecutive synchronization signals are lost.

In practice many devices allow three possible uses of the terminal: clear mode, secure mode and standby mode.

The term *clear mode* is self-explanatory and this mode is very useful if the network contains some devices which do not incorporate scrambling. If all the devices incorporate scrambling then the clear mode may be disabled. Similarly *standby*, which is the normal mode in which clear voice override is used, is of no value if all the devices are secured. If the network is such that the standby mode is used, then, when a secure transmission is received, the user will normally be given some 'prompt' to tell him and he will then manually switch himself to secure and avoid clear voice override. The biggest advantage of standby mode is that it is normally a mode in which the radio requires only a nominal amount of power. If the system is such that every device is secured then there is no need for any mode other than secure.

Initial synchronization only also has some advantages. If, for instance, the channel is very poor or if it is likely that someone will try to jam the signal, then this method may be more suitable. The reason for this is that, since it is the only chance for the transmitter and receiver to get in step, the initial synchronization signal tends to be more robust than those used for continuous synchronization. Some systems try to get the best of both methods by combining a robust initialization synchronization with a less robust continuous synchronization.

Another advantage of initial synchronization only is that it is obvious where to put the signal, i.e., at the beginning of the message. We have not yet discussed the problem of how often we should include synchronization updates when using continuous synchronization, nor have we looked at the effect that these updates may have on the quality of the recovered speech. We will postpone our discussion of these problems until we have discussed the forms which our synchronization signals may take. For the moment we will end our overall comparison of the two methods by saying that, in general, initial synchronization only (using the same TOD for the entire transmission) is often preferred for fixed point-to-point communications involving two stations, while continuous synchronization tends to be recommended for mobile, multi-station radio networks.

The form taken by the synchronization signal is greatly dependent on whether or not TOD information is to be transmitted. In other words, whether we are merely sending timing information or are also transmitting data. Another crucial factor is the type of channel over which the system operates. The simpler situation is, obviously, when we require only timing information. One simple technique, for instance, is to send a pair of tones, which the receiver is expecting, and use the transition from one tone to the other as the timing information. This is exceptionally easy to implement and can be very effective. However, if the channel is bad then the frequency offsets which occur can render the system inoperable. Furthermore, there is always a danger that the speaker at the transmit terminal will produce the same pair of tones during normal speech and, as a result, send the receiver out of synchronization.

An alternative technique for sending timing information is to send a data sequence which the receiver is expecting. The receiver then, at each instant in time, compares the data he is receiving with his next expected synchronization update. When the two agree he knows he has his timing information. If this method is adopted, then the data sequence must be chosen carefully. If, for instance, we use a sequence which might regularly occur as noise then the receiver is likely to obtain a number of false synchronizations. We also need to avoid sequences with bad autocorrelation functions. Although we introduced the autocorrelation function in Chapter 3 we did not say much about it. In order to see why our data sequence must have a good autocorrelation function we will work through an extreme example.

Suppose that we select the data sequence 00 ... 0 of length n as our synchronizing sequence. Then the arrangement at the receiver might be as shown in Fig. 6.11. The received signal is fed into an n-stage shift register while a second register holds the reference sequence; in this case 00 ... 0. As each new bit arrives the two registers are compared. In the scheme of Fig. 6.11 this is accomplished by modulo-2 adding the two sequences, of length n, bit-by-bit. If the bits agree the output from the XOR will be 0 and if they disagree it will be 1. The outputs from the n XORs are summed in the accumulator

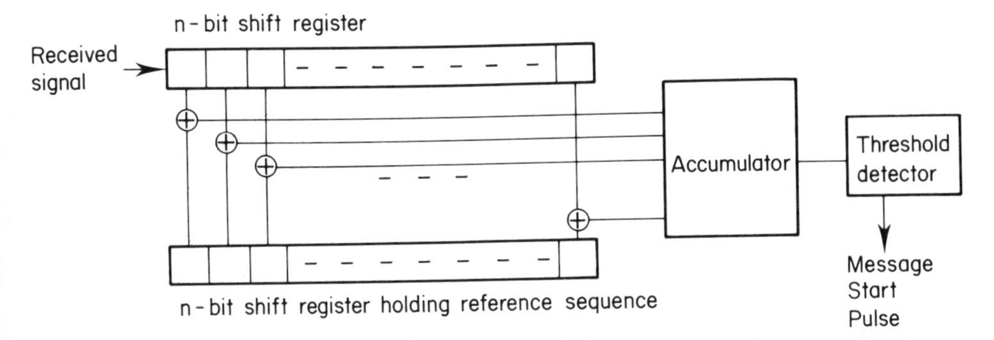

FIG. 6.11. Correlator.

and then passed to a threshold detector. For a perfect match we expect the accumulator to output 0. Thus, if the threshold factor is set at 0 and the output from the accumulator is also 0, a message start pulse will be sent to the rest of the system.

In order to illustrate the importance of the autocorrelation we will now return to our situation where the synchronization is 00 ... 0, and assume that the first $n - 1$ terms of this sequence have already arrived. To simplify this discussion we will, for the moment, also assume that the channel is error-free. Since our n-bit shift register for the received channel has received the first $n - 1$ bits of the synchronization signal, it will contain 0s in the $n - 1$ positions on the left and either 0 or 1 in the position on the right. So, even though *not one* of the received bits of the synchronization pattern is yet in its correct position, the two shift registers agree in every position except, possibly, one. Thus, we have a 50% chance of complete agreement one bit before the intended synchronization time and the accumulator will output 0 or 1 depending on this last bit. In any practical situation the users have to allow for the possibility of errors occurring during transmission and, consequently, the detector will almost certainly not be set at 0. Clearly, from our discussion, as soon as it is set at 1 or more such a system with a synchronization sequence of 00 ... 0 will always synchronize early. In other words, to emphasize the point, this system cannot possibly synchronize properly (unless, of course, sufficient errors occur to prevent it synchronizing early!).

Although the example just discussed is obviously extreme, it is nevertheless clear that we must take care in selecting our synchronization sequences. If we ignore the possibility of errors in transmission then one property that we require is that comparing a synchronization sequence with a translate of itself should be equivalent to comparing it with random data, (unless, of course, the shift is equal to the period). If this is not so, then certain translates may be misinterpreted as the synchronization sequences and, as in our extreme example, the system will synchronize too early. By looking back at Chapter 3, where all these terms were first introduced, we can see that this is one of the properties exhibited by maximal length linear feedback shift register sequences. For these m-sequences the out-of-phase autocorrelation is always $-1/(2^r - 1)$, where the period is $2^r - 1$. Furthermore if an m-sequence is compared with random data we would also expect roughly the same number of agreements and disagreements. So we would expect the autocorrelation to be about $-1/(2^r - 1)$ in that case also. For a number of other sequences, like for instance our extreme example $00\ldots0$, the autocorrelation with random data is likely to be much lower than its out-of-phase autocorrelation. If such a sequence is used then the probability of synchronizing early by obtaining part of the synchronization signal is likely to be much higher than we can accept. In view of their good autocorrelation properties, m-sequences appear to be suitable candidates for synchronizing sequences although, of course, they are not the only ones.

We will now assume that we are able to use a complete cycle of an m-sequence of length n as our synchronizing sequence and consider its performance in noisy conditions. (Note that this implies $n = 2^l - 1$ for some positive integer l). To do this we assume we have a probability p that a bit will be received in error. If we let P_i denote the probability that exactly i errors occur during transmission then, clearly, P_0 is the probability that the first bit is error free, then the second bit is error free, then the third and so on to the nth bit. Thus $P_0 = (1 - p)^n$. The probability that one particular bit is in error but the remaining $n - 1$ are not is $p(1 - p)^{n-1}$ and thus, since there are n possibilities for the position of the erroneous bit, $P_1 = np(1 - p)^{n-1}$. In general, if we let $\binom{n}{t}$ denote the number of ways of choosing t elements from n, (so $\binom{n}{t} = n!/t!(n - t)!$), we have

$$P_i = \binom{n}{i}p^i(1 - p)^{n-i}$$

If we let P_{r^-} be the probability of at most r errors occurring during transmission then $P_{r^-} = P_0 + P_1 + P_2 + \cdots + P_r$. Thus

$$P_{r^-} = \sum_{i=0}^{r} \binom{n}{i}p^i(1 - p)^{n-i}$$

So, for example, if we had a 15-bit sequence then the probability of at most 2 errors during transmission would be $(1 - p)^{15} + 15p(1 - p)^{14} + 105p^2(1 - p)^{13}$. Thus, in a channel where $p \cong 0.1$ we have $P_{2^-} \cong 0.816$. This means that if, for instance, we use a 15-bit sequence and arrange for our threshold detector to allow up to two errors then we would, over a channel with a $\frac{1}{10}$ mean bit error rate, expect to receive 81.6% of the synchronization sequences transmitted. This, of course, is true no matter how we choose the synchronization sequence. Furthermore, we can obviously increase the success rate by allowing more errors. Unfortunately as we increase the number of acceptable errors we also increase the number of sequences which may be mistakenly identified as synchronization signals. So, in particular, we are more likely to accept noise as a synchronization signal.

The normal method for measuring the false synchronization rate is to assume that the receiver is continually looking for a synchronization sequence and to estimate the probable number of false triggers per day. For this estimation we assume that the introduction of noise implies that totally random sequences are received (which of course is a slight oversimplification!) and determine the likelihood of accepting one of them. To do this we will work with our example of a 15-bit sequence and allow up to two errors. First we note that the total number of possible 15-bit sequences is 2^{15}. Then we observe that, if we are accepting two errors, a sequence will be accepted if it is the genuine one or the genuine one with one or two positions inverted. The number of sequences satisfying this is $1 + \binom{15}{1} + \binom{15}{2} = 1 + 15 + 105 = 121$. The probability of a random sequence being accepted as a synchronization signal is now given by dividing the number of 15-bit sequences which we will accept by the total number of 15-bit sequences. This gives $121/2^{15} \cong 0.0037$. In general if r errors are being allowed and if P_f denotes the probability of false synchronization then we have $P_f = \sum_{i=0}^{r} \binom{n}{i}/2^n$. To calculate the number of false synchronizations per day we now merely have to multiply P_f by the number of comparisons which will be made per day. If the signalling rate is s bits/sec, then the number of comparisons per day is $s \times 60 \times 60 \times 24$ and the number of false synchronizations per day is equal to $86400s \sum_{i=0}^{r} \binom{n}{i}/2^n$.

Table 6.3 shows some values for P_{r^-}, i.e., the probability of accepting the synchronization sequence, and the number of false synchronizations per day on the assumption that a 31-bit synchronization is used, the mean bit error

TABLE 6.3

A Probability Table

Number of errors allowed (r)	Probability of accepting the synchronization sequence (P_{r^-})	Expected number of false synchronizations per day
0	0.7323	0.002
1	0.9616	0.064
2	0.9964	1.00
3	0.9997	10.04
4	0.9999	73.34

rate is 0.01 and the transmission speed is 50 bits/sec. The table shows quite clearly the trade-off between obtaining a good value for P_{r^-} and obtaining a large number of false synchronization signals. If, for example, a user instructed the designer that he wanted P_{r^-} to be 0.99 but would not tolerate more than one false synchronization per day, then the designer would, on the evidence of Table 6.3, use a system allowing two errors. But if, on the other hand, he had to achieve $P_{r^-} = 0.999$ and no more than one false synchronization per day the designer would consider a longer sequence. If, to consider another possibility, he had to achieve $P_{r^-} = 0.999$, no more than one false synchronization signal per day and a transmission time of at most 0.6 sec, then the designer would conclude that these specifications could not be met using this method over this channel. His only options would be to find a different method, persuade the user to change his specification or resign!

There are many other techniques for transmitting start of message information. We will not discuss them here. However the example above should be sufficient to illustrate the kind of technique involved. Instead we now consider possibilities for transmitting some TOD information with these synchronization sequences. The simplest system is, possibly, to append the TOD information to the message start sequence. The receiver then knows that, as soon as it accepts a data sequence as synchronization, the data for TOD will follow immediately. If this type of system is used then it is important to appreciate that the TOD information will also be subject to errors and must also be error protected. In fact, in many ways, it is far more important to protect the TOD than to protect the synchronization sequence. To illustrate why, we will assume that we have a continuous synchronization system. If we miss the synchronization update then we can flywheel. The worst that is likely to happen is that someone trying to join the network might find that it took longer than normal. However, if we receive the synchronization sequence but then get the data wrong we will repeatedly load our sequence generator with wrong keys and hence fail to unscramble the cryptogram. Suppose, for example, that we have a system where, once the synchronization has been obtained correctly, there is a 95% chance of getting the correct data. This may appear to be reasonable, but it must be appreciated that it means that if the updates came at the rate of one per second then the descrambler would fail to descramble 5 sec of speech in every 100 sec. Of course, as we explained earlier in the chapter, the possibility of introducing flywheeling and the fact that we do not automatically accept a data block which disagrees with the expected data mean that the situation need not be quite as bad as this. Nevertheless it is obviously desirable to have a system which offers virtually 100% likelihood of correct data once synchronization has been obtained. In order to increase this likelihood we need to introduce some form of error protection. We will not enter into a discussion of error protection here. Instead, as in Chapter 2, we refer the reader to one of the many excellent books on coding theory. (See, for example, MacWilliams and Sloane, 1978; Peterson and Weldon, 1972).

Once we have decided on the form of synchronization which we intend to use we then have to decide how to transmit it. If we are in a situation where initial synchronization only is sufficient, then the decision may be easy. We may be able to use the entire speech band for this synchronization data transmission and perhaps use the data to modulate a carrier using *FSK* (*frequency shift keying*) or some other technique. In choosing a modulation scheme we will want one which restricts the data to the band available and does not interfere with other data on the band. We will also need to find a balance between the signalling rate and the ensuing bit error rate. As a general rule one may assume that increasing the data rate makes the data more prone to error. This, of course, suggests using a slow bit rate. But the slower the bit rate the longer the system takes to synchronize which means there is a corresponding increase in the delay between the user picking up his handset or pressing his PTT (press to talk) before he can commence speaking. The length of this delay depends on the type of channel for which the scrambler is being designed but, in currently available equipment varies from a few milliseconds to several seconds.

If we wish to use a continuous synchronization system then our choice is, essentially, between sending the synchronization information on a separate channel from the speech, which usually entails some bandwidth expansion and is consequently often unacceptable, or sharing the band between the synchronization information and the speech. If the latter technique is chosen then we must decide how to share the channel. An obvious possibility is to assign the synchronization information to the edges of the band where the speech energy is lowest and where, as a consequence, minimum interference will occur. However this is not necessarily a good idea because, as we saw in Chapter 2, the greatest distortion occurs at the band edge.

One popular technique for band sharing is to use a band stop filter to create a notch in the frequency band of the speech signal, typically somewhere between 1800 and 2000 Hz. This notch is then used for the synchronization information. With this technique a width of 100–200 Hz is normally sufficient for the size of the notch and does not normally cause any appreciable degradation in the speech quality. The synchronization data may then be transmitted in this small band using FSK, or some other modulation technique, at a low data rate. This data rate is often chosen so that the synchronization information, including any TOD data, can be transmitted during a single, or possibly two, frames of the speech. Thus the sequence generator at the transmitter can be loaded and used to select just one or two permutations before being reloaded and so on. So suppose, for example, that a time element scrambler used 1-sec frames and that synchronization plus TOD was 50 bits. If a signalling rate of 50 bits/sec were selected, the system would resynchronize every frame and, provided that the error rate was at an acceptable level, anyone joining the net would not have to wait more than 1 sec to synchronize.

When transmitting the synchronization data in this small band, it is customary to send it at a power level which is considerably lower than that of the speech signal. This restricts the power used for synchronization, as opposed to speech, and also ensures that if the receiver fails to completely remove this data band from the signal then the level of interference heard is minimal.

The technique which we have just described for combining synchronization and speech is essentially just a frequency multiplexing system. In other words all we do is remove part of the speech band and insert synchronization information. An alternative method is to time multiplex the synchronization and speech. We will consider this approach in the context of a time element scrambler. In this case we could remove part of the time spectrum, possibly 1 segment/frame, and then use this time to transmit the synchronization data. This has the advantage that the whole frequency band can be utilized and hence higher transmission rates can be obtained. However if we are to adopt this approach then we must decide what to do at the receiver. When we were withdrawing part of the frequency spectrum we were, nevertheless, continuously transmitting. Thus, the receiver always heard something, even if part of the spectrum was missing. This is usually tolerated but to have time sections of the speech missing might not be so acceptable. One possible way of avoiding these intervals, with no speech, is for the receiver to replay a segment in place of the missing one. For instance suppose that, in an 8-segment/frame hopping window system, we are transmitting two frames of speech and that segment 4 is being replaced by synchronization information. So, for instance, we might be in the situation shown in Fig. 6.12 where we have assumed that the receiver who has 'lost' segment 4 simply repeats segment 3. Clearly this type of arrangement inevitably causes some degradation. However, as we saw in Chapter 2, speech changes relatively

Input	1	2	3	4	5	6	7	8	1	2	3	4	5	6	7	8
Transmission	Sync	1	8	5	7	3	6	2	8	1	7	5	3	6	2	Sync
Output	1	2	3	3	5	6	7	8	1	2	3	3	5	6	7	8

FIG. 6.12. Time multiplexing speech and synchronization.

slowly and so, particularly if the time segments are short, this technique is usually acceptable. Since segment 4 is likely to be transmitted in any position within a frame, if we adopt this technique then synchronization is not sent at regular time intervals. However, once the receiver has found one synchronization burst he can then load his sequence generator, determine the next permutation to be used and, hence, when the next synchronization burst will be.

With the frequency multiplex system for transmitting synchronization information, an enemy can jam all communications simply by sending a high power tone continuously at the frequency used for the synchronization data. From the point of view of protection against jamming the time multiplex system has a definite advantage. Since, with time multiplexing, the time slot moves around the enemy cannot simply use a *pulse jammer*, i.e., a jammer which sends out jamming tones at regular time intervals. If he wants to be sure that he prevents all communications then he must continually blot out virtually all the band. We will return to this type of problem when we discuss digital speech.

In this section we have attempted to give an overall feeling for the synchronization problem. We have by no means given a complete treatment of the subject and have merely provided a brief introduction.

VII. Radio Range

One of the problems which we have repeatedly encountered is that of the reduction in the range of a radio, which might arise as a consequence of incorporating a scrambler into the communications system. In this short section we will simply summarize some of the more important aspect of the range.

For a clear radio transmission the range achieved is a function of many parameters which include the transmitting power, the transmitting and receiving aerial systems, the transmission path and its propagation characteristics, the receiver sensitivity and noise performance. In order to appreciate how the range may be affected when a scrambler is introduced we must consider (i) any additional noise which may be introduced by the scrambling/descrambling operation, (ii) the proportion of the transmitter power which is not used for the signal (e.g., it might be used for sending synchronization and TOD) and (iii) whether the synchronization data can still be recovered at a range where the clear voice signal would only just be acceptable.

With regard to (i) we must accept that almost anything we do to the clear signal, in order to scramble it, will introduce noise. The level of this noise will vary and the techniques which require most processing will probably introduce most noise. There are even some particular schemes, like amplitude masking, which deliberately introduce noise and then use power to transmit this noise rather than the wanted signal. With regard to (ii), once again we just have to accept that, in order to transmit synchronization and TOD information, we have to spend power on a signal other than the wanted speech signal. All we can do is keep this power to a minimum. The third point (iii) essentially recommends that the synchronization signal should be at least as robust as the speech signal. Speech is very redundant and can be intelligible with remarkably large volumes of noise added to it. (Indeed, if this were not so, many of the scramblers which we have discussed would not work!) We must ensure that the synchronization signal is at least as robust.

We end this chapter by noting that we have not yet discussed the problems associated with key handling for these analogue systems. However, these problems are very similar to those for digital systems and we will postpone that discussion until the next chapter.

7. Digital Scramblers

I. Introduction and Basic Concepts

In this, the final chapter, we look at digital scramblers. Although, in Chapter 1, we have already explained the difference between analogue and digital scramblers, we will begin by repeating our description of the typical digital scrambling and descrambling methods. In order to encipher speech using a digital scrambler we first input the analogue speech signal to an A/D converter to produce a binary data stream. We then encipher the binary data stream, essentially ignoring the fact that it was derived from speech and, finally, we transmit the resulting binary stream. It is not, of course, necessary for the A/D converter to produce binary data, however it certainly makes the situation easier and simplifies the discussion. Consequently we shall restrict our attention to the binary case. At the receiver the opposite operations are carried out in reverse order. Thus, the descrambler interprets the received signal as a binary stream, deciphers that stream and then uses a D/A converter to produce an analogue speech waveform.

Of course the above description is very simplistic and ignores most of the practical problems associated with such a technique. It does not, for example, mention synchronization. As we saw in the last chapter, achieving a robust method of synchronization is certainly not a trivial task and it is one of the many problems which we shall need to discuss.

In practice a simplex digital system is likely to be as shown in Fig. 7.1. One of the hardest tasks in designing such a system is to match the A/D converter and modulation system to the transmission channel. Fortunately, at least from the scrambler designer's point of view, digital communications systems, i.e., systems like Fig. 7.1 but without the scrambler and descrambler, are becoming more popular and, as a consequence, retrofitting security to this type of network is becoming much easier. It is not, however, a trivial matter because there are a number of important considerations, such as

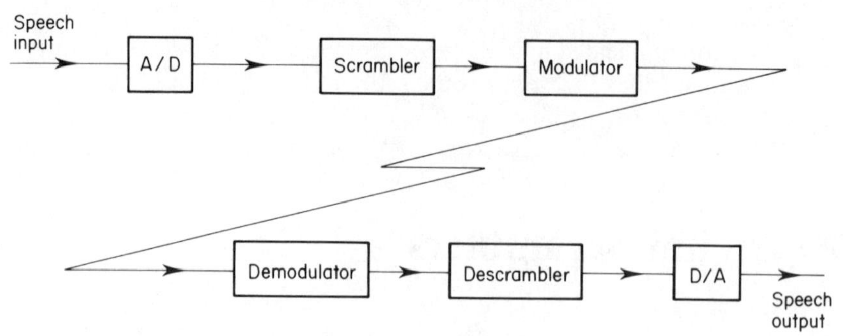

FIG. 7.1. Digital system.

synchronization and key management, which arise as a result of introducing the scrambler.

As we mentioned in the earlier chapters, recent advances in digital signal processing together with the advent of low-cost microprocesser-based technology mean that acceptable-quality, relatively low-bandwidth, real-time digital voice communications are becoming a reality. For instance there now exist modems capable of transmitting 16-kbit/sec data over a telephone system. Admittedly their performance is still slightly questionable, but they are definitely becoming more reliable. There also exist 2.4-kbit/sec duplex modems which operate over two-wire telephones. It is even expected that, in the near future, these will extend to 9.6 kbit/sec, by the use of sophisticated echo cancelling techniques. It is perhaps worth noting, in this context, that the quality of telephone systems varies dramatically from country to country. Consequently the user should not assume that a system which he sees working perfectly in one country will necessarily work as well elsewhere.

For radio communications the situation is somewhat different. Here the signalling rate which can be used is highly dependent on the choice of frequency. For instance, until very recently, hf communications which use a standard voice channel have been restricted to rates of little more than 300 bits/sec. This is certainly not enough to support digital speech at the present time. However the recent emergence of sophisticated parallel-tone hf modems now means that 2.4-kbit/sec communications are possible over hf. A parallel-tone hf modem utilizes a number of carriers within the speech band, each of which carries data at up to 75 bits/sec. Recent research suggests that, using sophisticated channel equalization techniques, a serial (i.e., a single carrier) 2.4-kbit/sec modem should soon be feasible. At vhf, which usually employs 25-kHz channel spacing, 12.5- or even 16-kbit/sec data can be supported. At higher frequencies the amount of total bandwidth increases and, as a result, the restrictions become easier. However, we must stress that digital data communicated by radio is susceptible to errors occurring during transmission and that this tends to be especially bad in the hf band. The problems of errors occurring is one of the principal factors to be considered when choosing the ciphering technique for digital voice encryption.

II. Encryption and Synchronization

We begin this section by discussing a scrambling technique which has been widely used for digital speech scrambling. It is an error propagating system and therefore, in our opinion, unsuitable for this application. Furthermore, most modern digital scramblers are moving away from this technique to the non-error propagating stream ciphers. The technique relies on the so-called cipher feedback or self-synchronizing sequence generator. We did not discuss it in Chapter 3 but feel we must say a little about it now. There are two reasons. One is for completeness and the other is to emphasize the (probably unacceptable) disadvantages which have to be tolerated as the price for obtaining self-synchronization.

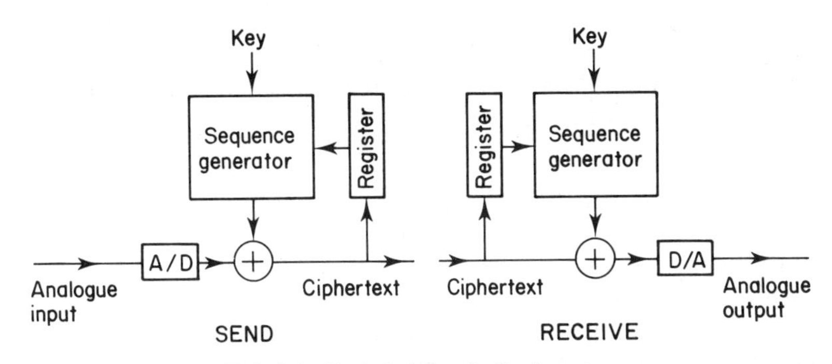

FIG. 7.2. Typical cipher feedback system.

The basic idea of a *cipher feedback system* is shown in Fig. 7.2. From the diagram we can see that the ciphertext is continuously providing one of the inputs to the sequence generator and, consequently, affecting the resulting encipherment. In order to illustrate how it works we will consider a specific example in which the sequence generator is a linear shift register. In Fig. 7.3 we illustrate one possibility for such a system. Here, as well as being transmitted, the ciphertext is fed back into the n-stage shift register. (This type of system is, in many ways, a 'cross' between a block and stream cipher, and it is often classified in either category.)

Suppose that we have such a system and that our key determines the feedback coefficients $c_0, c_1, \ldots, c_{n-1}$. If we let the binary message be

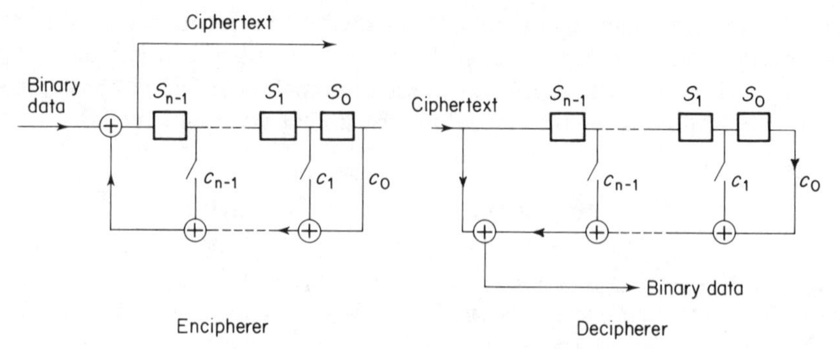

FIG. 7.3. Cipher system using a linear shift register.

$m_0 m_1 m_2 \ldots$ and the corresponding ciphertext bits be $e_0 e_1 e_2 \ldots$ then, if the initial contents of the registers are $s_0, s_1, \ldots, s_{n-1}$, when m_0 is fed in, the output e_0 will be given by:

$$e_0 = m_0 + \sum_{i=0}^{n-1} c_i s_i$$

where, of course, all additions are modulo 2. But now s_0 is no longer in the register. In fact, for $1 \leqslant i \leqslant n - 1$, s_i is now in stage S_{i-1} and e_0 is the new entry in S_{n-1}. Thus, when m_1 is input we get

$$e_1 = m_1 + \sum_{i=0}^{n-2} c_i s_{i+1} + c_{n-1} e_0$$

Thus, the preceding ciphertext is already affecting the encryption of the second message bit. As the process continues the initial entries in the register will eventually 'disappear' from the register and, after n outputs, each ciphertext bit e_j will depend only on m_j and the n previous ciphertext bits. In general, for $h \geqslant 0$, the enciphering equation is

$$e_{n+h} = m_{n+h} + \sum_{i=0}^{n-1} c_i e_{i+h} \tag{1}$$

In order to perform a similar calculation for the deciphering process we must assume that the receiver has the correct key, and hence the same feedback coefficients, as the transmitter. Since we have no reason to assume that they will be the same as the transmitter's, we let $s_0^*, s_1^*, \ldots, s_{n-1}^*$ denote the initial entries in the receiver's register. If we denote the receiver's input by $e_0^*, e_1^*, e_2^*, \ldots$, then, of course, for an error-free channel we will have $e_j^* = e_j$ for all j. If we denote the receiver's output by $m_0^*, m_1^*, m_2^*, \ldots$, then, clearly, for correct decipherment we want $m_j^* = m_j$ for all j.

In precisely the same way as at the transmitter, at each of the first n inputs one of the initial entries disappears from the register and does not affect the later decipherment. Thus, apart from the first n bits, each m_j^* depends only on e_j^* and the previous n received bits. More precisely we have

$$m_{n+h}^* = e_{n+h}^* + \sum_{i=0}^{n-1} c_i e_{i+h}^* \qquad \text{for all} \qquad h \geqslant 0 \tag{2}$$

Thus, if $e_i^* = e_i$ for all i, i.e., if there are no errors during the transmission, from Eq. (1) we get

$$m_{n+h}^* = e_{n+h} + \sum_{i=0}^{n-1} c_i e_{i+h} = m_{n+h}$$

In other words the ciphertext is deciphered correctly except that, unless the registers at the transmit and receive ends have the same initial contents, the first n bits of the message are lost.

As well as establishing that our cipher feedback system works, the preceding discussion also establishes that the system automatically synchronizes. In other words it shows that, without transmitting any particular synchronization bits, the system "self-synchronizes". Furthermore, if a bit is somehow lost or gained during transmission, as opposed to being altered, then the situation is merely equivalent to the initialisation process when the two registers have different initial entries. Thus, we would lose up to n bits and then come back into synchronization. There is, however, a price to be paid for the self-synchronization. The first disadvantage is the loss of the first n message bits; but, for highly redundant digital speech, this is not too great a problem. A second, and much more important, drawback is that error propagation occurs. Suppose, for example, that an error occurs during the transmission and a bit is altered. If we assume this bit is e_{n+k} then this means that $e_{n+k}^* \neq e_{n+k}$ which in turn means that, unless some other error occurs to compensate, m_{n+k}^* will not be the same as m_{n+k}. So, as we would expect, a transmission in error causes a bit to be deciphered incorrectly. Unfortunately, for this type of system, m_{n+k}^* is not the only bit of the deciphered message which is affected by e_{n+k}^*. Since e_{n+k}^* is in the register for n time pulses it affects a further n bits of the deciphered message (see Eq. (2)). So, on the assumption that each of these bits has a probability of about $\frac{1}{2}$ of being wrong, about $\frac{1}{2}n$ bits of the deciphered message will be affected by a single error in the transmission path.

Although we have only discussed cipher feedback in the context of our one shift register example, similar results hold for all other algorithms (even if they are non-linear). This has important consequences. Suppose, for instance, that we wish to transmit a 16-kbit/sec digital voice signal over a noisy channel with a 10% mean error rate. If we are transmitting clear speech then, surprising though it may seem, the redundancy of the speech is sufficient that this is workable although, in all probability, the resulting signal will not sound particularly pleasant. But if we want to use a cipher feedback system then, as we have just seen, we are introducing error propagation. This implies a significant increase in the error rate at the descrambler with the almost inevitable consequence that the output will be unintelligible. So, for this particular example, the introduction of a scrambler makes a workable, albeit noisy, channel totally unusable. If a radio system is being used then the effect will be a significant reduction in the range of the radio. Clearly, from the user's point of view, this is undesirable.

The disastrous consequences of error propagation are one of the major reasons why most modern systems tend to use a non-error-propagating stream cipher. Unfortunately stream ciphers are not self-synchronizing and thus a separate synchronization signal is required. Stream ciphers are also not as able to cope with bits being added or lost in the stream. However within most communications systems this is not very likely to happen. Furthermore if continuous synchronization is used then a stream cipher does, periodically, have the opportunity to recover from this problem.

There is another disadvantage of cipher feedback systems. It arises from the fact that, when using such a system, we have two inputs to the sequence generator: the key and the last n bits of ciphertext. Unfortunately, since he is monitoring the transmission medium, the interceptor knows these ciphertext bits and it is certainly conceivable that he will be able to use this information. With most current sequence generators it is very difficult to guarantee that the equations representing the algorithm will not be reduced in complexity for some particular sets of input variables. As a consequence it is generally recognised that any given algorithm's vulnerability to attack might be increased by using a cipher feedback. We will say no more about cipher feedback systems and refer the interested reader to Beker and Piper (1982d).

When we reviewed data equipment in Chapter 3 we discussed the worst-case conditions which we felt all designers should accept. They were that the cryptanalyst

(WC1) has a complete knowledge of the cipher system,
(WC2) has obtained a considerable amount of ciphertext,
(WC3) knows the plaintext equivalent of a certain amount of the ciphertext.

We must now consider these conditions in the context of digital speech scramblers. The first two conditions are self-explanatory. We have always assumed that an interceptor will be able to obtain complete information about our equipment and that he can intercept all communications. Since, in most cases, all he needs is an antenna the interception of communications is often particularly easy in the context of radio communications. There are, however, techniques which are often employed to try to make interception more difficult. One possibility is in the use of some form of frequency hopping, as discussed in Chapter 4, and another is to use *traffic flow security*, which we mentioned very briefly in Chapter 1. In order to define traffic flow security and to see why it 'works' we must consider the form of the intercepted signal. If we are using a stream cipher technique, or even a cipher feedback system, then provided that the sequence generator produces a good pseudo-random sequence the intercept will sound like white noise. With traffic flow security, random binary pulses are sent down the line whenever no message is being transmitted. So, in this case, the interceptor is always obtaining a stream of pulses which appear to be random and will not know if a message is being transmitted. (The reader may be interested to know that if a stream of random binary pulses is input directly to a loudspeaker, the result sounds like white noise. Thus, the interceptor is, in principle, unable to distinguish between traffic or noise modulation and this gives rise to the improvement in security.)

It is not quite so clear what condition WC3 means for a digital speech system. Indeed, given the way that the system is set up, even the encipherer does not know the plaintext for his message, i.e., he does not know the sequence of binary digits being enciphered. However, we must not forget that the digital encoder is a fixed process and will, consequently, produce a fixed output pattern of bits for any fixed input pattern, (apart, perhaps, for a few bits at the beginning of the message while the machine is stabilising). Now suppose, for instance, that there is an air-conditioner whine, (or some other well-known noise), in the background while someone is speaking. Then whenever they pause the bit pattern produced will be the response of the A/D converter to the air conditioner. But this is likely to be recognised, particularly in a long speech with many pauses. This illustrates one way in which known plaintext may be obtained. There is, however, another and much more important source of plaintext.

Throughout this book we have highlighted the extent of the redundancy in human speech. Although this is an advantage when considering transmission errors it has the disadvantage of enabling the interceptor to utilize the statistical tests described in Chapter 3. Rather than give a detailed discussion we merely record some of the results of applying them to a portion of digitized speech from a delta modulator. The input to the delta modulator consisted of English speech with rather exaggerated pauses and relatively little background noise. The modulator sampled at 16,000 bits/sec and the sample contained 7,110,496 bits.

First we applied the frequency test which, in this example, means nothing more than counting the number of zeros (n_0) and the number of ones (n_1). The results were $n_0 = 3{,}546{,}365$ and $n_1 = 3{,}564{,}131$. This gives 95% confidence intervals for the probability of occurrence of a 0 or 1 (p_0 and p_1, respectively) as $0.4984 \leqslant p_0 \leqslant 0.4991$ and $0.5009 \leqslant p_1 \leqslant 0.5016$. From this we see that there is a reasonably even distribution of zeros and ones and the probabilities are "roughly" as expected.

Next we applied a serial test considering every consecutive pair of bits. The results are shown in the following tabulation.

pair	frequency	
00	1,086,972	$(= n_{00})$
01	2,459,393	$(= n_{01})$
10	2,459,392	$(= n_{10})$
11	1,104,739	$(= n_{11})$

These give 95% confidence intervals for the probabilities p_{ij} (where p_{ij} is the probability that j follows i)

$$0.3030 \leqslant p_{00} \leqslant 0.3070 \qquad 0.3095 \leqslant p_{11} \leqslant 0.3104$$

$$0.6930 \leqslant p_{01} \leqslant 0.6940 \qquad 0.6896 \leqslant p_{10} \leqslant 0.6905$$

These probabilities p_{ij} are called the transition probabilities. It is clear that there is a far greater probability of making a transition than of remaining in the same state. For instance if the last bit produced was a 0 the next one is much more likely to be a 1 than a 0.

Next we considered a particular case of the poker test. For the poker test the bits are arranged in blocks of some fixed length, k say, and the observed frequencies of occurrence of the different possibilities for the k-bit blocks are recorded. Each block of k bits can be regarded as a binary number in the range 0 to $2^k - 1$ and this gives us a natural way in which to order the possibilities. For our test we took $k = 6$ and the results are shown in the Table 7.1. With a random sequence each of the 2^k possibilities is equally likely but the distribution we obtained is obviously not uniform and has two definite peaks at numbers 21 and 42 corresponding to 010101 and 101010 which are, of course, the idling patterns for the modulator. What appears to have happened is that, since there was virtually no background noise, each time the speaker paused, the delta modulator reverted to its idling state. Although these pauses were hardly perceptible to a listener, the relatively high sampling rate meant that even a pause of only 2 or 3 msec led to a

TABLE 7.1

Results of Poker Test for $k = 6$

0	6004.0	22	34928.0	44	18435.0
1	7276.0	23	7526.0	45	21168.0
2	2345.0	24	10859.0	46	7334.0
3	11781.0	25	24094.0	47	3109.0
4	2456.0	26	34235.0	48	10314.0
5	7550.0	27	5286.0	49	20831.0
6	11758.0	28	20726.0	50	19683.0
7	18574.0	29	5816.0	51	17310.0
8	2466.0	30	8215.0	52	14964.0
9	5256.0	31	6699.0	53	24830.0
10	23462.0	32	7425.0	54	4992.0
11	17055.0	33	6576.0	55	2857.0
12	16540.0	34	7626.0	56	20562.0
13	18211.0	35	18196.0	57	12834.0
14	19356.0	36	5253.0	58	5675.0
15	11525.0	37	32656.0	59	2284.0
16	11525.0	38	23320.0	60	12410.0
17	5240.0	39	12212.0	61	2369.0
18	18383.0	40	6348.0	62	6458.0
19	18334.0	41	31441.0	63	5804.0
20	22525.0	42	182459.0		
21	183784.0	43	25453.0		

Total number of characters = 1185082.0
Expected character total = 18516.9
5% confidence interval = 18252.3 – 18781.5
1% confidence interval = 18169.1 – 18864.7

30–50-bit idling pattern. Of course, in any environment there will be some background noise and, although the pattern may not be perfect every time, it certainly means that guessing some plaintext is much easier than we might have expected.

If a cryptanalyst is trying to break a system then he will repeatedly try to assess the difficulty of determining a large part, or maybe all, of the message on the assumption that he knows the cryptogram plus a certain portion, m bits say, of the plaintext equivalent. Clearly the answer will depend on many parameters including, in particular, the system being used and the size of m. For any given system, it seems reasonable to assume that the time necessary to break it decreases as m increases. (It certainly cannot increase as m increases!) Even when the cryptanalyst knows no plaintext at all he may still be interested in this assessment. He may need to decide whether or not it is worthwhile to try to guess some of the plaintext, m bits say, before trying to break the scrambler systematically. For any given integer m, the total time needed to break a given system using this type of attack depends on the number of trials necessary to guess m bits of plaintext and the time taken to break the system given m bits of plaintext. It may well happen that there is an optimum value of m, or range of values for m, for this method and the cryptanalyst will carry out a number of tests to try to find it. One such test is the poker test which he will apply for varying choices of k. As we observed after discussing our own statistical tests on the digitized speech from a delta modulator, it can be frighteningly easy to guess some of the plaintext.

Obviously this property of delta modulators is undesirable from the cryptographer's point of view. However delta modulators are not the only A/D converters which yield information when subjected to some simple statistical tests. In fact each of the digitization techniques which we have discussed has this type of weakness. The main reason is, usually, the highly redundant nature of speech. For our particular example, these properties were exaggerated by including reasonably long pauses in the speech and reducing the background noise. Nevertheless any user of a digital speech cipher system must continually be aware of both the highly redundant nature of the plaintext being ciphered and also of the vast quantities of ciphertext which the cryptanalyst is obtaining for analysis. For instance our sample of over 7,000,000 bits represented only seven minutes of speech. So, unless great confidence is held in the sequence generator being used, digitized cipher systems cannot be considered totally secure. Indeed it is partly for this reason that, at the present time, most messages of strategic importance, i.e., those requiring long-term security, are normally transmitted over data systems and do not use speech at all!

From now on we will accept our worst case conditions. Suppose that we are using a stream cipher to encrypt our digital speech and that the output resembles white noise. Since we are accepting the worst case conditions we are assuming that the cryptanalyst has complete details of the system and that our security depends on the key. This is, of course, also true for analogue scramblers and in both cases our security will be completely lost once the cryptanalyst knows the key. When we discussed analogue scramblers we saw that the cryptanalyst was often able to descramble the cryptogram without knowing the key, and in fact a direct attack on the scrambled speech was often the easiest method. Nevertheless, given the great importance of the key, it is obviously crucial to pay great attention to the problems of choosing, distributing and changing keys. This topic was mentioned briefly in Chapter 1 and, at the end of Chapter 6, we promised a further detailed discussion. We will now look at the various aspects of handling keys.

III. Keys

If a cryptanalyst wants to estimate how long it will take him to break a particular system, he can obtain an upper bound by calculating the time necessary to try all possible keys. Thus, when we are deciding a key size we must ensure that the resulting number of possibilities for the key is sufficient to inhibit any would-be cryptanalyst from trying them all. Unfortunately as we increase the number of possibilities for the key we also increase the difficulty of ensuring secure distribution and management. As we saw in Chapter 1 there are many practical situations where the operational constraints are very important and can affect the security and reliability of the system. If, for example, we are in a situation where the key is entered manually into the device and we increase the length of the key, then we increase the chance of the wrong key being used. In this case it is good practice to keep each key as small as possible. However as we have already said, the size of the individual keys influences the number of possible keys and in order to make this number large we need long keys. Thus, once again, we have conflicting requirements and must compromise.

If we use 64-bit keys then there are 2^{64} possibilities for the key and it is widely agreed that, with today's technology, this is sufficiently large to ensure that trying each key is not feasible in any reasonable time. However, any cipher equipment being designed today will presumably need to be secure for a number of years and, consequently, the key size must be large enough to allow for significant improvements in technology. One possibility for reaching the necessary compromise between the lengths of the keys and the total number of keys is to utilize a two-part key. This can be done is such a way that only one part needs changing at any given time and is one of the main reasons for the introduction of *customer option keys* or, as they are sometimes called, *family keys*. The main objective of these keys is to extend the number of possibilities for the key without increasing the work involved in changing the keys. As we have already seen, the key needs changing frequently and, consequently, is usually easily accessible. It may, for instance, be changed by means of front panel switches, a front panel keyboard or perhaps even automatically over a transmission channel. It is usually anticipated that the customer option keys will be changed much less frequently and they are likely to be much less accessible, possibly by means of wire links, plug-in modules or switches within the equipment. In practice the customer option key bits are often used as an algorithm modifier. Of course, if they are used in this way then the user must ensure that the security is not affected.

As an illustration of a possible customer option key we will consider the multiplexed sequences described in Chapter 3. Here we might use the key to provide the initial contents of the two shift registers plus the switch settings of each register. If this is the case then, provided that the all-zero state is avoided, any choice for the initial contents is satisfactory whereas the switch settings have to be carefully selected. (As we saw, the feedback polynomial must be primitive.) Thus, it is obviously easier to alter the overall key by changing the initial contents than by changing the switch settings. In this case we might choose to change the keys frequently by merely altering the initial states and our customer option key might be the appropriate primitive polynomials. Provided that the polynomials are carefully selected, the security of the system will be unaffected by the choice of customer option key.

The customer option key has the extra advantage that it gives the user some confidence that the algorithm he is using is unique to him. This may be particularly important if he is employing a commercially designed system, which is likely to have many other users.

As we saw in Chapter 3 one of the many difficult problems facing the user of any cipher system is deciding how often to change the key. If we do not change our key and accept our worst case conditions then we must assume that the cryptanalyst has obtained a number of messages enciphered with that key. For a stream cipher, if a fixed algorithm is used then the sequence it produces will be exactly the same every time the same key is entered. So if we were to use the same key for a number of messages, the cryptanalyst might obtain a set of n ciphered messages all utilizing the same sequence. As we saw when discussing A/D converters the cryptanalyst might also be able to deduce (or guess) part of the unenciphered data. He could then proceed as follows.

Let each of these n ciphered messages be denoted by a_i, $i = 1, \ldots, n$ and denote the bits of the ith ciphered message by $a_{i1}, a_{i2}, \ldots, a_{im_i}$, where m_i is the number of bits in the ith ciphered message. An array of ciphered bits of all the messages can be set out in the form shown in Fig. 7.4. The cryptanalyst may then notice that the rows of a number of the messages in a particular set of columns (for instance those between the broken vertical lines) have very similar characteristics which can be related to a particular speech signal after processing by the A/D converter. This particular signal may, of course, be a known sound such as the air conditioner whine that we mentioned earlier. Such knowledge could enable the cryptanalyst to deduce the sequence at that point and 'listen' to that section of all the messages. This type of attack is always possible whenever n is greater than one, and has proved very successful. In fact it is likely to lead to partial success in the cryptanalysis of most messages. Although we assumed that we were using a stream cipher, we did not use this fact in our argument and any system is prone to this attack.

This discussion seems to indicate that, irrespective of the algorithm used, the key should be changed after each individual message. If this were so, then

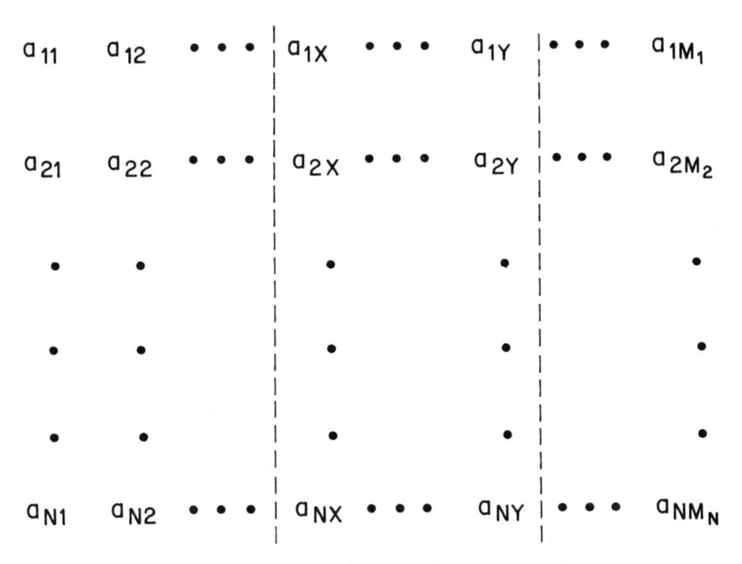

FIG. 7.4. Cryptanalysis—need for a message key.

it would be hard to see what genuine advantages the stream cipher, or any other cipher, has over the one-time pad. If, with all systems, the key should be changed after every single message, the only possible advantage of the stream cipher over the one-time pad is that the former has a fixed key size. To counteract this we have gone from a theoretically unbreakable system to one that is theoretically breakable. Fortunately the situation can be remedied and, in fact, we can avoid having to change the key so frequently. To avoid confusion, from now on we shall refer to our fundamental key, i.e., the key which is kept secret and can easily be changed on a regular basis, as the *base key*. The same key is often referred to as the *primary key*.

In order to demonstrate the essential function of a message key, we consider an analogy with the one-time pad system. In the traditional picture of this system, a pad is used and each page of this pad contains a random sequence of numbers. Each page is then used once as a key. However, if each page is numbered then there is no reason why the pages should be used in consecutive order. Each message could, for instance, be prefixed with a number telling the receiver which page to turn to. Thus these numbers would randomize the starting point for the enciphering sequence. This illustrates the role of our *message key*; it will alter the starting point of the pseudo-random sequence we are producing. To achieve this effect within a stream cipher, we generate a message key at the start of each message. For the moment we will not worry about the method of generation; it may be random, pseudo-random or even depend on the message itself. The base key is then mixed with

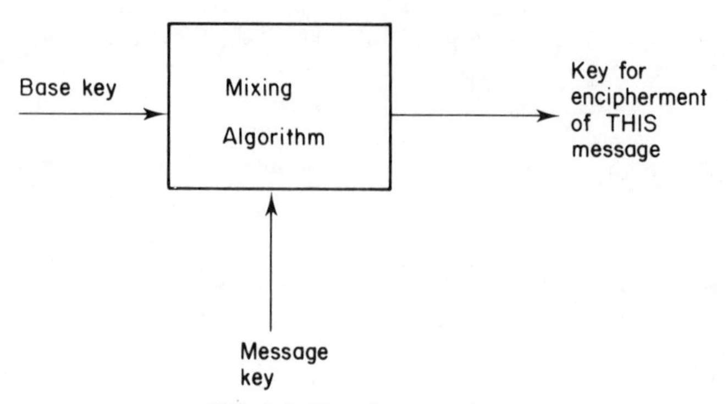

FIG. 7.5. Use of message key.

the message key in some way to produce a new key which is used to initialize the encipherment algorithm of that particular message only. At the start of the next message a new message key is generated and mixed with the base key in the same way. In this manner the algorithm for each message is initialized by its own individual key. The system is shown in Fig. 7.5.

It is important to remember that if we wish to use a message key, then that message key must be transmitted to the receiver. Furthermore, it is crucial that it be transmitted correctly, because if the receiver uses the wrong message key he will almost certainly decipher the ciphertext incorrectly. This incorrect decipherment would obviously cause a reduction in the effectiveness of the communications network and would, for a radio system, imply a reduction in the range. We have already seen, for instance, that 16-kbit/sec delta modulated speech is comprehensible over a channel with a 10% mean bit error rate. The message key should, therefore, have a high probability of being received even in these conditions. So, to avoid having to retransmit, it is obviously advantageous to apply an error correcting code to the message key. This code can then be chosen so that, for the type of link being used, it is highly unlikely that any errors will remain after the message has been transmitted and the error correction has been applied.

Looking back at Fig. 6.10 and comparing it with Fig. 7.5 we can see that the TOD is a message key. This shows that, as well as providing a method for changing the key, the message key can also aid synchronization.

We have still not decided how often the base key should be changed. Since our aim is to avoid the interceptor having two cryptograms which used the same enciphering system, the answer must depend on the number of possibilities and, hence, the size of the message key. For instance, to take a ridiculously small example, if we had a message key with just two bits then the message enciphered using a given base key would employ at most four different enciphering sequences. Thus if an interceptor obtained five enciphered messages he could be certain that at least two employed the same enciphering sequence. So, in this case, we would need to change our base key after at most four messages. Clearly, to avoid changing our base key too often, we need a reasonably large message key. But we must not forget that the message key also has to be transmitted to the receiver and, in the case of initial synchronization only, will extend the synchronization time. If we use continuous synchronization then we need to find a way of inserting both the synchronized sequence and the message key in the digital bit stream. Thus, as usual, we are faced with a trade-off between the length of message key which we really want and the length which the system can tolerate.

In practice, one normally begins by deciding the size of message key acceptable to the system, and then considers whether or not this allows the transmission of enough messages with a fixed base key. Thus, we must consider how, for a message key with m possibilities, the probability of using the same message key more than once varies as we increase either the number of messages being transmitted or, if we are using continuous synchronization, the number of reloadings. This is a routine statistical problem. To solve it we assume that r messages are transmitted and evaluate the probability that each one employs a different message key. For our first message we have m choices for the key. However, once we have made that choice, there will be only $m - 1$ choices for the second. Since any one of the original m choices can be followed by any of the remaining $m - 1$, the total number of choices for the first two message keys is $m(m - 1)$. Similarly there will now be $m - 2$ choices for the third message key and, by repeated use of the same argument, we see that the total number of ways of choosing our r keys is $m(m - 1)(m - 2) \cdots (m - r + 1)$. On the other hand if we do not insist that no key is used more than once then there are m^r ways of choosing r message keys. The ratio of these two numbers shows the proportion of the total number of possibilities which have all the message keys distinct, i.e., it is precisely the probability that all r message keys are different. But this ratio is

$$\frac{m(m - 1) \cdots (m - r + 1)}{m^r} = \left(\frac{m}{m}\right)\left(\frac{m - 1}{m}\right) \cdots \left(\frac{mm - r + 1}{m}\right)$$

$$= \left(1 - \frac{1}{m}\right)\left(1 - \frac{2}{m}\right) \cdots \left(1 - \frac{r - 1}{m}\right)$$

and thus, if we let p denote the probability that all r message keys are distinct, we have

$$p = \left(1 - \frac{1}{m}\right)\left(1 - \frac{2}{m}\right) \cdots \left(1 - \frac{r - 1}{m}\right)$$

To get some idea of what this means, suppose we use an 8-bit message key and transmit five messages employing the same base key. Then $r = 5$ and $m = 256$ which give a value for p of about 0.96. Thus the probability of two of our messages using the same message key is about 0.04. This means that, if we changed our base key after five messages, for about four base keys in every hundred we could expect to find a repeated message key. In practice, of course, the values for r and m will be much larger. However, r is also likely to be small compared with m and, on this assumption, we can use the approximation $\ln(1 - x) \cong -x$, for small x, to obtain a quick way of estimating p. Since

$$p = \left(1 - \frac{1}{m}\right)\left(1 - \frac{2}{m}\right)\cdots\left(1 - \frac{r-1}{m}\right)$$

$$\ln p = \ln\left(1 - \frac{1}{m}\right) + \ln\left(1 - \frac{2}{m}\right) + \cdots + \ln\left(1 - \frac{r-1}{m}\right)$$

$$\ln p \cong -\frac{1}{m} - \frac{2}{m} - \cdots - \frac{(r-1)}{m} = -\left(\frac{1}{m}\cdot\frac{r(r-1)}{2}\right)$$

Thus

$$\ln p \cong \frac{-r(r-1)}{2m} \quad \text{or} \quad p \cong e^{-[r(r-1)]/2m}$$

Although obviously important, the size chosen for the message key is certainly not the only decision to be taken. Other factors have to be considered. For instance, one practical consideration is that it is often physically impossible to send a new base key within a certain time interval. Another relevant factor is the amount of use made of the system. Clearly, for any single base key, we want to keep the length of ciphertext available to an interceptor as small as possible. An absolutely crucial consideration is that we must ensure that any base key is changed before it has been used for the duration of its break time. By this we mean that for any given base key, we will have our own estimate of the time needed to discover it, and we must not use it for anywhere approaching this length of time. If, for instance, we believe we have a system with a break time of one year and we change the key weekly, a would-be cryptanalyst trying to read all the communications will very quickly be hopelessly behind.

Another problem with key change involves the actual physical changing of keys within a network. If, for example, it is decided to change all the keys in a given network at midnight this will almost certainly result in the disruption of all transmissions in a short time interval around midnight. As an illustration, all messages en route at midnight are likely to be lost because, by the time they reach their destinations, the key may have changed. Furthermore any errors incurred during the change of keys may be catastrophic. Not only will they lead to confusion, but they may also offer the interceptor useful information. Each of the above problems can be partially overcome by allowing the equipment to store a small number of base keys. We can then include an identifier at the start of each message to signify which store is being used. If, when this is done, the key is changed during a transmission it can be ensured that the old key is still available in the receiving equipment. In practice the storage of too many keys can lead to confusion and about ten keys are usually considered sufficient.

We have now introduced a key hierarchy which consists of customer option key, which is changed infrequently, the base key, which is changed reasonably often, and the message key which is automatically changed for every message. If continuous synchronization is used then the message key may even be changed many times during a message. Within many systems this is the only key structure offered and the user has to determine his own handling procedure for the base and customer option keys or, alternatively, to buy a separate system for their generation, distribution and management. The generation and distribution of the customer option keys tend to be considerably simpler than those of the base key, and so we will concentrate on the latter.

As far as the generation is concerned it is important that the keys be unpredictable to any interceptor. This means, ideally, a random number generator, which is usually a purpose-built device, should be used. In this case tests must be performed regularly to test the randomness of the generation. For this, one can develop a series of tests similar to those which we introduced in Chapter 3 and use them to assess the randomness properties of a sequence generator. In many tactical situations, when the key is entered via an alphanumeric keyboard, there are obvious advantages in using phrases for the key. Although this significantly reduces the number of possible keys available to the user, the advantage that he can easily remember it without writing it down is likely to be the overriding factor. Since the secrecy of the key phrases is so important, their choice must not be left to the user; he is too likely (without realising it) to choose a key which has a special relevance to him, e.g., an address, telephone number or name. Such an association between the key phrase and the user is likely to be noticed by a clever cryptanalyst.

The distribution of key information is probably the hardest problem in key management. Traditionally the safest method is the use of couriers. Another popular technique is the use of a second cipher system, perhaps even using a technique similar to the one-time pad. At the present time various other systems are becoming available. A number of them use one of the public key systems in order to transmit the keys securely over an insecure channel. However, such systems are only just beginning to be accepted by users. Military users, in particular, tend to be very wary of any new techniques, (too many mistakes have been made in the past!)

With skilled operators and good management procedure, the key structure described is sufficient for the establishment of a secure system. However, in many commercial systems and telephone networks it is essential that the operators do not even know that encryption is taking place. Furthermore the changing of the keys on a regular basis may be impracticable. But if we cannot rely on the operator to change the keys, we have no alternative but to look for ways of changing the base key automatically. Before considering the possibilities, we note that any automatic changes will involve the loss of some security. Perhaps the most obvious method is simply to encipher the new base key using the previous key, and then to transmit it to the rest of the network. This is obviously feasible but has the great disadvantage that, once an interceptor has deduced one base key, he will be able to decipher all later keys as they are transmitted. A better method, which is used in many computer networks, involves the concept of key-encrypting keys and data-encrypting keys. The base key becomes a *master key*, which is our *key-encrypting key*, and at the start of each session a master equipment somewhere within the network (often the central processor) generates a new key. This key is then enciphered under the control of the master key. It is transmitted to all other equipment and initializes a sequence generator. This is now the only purpose which our master key has: to encrypt other keys. The new key, often called the *session key*, is then decrypted by the receiving equipments and loaded into a store to be used for the encryption and decryption of data until the end of that session. Thus, while our master key is a key-encrypting key, the session key is a *data-encrypting key*. (We have not formally defined a *session*. It can be defined in a number of ways, e.g., in terms of a fixed number of characters or messages or as a certain time interval.)

If our master key is only used for enciphering session keys then, if session keys are generated randomly, it is only used to encipher random information. Thus, the only way in which a cryptanalyst can obtain plaintext for an attack on the master key is by discovering a number of session keys. By carefully designing the key-encrypting sequence generator, we can ensure that the number of session keys which must be discovered, in order to mount such an attack, will be large. Furthermore, despite the automatic change of keys, even if after a certain amount of work a cryptanalyst manages to discover one session key, he will almost certainly need to do the same amount of work to discover the next one. Note, by the way, that apart from hardware constraints there is no reason why the key-encrypting sequence generator and data-encrypting sequence generator should be the same.

We could now go on to complicate our system by extending the key hierarchy and introducing further key-encrypting keys. In this way we could ensure that, apart from inside a secure area within the equipment, unciphered keys are never stored. This should certainly increase the security. Later in this chapter we will consider how one particular key hierarchy of this type may be applied to a digital telephone network using DES as the sequence generator.

No matter how complex and apparently secure we make our system we must not forget that, at least in theory, an automatic key system is not as secure as a system which uses individually generated and distributed keys. But, as we have seen, in practice it is not usually possible for the generation and distribution of base keys to be totally secure and, when this is so, an automatic system may be advantageous. Even within an automatic system the base key will need changing occasionally. The frequency with which it is changed will be influenced by the volume of traffic within the network and the practical difficulties involved in the actual change.

Now that we have discussed digital systems in general we will devote the rest of the chapter to three particular examples of digital scramblers. The first will be a simple, low-security system which is similar to the time sample scrambler of Chapter 5. The second will be a high-security vhf radio system and the third will be a digital four-wire telephone network.

IV. Permuting LPC Parameters

In Chapters 4–6 we discussed a number of techniques which use A/D and D/A conversion before and after processing. This first example is included to emphasize that, by simply omitting the final D/A conversion, almost all those techniques can be used in a digital scrambler. Of course, when they are, the data rate required will depend on the A/D converter.

We have repeatedly observed that one of the biggest advantages of digital communications is that they permit the use of data encipherment techniques for voice as opposed to the analogue methods. In fact one of the principal motivating objectives behind the development of vocoders, i.e., low bit-rate voice coders, has been to provide true digital scrambling for voice over telephone, hf or narrowband vhf radio. Despite this we need not be confined to these data encipherment techniques, and the application of, for example, permutations to the digits representing the speech can be a very cost effective way of providing privacy against an eavesdropper.

In order to discuss an example we will suppose we have a telecommunications systems which utilizes an LPC vocoder together with an appropriate 2.4-kbit modem which provides suitable modulation for the digital system.

Our task is to retrofit some security to the system which, for our particular example, we will assume means to provide some privacy against an eavesdropper. For this discussion we will suppose that no security against 'real cryptanalysis' is required. We will, however, assume that the cost is a major factor and that our proposal must make only a negligible difference to the marginal cost of apparatus. Finally we will assume that we must not affect communications performance. So, for instance, any delay at the start of a transmission is unacceptable. Similarly, there must be no change in the format of bits transmitted or in the total number of bits. These latter constraints imply that we cannot send any form of synchronization and that, because of the errors at the start of transmission and the error propagation which would result, a cipher feedback system is also forbidden. Thus, our only chance of satisfying the design specification is to rely on the synchronization of the system which is already in place. We will remind ourselves of the principal properties of an LPC vocoder.

The basic vocoder elements are shown in Fig. 2.26. In an LPC vocoder the basic vocal-tract model utilizes a filter which is continually modified. So essentially, the speech is modelled as the output of a filter excited by a sequence of pulses which are separated by the pitch period for voiced sounds or pseudo-random noise for unvoiced sounds. To account for the non-stationary character of the speech waveform, the filter coefficients are periodically up-dated. This takes place on a frame-by-frame basis where, in this context, a frame is a portion of speech over which the signal can be regarded as stationary. This typically ranges from 10 to 30 msec. (For instance, one widely used LPC vocoder uses 54 bits to represent a frame which, at 2400 bits/sec, means that a frame corresponds to 22.5 msec.) As a result, the vocoder digital output is formatted into frames and part of each frame is devoted to synchronization to enable the receiver to 'frame synchronize' with the transmitter. Clearly it would be useful if the scrambler which we are going to retrofit to the system could utilize the frame synchronization already provided. With this in mind, we might consider a block cipher where the LPC frames are the data blocks for encipherment. If we were to do this then, of course, our plaintext blocks could not include any synchronization bits in the frame. This is because, since there is no synchronization transmitted specifically for the cipher and remembering that decipherment could only take place after synchronization, once any bits were enciphered they would be useless for synchronization.

If we try to use a block cipher of the DES type, then the diffusion will lead to error propagation and, once again, we will not be able to meet our criteria. So if we are to satisfy the criteria we must avoid error propagation, which means we must restrict ourselves to a block cipher with no diffusion, i.e., as we saw in Chapter 3, one for which the encipherment of any one message bit is independent of all others. One technique with this property is the use of permutations. We might, for instance, permute all the non-synchronization bits within each frame. Unfortunately, since we have no possibility for any synchronization, other than the simple frame synchronization provided by the vocoder system, we will not be able to change the permutation from frame to frame. Thus we will have to use a fixed permutation, dependent on the key.

Since we know of no detailed statistical tests which have been performed to determine the level of residual intelligibility in the signal, we cannot give an authoritative assessment of this technique's likely effectiveness. Sambur and Jayant (1976) have, however, carried out a few experiments in this area, permuting LPC parameters in blocks of 8 and 16. They conclude that the scheme was 'somewhat successful in distorting the original signal'.

V. A Secure VHF Radio System

In order to discuss this example we will begin by listing a number of assumptions. Each of these is, in our view, realistic in that it either represents a reasonable constraint on the channel or a reasonable demand from the user.

(a) The channel is capable of supporting 16-kbit/sec digital communications.
(b) A high level of security is required.
(c) A 'late entry' facility is required, with a maximum waiting time of 2 sec.
(d) No more than one false synchronization per day is acceptable.
(e) Traffic flow security will be utilised.
(f) The system must work under channel conditions of 10% error at 16-kbit/sec transmission.
(g) The base key will be changed once per day.

Our first decision concerns the type of A/D converter which we should use. From our discussion in Chapter 2, some form of delta modulation appears to be the most suitable. We also know that 16-kbit/sec delta modulated speech can tolerate a 10% mean bit error rate. If we did not have this knowledge and were concerned about this aspect of the system, we might consider the A/D converter working at a slower rate and using some error correction to compensate for the channel. In this case we would obviously have to investigate the reduction of voice quality caused by reducing the bit rate and see if it were acceptable. For our example however, we shall assume that error correction is unnecessary. Thus, provided that the synchronization system is also robust at a 10% error rate, we should, by restricting ourselves to a non-error propagating stream cipher, be able to satisfy criterion (f). This should also enable us to meet the high-security requirement. As we saw in Chapter 6, in order to meet the late entry we must use a continuous synchronization technique.

In order to utilize the provision of traffic flow security we might wish to include a random number generator in the terminal and use it to provide the output whenever there is no digitized speech present. But if we do this we must ensure that any synchronization signals which we send do not stand out like "sore thumbs". We must remember that the cryptanalyst knows our system and that, if we use a fixed sequence for the synchronization, he will be able to detect it as easily as the receiver. This would nullify the advantage gained by the traffic flow security. As well as varying it we should also send the synchronization sequence at irregular intervals. This would clearly make it even more difficult for an interceptor to detect. For our example we will assume that the synchronization sequence is of the type discussed in Chapter 6 although, as we explained, it is not the only technique available. By using it here we certainly do not wish to give the impression that it is the best technique. In most situations it is not. However, it is certainly one of the simplest and will serve for this example.

Our first problem is to decide upon the length of the synchronization sequence and the maximum number of errors which we can tolerate within it. To do this we adopt the method which we described in Chapter 6, i.e., we produce tables which, when r errors are allowed in an n-bit sequence, give the probabilities of acceptance and false synchronization. Since our specification contains nothing which relates to the acceptance probability we will aim at 0.99. In practice we would produce these tables for a number of different values for n. However, if we decide to use an m-sequence then we need only consider values for n of the form $2^t - 1$ for some t. (Once again we must point out that there are many sequences, other than m-sequences, which exhibit good autocorrelation properties.) It can be verified easily that $t = 6$ is too small to meet the specification and so we use $t = 7$, i.e., $n = 127$. Part of the resulting table is shown in Table 7.2 from which it is clear that we can meet the specification for the number of false synchronizations per

TABLE 7.2

The Probabilities for $n = 127$

Number of errors allowed	Probability of accepting the synchronization sequences	Expected number of false synchronizations per day
29	0.9999935	0.41
30	0.9999978	1.37

day and still achieve 0.99999 as the acceptance probability. This compares very favourably with the 0.99 upon which we decided. Although taking $t = 6$ is too small to satisfy our specification requirements, the value $n = 127$ is certainly not the smallest possibility for n. (The reader might like to try to find it!) But since we intend to use an m-sequence we shall use $n = 127$ and then, from Table 7.2, we know that at least 98 of the 127 bits must be correct.

In order to decide the time intervals at which to send our synchronization updates we must ensure that the waiting time for the late entry should not be more than 2 sec. If we send updates approximately every second then, if p is the acceptance probability, the probability of the receiver obtaining at least one of these every two seconds would be about $1 - (1 - p)^2$. This should be acceptable.

The next problem is to fix the size of the message key. Since the base key is to be changed once per day and a message key is to be sent every second, there will be up to $60 \times 60 \times 24$ message keys sent for each base key. However it is extremely unlikely that a radio will be operating continuously and it is probably sufficient to assume 1 hour's worth of messages/day. Once again we should now produce tables to show, for various values for the size of message key, the probability that no 2 sec of transmission will employ the same message key. If we take the number of message keys used per day to be $r = 3600$ then we must evaluate $\exp(-r(r - 1)/2m)$, where m is the number of possibilities for the message key, (see Section III). The results are shown in Table 7.3 from which it appears that a message key size of 32, i.e., having 2^{32} possible message keys should be more than adequate.

Once we have decided to have a message key of 32 bits we will use a shift register of length 32 with the switches set so as to generate an m-sequence.

TABLE 7.3

Estimating the message key size.

Message key size	Probability that all messages will use different message keys
24	0.462
25	0.680
26	0.824
27	0.908
28	0.953
29	0.976
30	0.988
31	0.994
32	0.997
33	0.998
34	0.999

We will probably choose to use a random message key at the start of transmission. We will then load this first message key into our shift register and use successive states of the register for the subsequent keys. In this way our message key will act as a TOD signal and the receiver will be able to flywheel.

With a message key length of this size it is necessary to think about the transmission problems. Obviously it is important that the message keys are received correctly, even in adverse conditions. But, in a channel with a 10% mean bit error rate, the probability of 32 consecutive bits being received correctly is $(0.9)^{32}$ which is about 0.03. Clearly this is unacceptable and we must provide some form of error correction. There are a number of ways of doing this. One simple, but certainly not very efficient, method is simply for the transmitter to repeat the 32 bit message key s times, where s is an odd number, and for the receiver to compare the s received versions of each bit and take a majority decision. In this case a bit will be received correctly provided that at most $(s - 1)/2$ errors occur in the s bits transmitted. Thus, in our particular situation, the probability q that a given bit will be received correctly is $q = \sum_{i=0}^{(s-1)/2} \binom{s}{i} (0.1)^i (0.9)^{s-i}$. The probability that all 32 bits of our synchronization update will be received correctly is then q^{32}. In Table 7.4 we show the values of q^{32} for various choices of s. If our criteria is a 99% chance of successfully receiving the message key then we must use 11-fold repetition. This means transmitting $32 \times 11 = 352$ bits for each message key and so, if we include the 127-bit synchronization sequence, we require a total of 479 bits at each synchronization update. (We must stress that a more sophisticated coding technique would considerably reduce this number. However, as we said earlier, we do not want to get involved in the theory of error correcting codes.)

For our particular example we will use a repetition code with $s = 11$. Our next problem is how to insert these 479 bits into the data stream every second. Since the transmission over the channel is at 16 kbit/sec we have, essentially, two options.

TABLE 7.4

Probability of Receiving the Message Key Using Majority Logic

s	q	q^{32}
3	0.972	0.403
5	0.991	0.759
7	0.997	0.916
9	0.9991	0.972
11	0.9997	0.991

(i) Arrange for the A/D converter to produce exactly (16,000 − 479) bits/sec.

(ii) Let the A/D converter produce 16,000 bits/sec and then discard 479 of them.

If we choose (ii) then this, in turn, allows two possibilities.

(iia) Discard a block of 479 bits and let the receiver try to interpolate for the missing bits, perhaps by repeating the last 479 bits. (We saw, when discussing the synchronization of analogue scramblers, that it is possible to treat a segment of speech in this way). Since 479 bits only represents about 30 msec, this method may be quite adequate.

(iib) Since 479 out of 16,000 is approximately 1 out of 32, we can make a 'hole' in the speech by removing one bit in every thirty two. If we do this the receiver has a number of small holes to fill in which he can do, for example, by merely changing state at the delta modulator, i.e., by making the 32nd bit the complement of the 31st. This should be virtually undetectable in the quality of the received signal.

For our particular example we choose, quite arbitrarily, (iia). We now have to decide how to disguise the synchronization signals and to arrange to send the synchronization at irregular intervals. It is theoretically, if not practically, very easy to disguise the signals. One possibility involves the use of (part of) the base key via the sequence generator, or possibly via a second sequence generator, to produce a 479-bit sequence. The sequence is then modulo-2 added to the synchronization/message key sequence before it is transmitted. If this method is adopted the receiver must, at every bit time, look at the previous 127 bits, strip off the first 127 bits of the masking sequence and then check for a synchronization sequence via his correlator. If he finds it, he must then strip off the remaining 352 bits before starting to recover the message key. We should point out that the synchronization sequence transmitted, (i.e. the masked version), will only change when the base key is changed. There are more sophisticated systems which allow the synchronization sequence to change each time the message key changes, but we will not discuss them here.

There are also a number of possible ways for arranging for synchronization to be transmitted at irregular intervals. One is to let the sequence generator which produces the enciphering sequence produce a number of extra bits per second and to use these to determine a time slot. This time slot is then the interval when the synchronization and message key will be transmitting during the next second of transmission. Clearly the receiver can generate the same bits and thus knows when to expect the next synchronization update.

We have now designed a system to meet the specifications! To summarise this system, we will briefly run through the transmitter operation. When a new base key is loaded, a 479-bit pseudo-random sequence, A say, is generated and stored. At the start of a transmission, a 32-bit random message key is generated and repeated 11 times. It is appended to the 127-bit synchronizing sequence and the result is masked by modulo-2 adding it to A. This is transmitted. Meanwhile the sequence generator is loaded with a mix of the base key and message key. A few bits are produced and these determine the next time slot during which synchronization will be sent. The sequence generator is then set to produce bits which will be modulo 2 added to the digitised speech until the time for the next synchronization burst. The message keys which will be used in future synchronization updates will be generated from a 32-stage linear feedback shift register, The initial contents of this register are the first 32-bit random message key and its feedback coefficients are selected so as to generate an m-sequence.

Before we discuss our third example we must point out that the specifications at the beginning of this section were far from complete. Many factors were missing, including, for example, the size, weight and environmental features. There was also no mention of the key management facilities which were required. These are all important considerations. Since, for instance, it is intended that the key should be changed daily, we should consider including, within the device, a store for several keys. Then we could load a number at the same time, perhaps sufficient for a week, and the operator could simply switch on to the next key each day. Furthermore, it may also be advantageous to design some *keyfill devices*. These are electronic devices into which the key can be entered manually or remotely, perhaps via a sophisticated key handling system. The keyfill device can then be connected to each scrambler in turn so that the keys are loaded automatically. This has many advantages. The first is that the operator who loads the keys does not see them which, of course, is one possible security weakness removed. Furthermore the radio operator's only involvement with the scrambler will be the daily switching to a new key. A second is that the probability of the keys being entered correctly is far higher than if each scrambler were loaded manually and independently. A third is that, if we are using a customer option key, it can be resident in the keyfill device as opposed to being entered in each separate unit. This not only removes electronics from each device but also adds to the reliability of the system.

Finally we must stress that the system designed in this section is not complete and, more importantly, by no means optimised. It is simply intended as an example of some of the factors which need consideration. The interested reader might like to decide which other features he would add to see how they might be incorporated. Having said that, we should point out that there are a number of commercially available devices of the type we have just discussed, (but almost certainly using a more sophisticated synchronization and message key system). They make use of modern electronics. Some of them are only a few cubic centimetres in volume and are built into standard radios.

VI. A Secure Digital Telephone System Based on DES

For this particular example we will assume the following:

(a) The telephone network is a fully duplex system.

(b) The scrambler must not require any user operations and should not degrade the service.

(c) The scrambler will embody digitization, modem, encryption, algorithms and control components. The A/D converters and modems are provided and their signalling and synchronization requirements are met independently of the scrambler function.

(d) As soon as the terminal senses that a connection has been made it should immediately enter a cipher mode, i.e., no clear speech should be permissible.

(e) The system must provide a high degree of key management and, to this end, it can be assumed that (i) all terminals are located at a number of sites and it is acceptable for all terminals on the same site to share a key; (ii) all terminals have sufficient memory to store a current key and a future key for each site and (iii) there is a network management centre where keys can be generated and encrypted.

(f) DES must form the basis for the encryption technique.

The system which we shall develop is based upon a paper by Orceyre and Heller (1978). As with all the examples which we have considered, our aim is to illustrate various concepts and problems which may arise. We would certainly not claim that this system is, in any sense, the best possible.

Since there is no requirement for late entry with a telephone network, we shall assume that initial synchronization only is sufficient for this system. We shall also use this example to illustrate the master key/session key which we described earlier in the chapter. We shall not, however, concern ourselves with the generation and distribution of master keys, but simply point out that this is, nevertheless, an important aspect of the system. Figure 7.6 shows a basic module for performing the DES function in a master key/session key system. Since we are assuming that we have a network centre for key generation and distribution all that we need within a module of each terminal is key decipherment. No clear keys should exist outside this module and, therefore, the process for key decipherment is that the master key MK is moved from the master key register to the session key register. The enciphered session key is then moved into the input register and DES is used in a standard block cipher decipherment mode to decrypt the session key which is then moved into the session key register, (all switches are held in position 1). The session key is then ready for DES encipherment/decipherment and can be used in either a stream cipher mode or a block chaining mode. In the stream

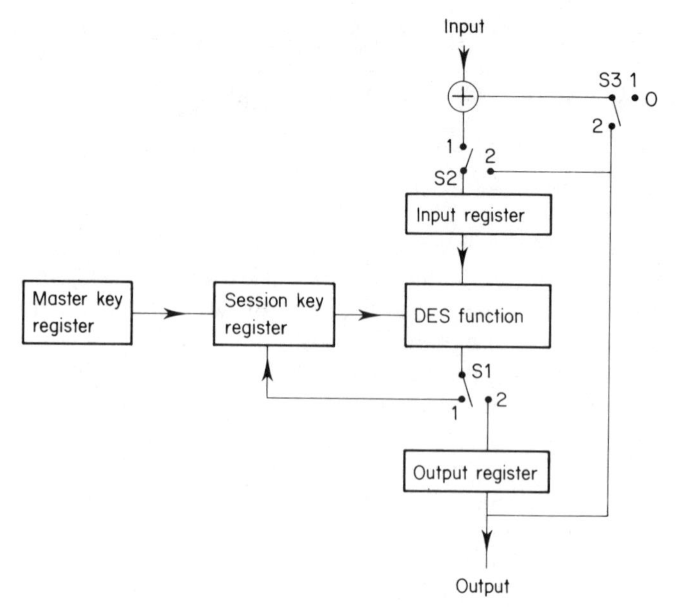

FIG. 7.6. DES module.

cipher mode, which is not exactly the same as in Chapter 3 but is the method suggested by Oceyre and Heller (1978), switches S1 and S2 are held in position 2 while S3 is set to position 1. Note that for this mode the receiver cannot produce the same sequence as the transmitter unless he knows the initial contents of the input register. A *block chaining mode* is a data-dependent mode which is often used for producing checksums, i.e., functions of the data. In the checksum context it has the advantage that each output bit depends on all the previous data bits. For the block chaining mode, switches S1 and S3 are at position 2 and S2 is at position 1.

Before we consider how the speech will be scrambled we must discuss the distribution of the session keys. For this discussion we will assume that all the terminals at a site employ the same master and session keys. The session keys will be distributed as follows:

(1) The network management centre generates a session key for each site; this key will be called the *site key*. For each particular site it then uses DES in its block cipher mode to encipher all the keys required by that site under the site's master key.

(2) To ensure that errors do not occur during the distribution of these keys on the channel, the network management centre generates a verification vector. This is produced as follows. (a) A random 64-bit vector, r, is generated, (b) r is enciphered under the appropriate master key and appended

to the collection of enciphered site keys and (c) r is input to a DES module as both input and session key. With DES in its block chaining mode each enciphered site key is presented to the DES module in turn. Thus the first block to be enciphered is r, the second block is the first enciphered site key added modulo-2 to the result of the previous stage and so on. The final vector, which is the same length as the set of enciphered site keys, is called the *verification vector*.

(3) The set of enciphered site keys, together with r enciphered, are transmitted, either via a distribution centre or directly, to the scrambling terminal.

(4) The terminal stores the enciphered site keys as future keys.

(5) The terminal inputs r to its input register of the DES module.

(6) The terminal decrypts r with its master key. This is done with DES in its block cipher mode.

(7) The terminal can now produce the verification vector in exactly the way used by the network management centre.

(8) The terminal transmits the verification vector to the network management centre.

(9) The network management centre checks what it has received against the vector which it produced.

(10) When site keys have been distributed to all terminals in this way then, at any given time, the terminals can all be instructed to switch future site keys to current keys and a new cycle can begin.

The distribution scheme above is just one of many possibilities. There are many different schemes in operation and, as yet, no single standard exists. Now that we have a distribution scheme for the session keys we can look at the speech scrambling. Since we have to work in a fully duplex mode, we shall assume that both transmission directions use the called site's site key. We will also use a stream cipher for our speech encryption. From Fig. 7.6 we can see that both ends of the link must begin with the same contents in their input registers. To achieve this we use the initialization procedure shown in Fig. 7.7 which, for simplicity, shows one DES module being shared for transmit and receive. In the following procedure, the terminals are referred to as the originator and acceptor.

(1) All initial dialing and connection signaling are in clear and immediately followed by modem synchronization. As soon as this has been completed successfully, the crypto initialization will begin and thus prevent any clear transmissions between the terminals.

(2) The originating terminal causes the acceptor's terminal site key, (based on the dialed number), to be loaded from the memory store into the input register, i.e., S1 is at position 2. It is deciphered under the master key, in block cipher mode, and then placed in the session key register (S3 at

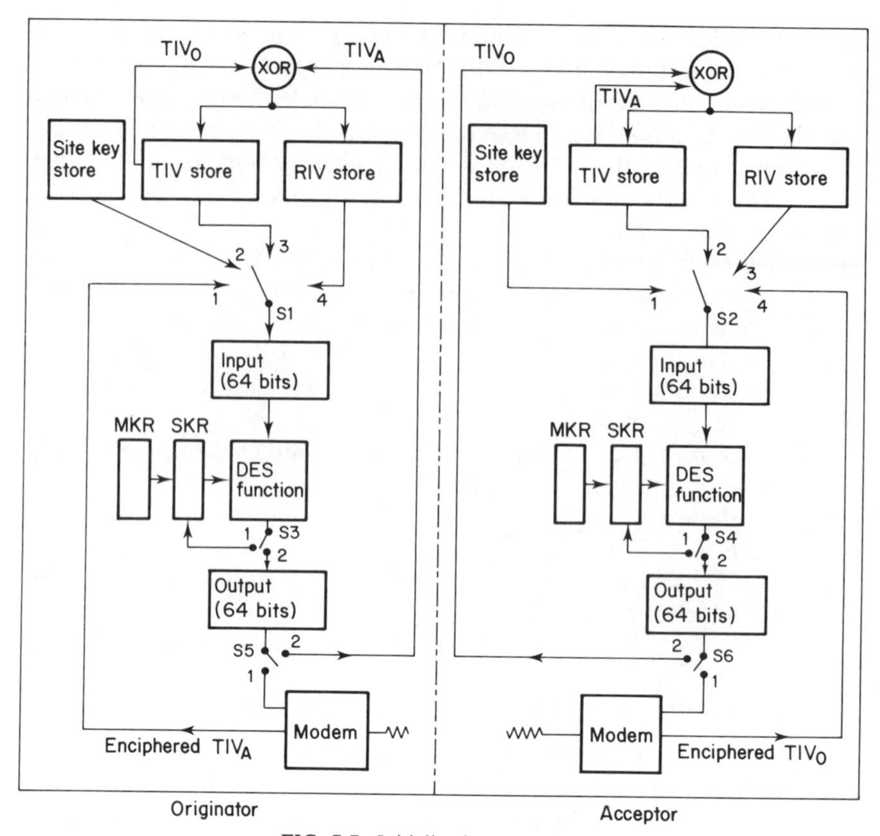

FIG. 7.7. Initialization procedure.

position 1). Similarly, the acceptor terminal loads its own site key into the input register (S2 at position 1), deciphers it under its master key and loads the result into its session key register (S4 at position 1). As a result of these two stages both terminals are now using the same session key.

(3) The originator terminal loads the current contents of its *transmit initialization vector* (TIV) store into the input register (S1 at position 3) and enciphers it, under the session key, in block cipher mode. This is then transmitted to the acceptor terminal (S3 at position 2 and S5 at position 1) appended to a synchronization sequence. This sequence would, probably, be of the type discussed earlier.

(4) The acceptor terminal receives the enciphered TIV_0, loads it into his input register (S2 at position 4) deciphers the result and, with both S4 and S6 at position 2, modulo-2 adds TIV_0 and TIV_A, where the latter is the current contents of its TIV store. At the same time, TIV_A is enciphered

(S2 and S4 at position 2, S6 at position 1) and is transmitted following a synchronization squence to the originator terminal. The result of adding TIV_0 and TIV_A, which we denote by IV, is loaded into both the TIV and RIV (*Receive initialization vector*) stores. The acceptor can now begin to transmit enciphered speech.

(5) The originator terminal receives the enciphered TIV_A and, in a way completely analogous to that above, can generate IV. It is now ready for steady state operation.

There are two observations to make about the above techniques. First, when the terminal is initially powered the TIV store should be filled in some random way. Second it precludes the possibility of an interceptor obtaining any information by recording an enciphered digital voice stream and simply playing it back later through a terminal at the recovery site.

The steady state operation, i.e., speech transmission, is shown in Fig. 7.8.

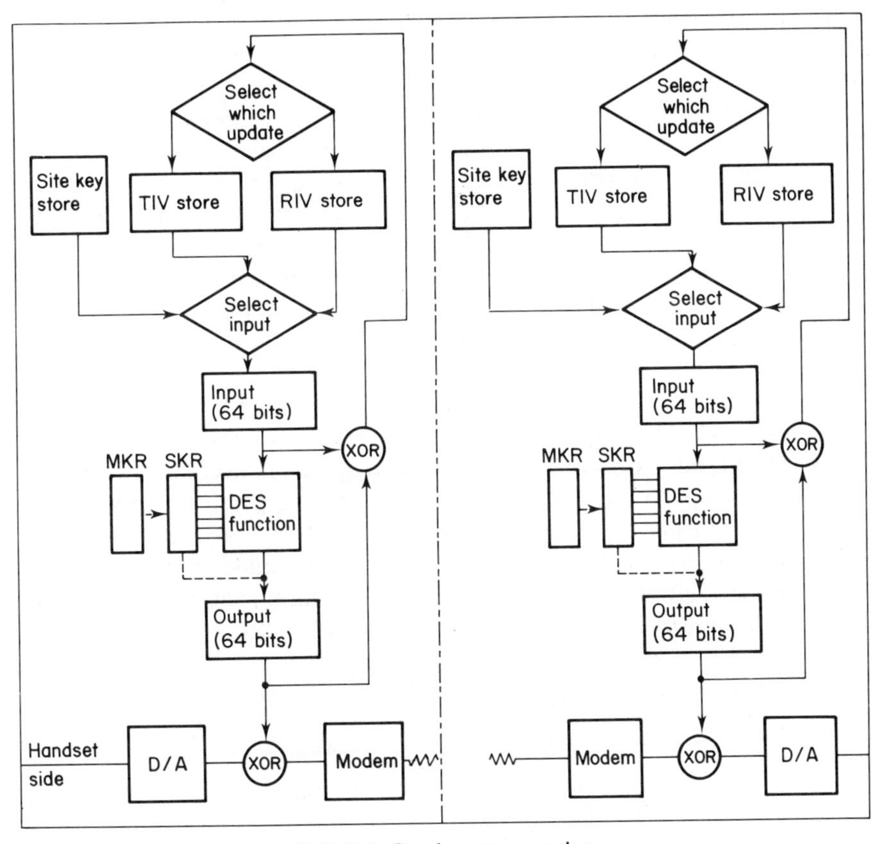

FIG. 7.8. Steady-state operation.

It is essentially the stream cipher mode which we described earlier. In this operation either the TIV or RIV store are updated every 64 bits and this process continues until one of the parties hangs up.

The system just described meets the criteria in the sense that it employs DES, is transparent to the user, i.e., the user is unaware that a scrambler is used, and only the cipher mode can be utilized. However, although we have looked at certain aspects of the key management, we have not discussed the distribution of the master keys. One possibility suggested by Oceyre and Heller (1978) is for the master key to be held on a separate, pluggable unit within each terminal, and that replacements could then be held, under strict physical security, at each site. It must not be forgotten that each terminal also has to hold two site keys for each site and, although the cost of memory is decreasing rapidly, this is obviously going to place a constraint on the size of the network. Oceyre and Heller, in 1978, predicted a price of several thousand dollars per terminal, which would certainly deter the casual use of this type of device.

We conclude this discussion of digital systems by noting that there is little doubt that a digital scrambler can achieve a high level of security. In fact, in general, at present it can achieve a higher level than that obtainable by an analogue system. Nevertheless, today, analogue systems are more widely used. This is due to the fact that they can more easily be retrofitted to telecommunications systems, that they usually imply virtually no increase in the bandwidth and that they tend to be well proven and highly robust. However, digital speech networks are becoming more popular and we can expect to see a dramatic increase in the number of digital scramblers being used. Then, as the usage increases, the cost of these systems should decrease.

As we remarked at the beginning of Chapter 1, speech is our most fundamental form of communication. The importance of speech is unlikely to diminish and, consequently, the use of speech scramblers is likely to grow. This will certainly be true if the transmission of speech over channels which are easy to intercept, e.g., satellite communications, continues to increase.

Hopefully this book has provided a would-be user of a speech scrambler with the appropriate background knowledge for making his decisions. However, reading the book may be just the beginning and he may now be faced with a lot of hard work. We wish you luck!

Bibliography

Bailey, R. E. (1977). A digitally encoded voice encryption system, *Proc. Int. Conf. Crime Countermeasures*, University of Kentucky, pp. 1-4.

Baker, H. C. (1972). Voice privacy transmission techniques, *Commun. News*, (June) 38-42.

Baschlin, W. (1977). The integration of time division speech scrambling into police telecommunication networks, *Proc. Carnahan Conf. Crime Countermeasures*, University of Kentucky, pp. 141-145.

Beker, H. J. (1980a). Cryptographic requirements for digital secure speech systems, *Elect. Eng.* **52** (634), 37-46.

Beker, H. J. (1980b). Cryptography for radio communications applications, *Commun. Eng. Int.* **2** (4), 36-41.

Beker, H. J. (1980c). Cryptography—what is a cipher system, *New Elect.* **13** (23), 29-31.

Beker, H. J. (1980d). Cryptography—modern cipher systems, *New Elect.* **13** (24), 29-33.

Beker, H. J. (1981). Digital secure speech systems, *IERE Conf. Proc.* **50**, 237-246.

Beker, H. J. (1984). Options available for speech encryption, *Radio Electron Eng.* **54**, (1), 35-40.

Beker, H. J. and Mitchell, C. J. The enumeration of permutations with limited displacement, (to be submitted).

Beker, H. J. and Piper, F. C. (1981). Shift register sequences, *Proc. British Comb. Conf. 8th*, pp. 56-79.

Beker, H. J. and Piper, F. C. (1982a). Analogue speech scrambling, *New Elect.* **15** (17), 28-32.

Beker, H. J. and Piper, F. C. (1982b). Digital speech scrambling, *New Elect.* **15** (18), 94-100.

Beker, H. J. and Piper, F. C. (1982c). Communications security: A survey of cryptography, *Proc. IEE* **129** Part A, 357-376.

Beker, H. J. and Piper, F. C. (1982d). "Cipher Systems: The Protection of Communications". Van Nostrand-Reinhold, Princeton, New Jersey and Wokingham, Berks, England.

Belland, E. and Bryg, N. (1978). Speech signal privacy system based on time manipulation, *Proc. Carnahan Conf. Crime Countermeasures*, University of Kentucky, pp. 37-40.

Beth, T., Hess, P. and Wirl, K. (1983). "Kryptographie". B. G. Teubner, Stuttgart.

Blesser, S. (1972). Speech perception under conditions of spectral transformation: I phonetic characteristics, *J. Speech Hear. Res.* **15**, 5-41.

Bromfield, A. J. and Mitchell, C. J. Permutation selector for a sliding window time element scrambler, (to be submitted).

Brown, J. and Glazier, E. V. D. (1964). "Telecommunications". Chapman and Hall, London.

Brunner, E. R. (1976). Efficient speech scrambling: an economic solution to the secure voice communication problem, *Proc. Int. Conf. Commun. Equip. Sys.*, Brighton, pp. 336-339.

Brunner, E. R. (1980a). Efficient scrambling techniques for speech signals, *Proc. IEEE Int. Conf. Commun.* Seattle, pp. 16.1.1–16.1.6.

Brunner, E. R. (1980b). Speech security systems today and tomorrow, Gretag Report.

Carlson, R. L., Telley, J. M. and Schreiber, W. L. (1972). Privacy of voice communication, *Security World*, (May) 49–53.

Cox, R. V. and Tribolet, J. M. (1983). Analog voice privacy systems using TFSP scrambling: full duplex and half duplex, *Bell Syst. Tech. J.* **62** (1), 47–61.

Davies, D. W. (1980). Limits to computation. Note from NPL.

Davis, R. M. (1978). The data encryption standard in perspective, *IEEE Commun. Soc. Mag.* **16** (6), 5–10.

Diffie, W. and Hellman, M. E. (1976a). Cryptanalysis of the NBS data encryption standard. Stanford University Report MEH-76-2.

Diffie, W. and Hellman, M. E. (1976b). A critique of the proposed data encryption standard, *Comm. ACM*, **19**, (3), 164–165.

Diffie, W. and Hellman, M. E. (1976c). New directions in cryptography, *Trans. Inform. Theory* **IT-22** (6), 644–654.

Flanagan, J. L. (1972). "Speech analysis, synthesis and perception". Springer-Verlag, Berlin and New York.

Flanagan, J. L., Schroeder, M. R., Atal, B. S., Crochiere, R. E., Jayant, N. S. and Tribolet, J. M. (1979). Speech coding, *IEEE Trans. Commun.* **COM-27** (4), 710–737.

French, R. C. (1972). Speech scrambling, *Electron. Power* (July) 263–264.

French, R. C. (1973). Speech scrambling and synchronization, Philips Research Report No. 9, pp. 1–115.

Gallois, A. P. (1976). Communications privacy using digital techniques, *Electron. Power* **22**, 777–780.

Gold, B. (1977). Digital speech networks, *Proc. IEEE* **65**, 1636–1638.

Gold, B. and Rader, C. M. (1967). The channel vocoder, *IEEE Trans. Audio Electroacoust.* **AU-15** (4), 148–160.

Golomb, S. W. (1967). "Shift Register Sequences", Holden-Day, San Francisco, California.

Good, I. J. (1957). On the serial test for random sequences, *Ann. Math. Statist.* **28**, 262–64.

Guanella, G. (1973). Automatic speech scrambling, Publication CH-E7.30038.2E, Brown, Boveri and Co. Ltd.

Gunawardana, R. (1980). Using the LPC speech synthesis circuits, *Elect. Prod. Design* 35–37.

Hartmann, H. P. (1978). Analog scrambling vs. digital scrambling in police communication networks, *Proc. Carnahan Conf. Crime Countermeasures*, University of Kentucky, pp. 47–51.

Hong, S. T. and Keubler, W. (1981). An analysis of time segment permutation methods in analog voice privacy systems, *Proc. Carnahan Conf. Crime Countermeasures*, University of Kentucky.

Houghton, M. R. (1980). Developments in speech security, *Commun. Int.* (Feb.) 22–23.

Jayant, N. S. (1982). Analog scramblers for speech privacy, *Comput. Security*, **1**, 275–289.

Jayant, N. S., Cox, R. V., McDermott, B. J. and Quinn, A. M. (1983). Analog scramblers for speech based on sequential permutations in time and frequency, *Bell Syst. Tech. J.* **62** (1), 25–45.

Jayant, N. S., McDermott, B. J., Christensen, S. W. and Quinn, A. M. S. (1981). A comparison of four methods for analog speech privacy, *IEEE Trans. Commun.* **COM-29** (1), 18–23.

Jennings, S. M. (1980). A special class of binary sequences, PhD Thesis, University of London.

Kahn, D. (1967). "The Codebreakers". MacMillan, New York.

Kak, S. C. (1983). An overview of analog signal encryption, *IEE Proc.* **130**, Part F, 399–404.

Kak, S. C. and Jayant, N. S. (1977). On speech encryption using waveform scrambling, *Bell Syst. Tech. J.* **56** (5), 781–808.

Kirchhofer, K. H. (1976). Secure voice communication–cryptophony, Int. Defence Rev. No. 9, pp. 761–767.

Konheim, A. G. (1981). "Cryptography, A Primer". Wiley, New York.

Lamba, T. S. and Faruqui, M. N. (1978). Intelligible voice communications through adaptive delta modulation at bit rates lower than 10 kbit/s, *Radio Electron. Eng.* **48** (4), 169–175.

Leitich, A. J. (1977). Scrambler design criteria, *Proc. Int. Conf. Crime Countermeasures*, University of Kentucky, pp. 5–9.

MacKinnon, N. R. F. (1980). The development of speech encipherment, *Radio Electron. Eng.* **50** (4), 147–155.

MacWilliams, F. J. and Sloane, N. J. A. (1978). "The Theory of Error-Correcting Codes", North-Holland Publ. Amsterdam.

Markel, J. D. and Gray, A. H. (1976). "Linear Prediction of Speech", Springer-Verlag, Berlin and New York.

McCalmont, A. M. (1973). Communications security for voice techniques, systems and operations, *Telecommun.* (Apr.) 35–42.

McCalmont, A. M. (1974). How to select and apply various voice scrambling techniques, *Commun. News* (Jan.) 34–37.

McCalmont, A. M. (1980). Measuring security in analog speech communications security devices, *Proc. IEEE Int. Conf. Commun.*, Seattle, pp. 16.5.1–16.5.4.

McGonegal, C. A., Berkley, D. A. and Jayant, N. S. (1981). Private communications, *Bell Syst. Tech. J.* **60** (7), 1563–1572.

Meyer, C. H. (1972). Voice scramblers in two-way systems, *Commun. News* (Aug.) 32–33.

Meyer, C. H. (1974). Enciphering data for secure transmission, *Comput. Design*, 129–34.

Mood, A. M. (1940). The distribution theory of runs, *Ann. Math. Statist.* **11,** 367–392.

National Bureau of Standards (1977). Data encryption standard, Federal Information Processing Standard (FIPS) Publication No. 46.

National Bureau of Standards (1978). Computer security and the data encryption standard, NBS Publication 500–7.

National Bureau of Standards (1981). Guidelines for implementing and using the DES, FIPS Publication 74.

Nelson, R. E. (1976). A guide to voice scramblers for law enforcement agencies, NBS Special Publication 480–8.

Nicolai, C. R. (1980). Spread spectrum techniques for narrowband scrambling, *Proc. IEEE Int. Conf. Commun.*, Seattle, pp. 16.3.1–16.3.4.

Nye, J. M. (1981). "Who, what and where in communications security". Marketing Consultants Int.

Nye, J. M. (1982). Satellite communications and vulnerability, *Comput. World*, (May).

Orceyre, M. V. and Heller, R. M. (1978). An approach to secure voice communication based on the data encryption standard, *IEEE Commun. Soc. Mag.* **16** (6), 41–52.

Papoulis, A. (1977). "Signal Analysis". McGraw Hill, New York.

Peterson, W. W. and Weldon, E. J. (1972). "Error-correcting Codes", 2nd Ed. MIT Press, Cambridge, Massachusetts.

Phillips, V. J., Lee, M. H. and Thomas, J. E. (1971). Speech scrambling by the re-ordering of amplitude samples, *Radio Electron. Eng.* **41** (3), 99–112.

Phillips, V. J. and Watkins, J. R. (1973). Speech scrambling by the matrixing of amplitude samples, *Radio Electron. Eng.* **43,** (8), 459–470.

Pichler, F. (1982). Analog scrambling by the general fast Fourier transform, *in* "Cryptography, Lecture Notes in Computer Science", Vol. 149 pp. 173–178. Springer-Verlag, Berlin and New York.

Rivest, R. L., Shamir, A. and Adleman, L. (1978). A method for obtaining digital signatures and public key cryptosystems, *Commun. ACM*, **21** (2), 120–126.

Rosie, A. M. (1973). "Information and Communication Theory", 2nd Ed. Van Nostrand-Rheinhold, Princeton, New Jersey.

Sambur, M. R. and Jayant, N. S. (1976). Speech encryption by manipulations of LPC parameters, *Bell Syst. Tech. J.* **55** (9), 1373–1388.

Shannon, C. E. (1949). Communications theory of secrecy systems, *Bell Syst. Tech. J.* **28,** 656–715.

Sloane, N. J. A. (1982). Encrypting by random rotations *in* "Cryptography, Lecture Notes in Computer Science", Vol. 149, pp. 71–128, Springer-Verlag, Berlin and New York.

Smol, G., Hamer, M. P. R. and Hills, M. T. (1976). "Telecommunications: A Systems Approach". George Allen and Unwin Ltd., London.

Steele, R. (1975). "Delta Modulation Systems". Pentech Press, London.

Taub, H. and Schilling, D. L. (1971). "Principles of Communication Systems". McGraw-Hill, New York.

Telsy Systems (1979). "Secure voice: reality and myth".

Timmann, K. P. (1982). 'The rating of understanding in secure voice communication systems *in* "Cryptography, Lecture Notes in Computer Science", Vol. 149, pp. 157–164.

Udalov, S. (1980). Microprocessor-based techniques for analog voice privacy, *Proc. IEEE Int. Conf. Commun.*, Seattle, pp. 16.4.1–16.4.5.

Vernam, G. S. (1926). Cipher printing telegraph systems for secret wire and radio telegraphic communications, *J. AIEE* **45,** 109–115.

Vouga, C. A. (1973). Speech scrambling in radio communication, 1st *Int. Conf. Electron. Crime Countermeasures, 1st*, Edinburgh.

Weinstein, S. B. (1980). Sampling-based techniques for voice scrambling, *Proc. IEEE Int. Conf. Commun.*, Seattle, pp. 16.2.1–16.2.6.

Wyner, A. D. (1979a). An analog scrambling scheme which does not expand bandwidth, Part I: Discrete time, *IEEE Trans. Inform. Theory* **IT-25** (3), 261–274.

Wyner, A. D. (1979b). An analog scrambling scheme which does not expand bandwidth, Part II: Continuous time, *IEEE Trans. Inform. Theory* **IT**-25 (4), 415–425.

Index

I

J

K

L

M

N

O

P

Q

R

S